# THE
# **30**-DAY
# HEART
# TUNE-UP

# THE 30-DAY HEART TUNE-UP

**A BREAKTHROUGH MEDICAL PLAN
TO PREVENT AND REVERSE
HEART DISEASE**

## STEVEN MASLEY, MD

**Fellow, American Heart Association**

CENTER
STREET

NEW YORK   BOSTON   NASHVILLE

The instructions for the Bruce Protocol and exercise instructions in Chapter 5 have been adapted from my previous book, *Ten Years Younger.*

Copyright © 2014 by Steven Masley, MD

Foreword copyright © 2014 by Douglas D. Schocken, MD

Center Street
Hachette Book Group
237 Park Avenue
New York, NY 10017

www.CenterStreet.com

Printed in the United States of America

RRD-C

First edition: February 2014
10 9 8 7 6 5 4 3 2 1

Center Street is a division of Hachette Book Group, Inc.
The Center Street name and logo are trademarks of Hachette Book Group, Inc.

The Hachette Speakers Bureau provides a wide range of authors for speaking events. To find out more, go to www.HachetteSpeakersBureau.com or call (866) 376-6591.

The publisher is not responsible for websites (or their content) that are not owned by the publisher.

Library of Congress Cataloging-in-Publication Data

Masley, Steven.
    The 30-day heart tune-up : a breakthrough medical plan to prevent and reverse heart disease / Steven Masley, MD — First edition.
        pages cm
    Includes bibliographical references and index.
    ISBN 978-1-4555-4713-5 (hardback) — ISBN 978-1-4555-4712-8 (ebook) — ISBN 978-1-4789-2532-3 (audio download)   1. Heart—Diseases—Treatment.   2. Atherosclerotic plaque.   3. Blood sugar monitoring.   4. Diet therapy.   I. Title.   II. Title: Thirty day heart tune up.
    RC683.8.M37 2014
    616.1'2—dc23
                                                                              2013027841

# Contents

# Foreword

*by Douglas D. Schocken, MD*

This book can actually change your life. Sounds crazy? Read on. Science has made great progress in the war on heart disease, yet heart disease remains a leading cause of death and disability throughout the developed world, and the evolving pandemic of coronary artery disease is now sweeping into the developing nations of the world. As Western civilization appears in emerging countries and cultures, the incidence of heart disease, hypertension, obesity, diabetes, and stroke is soaring. In the United States, the epidemic of obesity and adult onset diabetes is one important area where the battle remains to be won. Because of the wonders of modern living, we have become a largely fast-food and sedentary society. To quote Pogo, a twentieth-century cartoon character and philosopher, "We have met the enemy, and he is us."

Dr. Steven Masley has been leading the fight against heart disease for many years, and in his new book, he provides excellent practical advice for heart health. Dr. Masley draws liberally on the evidence base of medical literature on heart disease and prevention, along with real-life examples from his own medical practice, years of research, and his personal family journey.

In *The 30-Day Heart Tune-Up,* Dr. Masley teaches readers how to discover potential and real threats to their cardiovascular health and, as a result, possibly prevent a destructive heart event. The book provides well-structured, practical, and achievable goals to achieve better heart health. These goals are admirable and attainable. However, there is no single route on the road to heart health success. This is not a one-size-fits-all tactical approach. Each of us brings our own set of both reversible and nonmodifiable risk factors for heart disease.

When I was 12 years old, my grandfather died from a heart attack, his first, at age 67. Barely eight years later, at the peak of his successful career as a naval officer, my father suffered a life-changing and career-ending heart attack at age 49. That experience, while I was a college sophomore, gave me pause to examine my own genetic roots and look toward my personal and professional future. I decided that if I was going to acquire this terrible illness that was striking men in my family at younger and younger ages, I'd better learn as much as I could to avoid the fate of my father and grandfather. I focused my professional goals on going to medical school to help those with heart disease. In addition, however, I decided to help people keep from getting heart disease in the first place. Adopting an adage of Benjamin Franklin's alter ego, Poor Richard, I became a strong advocate for the philosophy that an ounce of prevention is worth a pound of cure. His philosophy has been a guide to me throughout my entire life.

So throughout our careers, both Dr. Masley and I have worked to answer the question "How can we prevent this growing epidemic of heart disease?" The United States Department of Health and Human Services in its Healthy People 2020 program has set aggressive goals for weight standards and enhanced diet for both adults and children. The concepts proposed by the American Heart Association and its Simple 7 Program are all focused on prevention at the individual level. Dr. Masley's book is a great tool in this prevention effort.

Dr. Masley has drawn from his own singular professional and personal background to bring into one volume a combination of risk assessment and intervention tools that anyone can adopt to create real change in his or her life. For example, the use of carotid intimal medial thickness (IMT) as an assessment tool for determining the pathological "age" of arteries also can be used to measure response to prevention programs. Dr. Masley is on the leading edge of early adopters of this technology to assess the arterial wall thickness and its response to aggressive approaches to slowing or reversing the progress of plaque growth.

No one can speak for the potential of self-help books for the millions who are in need but who have not taken the first step. You have already taken the first and most important step: You have picked up this book. You have already expressed that you are ready to make a change in your life. In his classic work addressing stages of change, Dr. James Prochaska described the critical early stage, that of precontemplation. You have already moved to the next stage. You have decided to get engaged. That decision could mean a life change for your health and much more. I encourage you to keep reading Dr. Masley's work and to put his plan into action in your life. His book brings to the lay public a special approach. Self-help books are usually short on assessment and long on opinion, with highly variable evidence bases. In contrast, *The 30-Day Heart Tune-Up* provides both assessment tools and practical guides to therapeutic lifestyle change (TLC) for addressing both a sedentary lifestyle and unhealthy diet choices.

Much of our population views doctors as purveyors of pills and other invasive interventions. All too often, we as physicians forget that therapeutic lifestyle changes such as those proposed by Dr. Masley ought to be the cornerstones of both prevention and treatment programs. His concrete dietary suggestions are well grounded in nutritional literature. His suggestions for aerobic exercise programs and training targets are based on the evidence supporting national guidelines established by the American Heart Association, the American College of Sports Medicine, and the Institute of Medicine. In this book, you'll find Dr. Masley's approach to measuring arterial aging and disease. He then describes his tools for measuring fitness, dietary and exercise plans to improve your heart and arteries. Your personal 30-Day Heart Tune-Up package can be accessed by your doctors and implemented by others involved in your care. You have taken the first step. Keep up the good work. Read on.

—Douglas D. Schocken, MD
Professor of Medicine/Cardiology
Duke University School of Medicine

# My Promise

In *The 30-Day Heart Tune-Up*, I offer you:

- an easy way to assess the real age of your heart and blood vessels so that you can clearly understand your risk for a heart attack or stroke
- a way to finally understand what those cholesterol numbers mean—and don't mean!
- a medically sound plan that will markedly reduce your cardiovascular risk without surgery, drugs, invasive tests, or frequent and expensive trips to the doctor
- a scientifically proven program that can reduce the plaque in your arteries—the main culprit behind heart attacks and strokes
- an eating plan based upon adding heart-healthy foods, *not deprivation*. It will feature foods that you can personalize to match your taste preferences and lifestyle, made with ingredients you can find at most local grocery stores
- 60 great recipes to get you on your way!
- a way to make your heart younger and stronger and at the same time make you feel healthier, sexier, trimmer, mentally sharper, and better than you have in over a decade

Best of all, with this heart-healthy tune-up you'll begin to see results in as little as 30 days.

That's my promise!

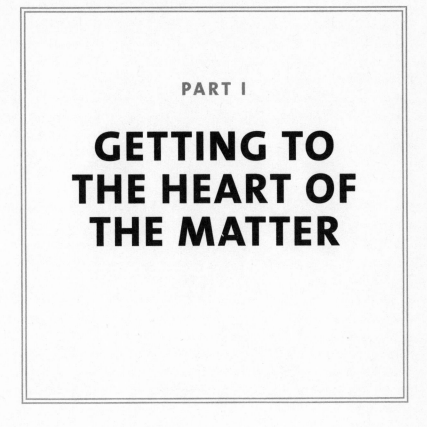

PART I

# GETTING TO THE HEART OF THE MATTER

*Chapter One*

# The 30-Day Heart Tune-Up Breakthrough

I've written *The 30-Day Heart Tune-Up* to enable you to prevent heart disease and strokes and, if you already have cardiovascular disease, to help you reverse it. In this book, you will find all the tools you need to succeed.

Cardiovascular disease remains the #1 killer of people in the United States today—accounting for more deaths than all forms of cancer combined. Cardiovascular disease causes heart attacks, strokes, sudden cardiac death, sexual dysfunction, and poor circulation. All stem from abnormal plaque growth within our arteries. Almost all of us have had experience with cardiovascular disease— if not personally, then with a family member, friend, or coworker. *But are you aware that 20% of people who have suffered a heart attack actually have a normal cholesterol profile?* Even if your cholesterol level is low, this doesn't mean that you're free of the risk of heart disease. And even if your doctor has "passed" you on a treadmill stress test, or by all outward appearances you're fit, you may not really know what's going on in your heart or blood vessels. If you've been diagnosed with high cholesterol, that makes understanding your heart's condition even more challenging and important. The true state of the cardiovascular system is a mystery to most everyone, including many of our doctors. Because of this uncertainty, as we age, it is justifiable to fear an unexpected heart attack or stroke.

## MY UNIQUE PERSPECTIVE

As a child growing up, I watched my father work miracles as a vascular surgeon. Although I was still too young to drive, I remember gingerly donning oversized scrubs and entering the inner sanctum—the operating room—where I watched my dad repair diseased arteries in patients with cardiovascular disease. After surgery, I walked the hospital floors with him and was amazed by the technology and tubes extending from every conceivable orifice in his patients' bodies. Obviously these treatments were needed, yet the ordeal of surviving these complex surgeries made a strong impression on my early development. I saw how, weeks later, people still needed dressing changes in their homes to recover from their hospital-acquired wounds. Yet, despite all the wonder surrounding this technology and a long list of my father's eternally grateful patients, as a child I dreamed that one day I might be able to help people avoid this type of invasive medical care.

Over the years, as a resident and then as a physician, I have been fortunate to volunteer in more than 15 impoverished countries. I discovered that most of the time, the human body has the capacity to heal itself without high technology, fancy drugs, or risky procedures and surgeries. I have witnessed that most people living in poverty in the underdeveloped world by necessity had to be fit and to eat unprocessed food. In fact, I was shocked to realize that, despite their difficult living conditions, if they weren't starving, they usually enjoyed better cardiovascular health than most of my patients back home in the United States. They were trimmer, fitter, and had fewer joint problems. They also had better blood sugar, cholesterol, and blood pressure control.

From these unique experiences, I view healing from a different perspective than many of my medical colleagues here in the United States. In truth, I have developed a different understanding as to why cardiovascular disease remains the #1 cause of death in the United States, despite the fact that it is preventable 90% of the time.[1]

## WHY IS CARDIOVASCULAR DISEASE STILL THE #1 KILLER OF AMERICANS?

For one thing, the traditional approach to assess cholesterol, blood sugar, and blood pressure that most physicians use today in order to evaluate heart disease does not address what is actually happening to the biochemistry within your arteries. Often, as I will explain, these tests are inadequate to figure out what's really going on.

Second, most physicians have become accustomed to treating so-called "high" cholesterol levels. This is natural, since some years ago we all learned that an abnormal cholesterol profile was the leading cause of heart attacks and strokes. However, today, the recent epidemic of elevated blood sugar levels, low fitness, expanding waistlines, and obesity (collectively called the metabolic syndrome, which I'll discuss in Chapter 2) has become the new #1 cause. This has rendered cholesterol-lowering drugs by themselves less effective, even though this therapy may play a decisive role for some people. Indeed, present-day solutions may be the answer for only a few.

Third, and perhaps the most important reason why cardiovascular events such as heart attacks or strokes remain the top cause of death in the United States: Most of us are unaware of the treatment options available to us before we get into trouble. For example, upon arrival in an emergency room with symptoms of heart disease and abnormal heart findings, we are often subjected to the least effective and the most dangerous treatment first. In that urgent situation, you're more likely to be diverted to a relatively invasive procedure such as an angiogram or angioplasty. We need to understand that cardiac procedures treat heart symptoms, such as angina, nicely but do not do a good job of preventing future heart attacks and strokes. Before we go ahead and learn more, let's define some terms that we'll need to use.

## Cardiovascular Disease Definitions

**Angina:** The classic symptoms are chest pressure (not always pain), shortness of breath, radiation of the discomfort into the neck or down either arm (some people only have jaw, neck, or arm discomfort without chest pain), nausea, sweating, indigestion, and maybe dizziness or fatigue. Angina symptoms signify a decreased blood supply to the heart, causing ischemia (a lack of oxygen to the tissues). Typically, exertion or exercise worsens the symptoms. When all of the symptoms occur together, the diagnosis of angina is easy. Women more often than men have just one or two of these symptoms, and may only have shortness of breath or fatigue, aggravated by activity.

**Heart Attack:** With prolonged angina, usually more than 30 minutes of decreased oxygen to heart cells, the cells begin to die. This results in either sudden death or in the formation of scar tissue and a weakened heart. A minimal heart attack does not weaken the heart significantly, but it leaves a permanent scar, which increases the lifetime risk for a worrisome or potentially fatal heart arrhythmia. If you have angina symptoms that last more than a few minutes despite rest, call 911. If you are having a heart attack, the sooner you receive treatment, the better. Minutes matter greatly.

**Transient Ischemic Attack (TIA):** An ischemic attack is the result of a decreased blood supply to the brain, causing sudden loss of oxygen to brain cells. If transient, this does not lead to cellular death. Symptoms include numbness or weakness on one side of the body, vision or speech loss, and balance problems. Typically, a doctor can identify from the patient's symptoms the region of the brain with diminished circulation. With a TIA, all symptoms resolve within 24 hours and sometimes last only minutes. If symptoms exceed 24 hours, the event is called a stroke. Once you have one TIA, there is a much higher risk of a subsequent stroke. With a TIA, brain-imaging studies, such as computerized tomography (CT) scans or magnetic resonance imaging (MRI) scans would show normal results, indicating that no permanent damage occurred, such as the death of brain cells. A TIA is the brain equivalent of angina.

**Stroke:** Stroke is a persistent loss of blood supply to the brain, causing the death of brain cells. With stroke, the same TIA symptoms noted above occur, but they last more than 24 hours, and they can be permanent. Varying degrees of recovery can occur over several months. If you have TIA or stroke symptoms, seek immediate attention and call 911; it is essential to be seen within 1 hour. Most doctors treat symptoms that exceed 60 minutes as if a stroke were occurring. Don't delay getting help, hoping the symptoms will resolve within 24 hours, because if they don't, recovery and treatment options can become very limited, resulting in a major disability.

**Sudden Cardiac Death:** Sudden cardiac death occurs as a result of a sudden change in the heart rhythm that makes it unable to maintain blood flow.

---

If you haven't had to face an urgent cardiac situation and you're diagnosed with some form of cardiovascular disease in a doctor's office, you'll typically be put on drugs to slow the progression of your disease. But medications don't solve the underlying problem. Hopefully, most doctors will also recommend that you eat better, exercise more, and lose weight, but you may not be given the right tools to succeed with these changes on your own. In that case, your condition may gradually worsen, and at some point, you could end up in the emergency room, facing a crisis and a major procedure.

Unfortunately, very few people will opt for lifestyle changes that can prevent or reverse cardiovascular disease. In fact, most people will falsely assume that their condition has been fixed with a medical procedure and/or drugs, and that a lifestyle change is no longer required.

Why? Because many doctors don't give their patients the tools they need to initiate the lifestyle choices that would eliminate their heart condition. They may say, "Lose weight, eat smarter, and exercise," but seldom do they provide the information and ongoing support their patients need to succeed. And, just as important, many people are unwilling to take responsibility for the damage they inflict on their own bodies. They want somebody else to fix their problem. Even with appropriate coaching, many will accept cholesterol-lowering medications but will still avoid substantial lifestyle changes.

As a physician, I find this state of affairs incredibly frustrating. Nationally, we spend far too much money on procedures for a problem that is preventable, should be diagnosed earlier, and is best treated with lifestyle changes. We often don't act until a heart attack or stroke occurs, and by then it's often too late! For too many people, the first symptom of heart disease is sudden death—they don't get another chance to change anything! Studies published in the *American Journal of Cardiology*[2] have shown that we devote less than 10% of our health-care dollars for cardiovascular disease to prevention and medical management and more than 90% to procedures and hospital care. We head down this wrong road because today's paradigm doesn't target the real cause of heart disease and cardiovascular events. The truth is, until now, we have not gotten to the heart of the matter. Yet despite the bleak scenario I've described above, there is a solution. The 30-Day Heart Tune-Up can save you and your loved ones from most forms of cardiovascular disease.

## THE REAL CULPRIT

The cause of cardiovascular disease is arterial plaque. Getting to the heart of the matter means getting to the plaque. A healthy young cardiovascular system has less of it. An unhealthy old one has more. It's as simple as that.

What is plaque? Where does it come from? Well, it's a fine layer of fatty material that is deposited in your arteries, mostly as a result of the kinds of food you eat and the degree of inflammation in your blood. As you age, arterial plaque thickens; eventually it hardens, much like cement. This older, more calcified plaque narrows the diameter of your arteries, gradually reduces blood flow, and causes symptoms like angina, but seldom in itself triggers life-threatening events.

On the other hand, newly formed, soft plaque can wreak havoc. It coats the inner lining of the arteries and can mound up in spots, like acne growing on your skin. The medical term for such a plaque lesion is *atheroma*, which in Greek means a "lump of gruel," as atheromas can have a soft, partly liquid center, like a pimple. These plaque lesions can pop into the bloodstream from within the artery wall (the medical term for this is *plaque rupture*). The inflammatory chemicals released from this arterial pimple cause large blood clots to form. These clots can then travel to the heart and brain, blocking the supply of oxygen and leading to a heart attack, stroke, or sudden death.

Even though these plaque lesions are too small to obstruct blood flow in an artery, their rupture is the cause of more than 80% of heart attacks, strokes, and sudden cardiac deaths today.[3] In my patients, I have observed that even while they're taking cholesterol medication and blood pressure medication, this soft plaque may continue to grow, undetected, within their arteries, silently endangering their lives without their ever knowing it—despite their belief that they're taking care of the problem.

## THE HEART TUNE-UP

In *The 30-Day Heart Tune-Up*, I propose to revolutionize the diagnosis and treatment of cardiovascular disease. Today, we can all benefit from a simple ultrasound test that diagnoses in just a few minutes the thickness of arterial plaque. This carotid intimal medial thickness (IMT) ultrasound testing measures the thickness of your arteries, allowing an estimate of your arterial age. This type of test is very different from standard carotid Doppler ultrasound, which looks for artery obstructions that qualify for surgery.

At the Masley Optimal Health Center in St. Petersburg, Florida, I have successfully utilized my approach to prevent heart attacks and strokes for years, yet most people don't get the advice or tools they need to save their own lives. The good news is that my 30-Day Heart Tune-Up provides the opportunity to help everyone. In this book, you'll discover that it is easy to make a U-turn on the road to heart disease in just 30 days.

Since arterial plaque growth is our enemy, the questions simply become:

- How do you prevent plaque from forming?
- How do you find out how much plaque has collected in your arteries?
- If you have plaque, how do you reduce it?

The answers to these questions are in this book! The good news is that everyone—regardless of body composition, genetics, gender, or age—can do a better job preventing heart attacks and strokes. Even people with advanced cardiovascular disease can show measurable improvement in a month with the 30-Day Heart Tune-Up. And if they maintain the program, they can shrink their arterial plaque over time, restore their cardiovascular function, and lower their risk for sudden heart attack.

What makes the 30-Day Heart Tune-Up different? Most doctors focus on lowering cholesterol and blood pressure to prevent heart disease. Their approach relies on drug therapy and laboratory testing, which have been a tremendous boon to the pharmaceutical and medical laboratory industries, but not necessarily to patients. Statins, a group of cholesterol-lowering medicines, still have an appropriate use in some patients, yet they actually increase the risk of diabetes, and unfortunately, their testosterone-lowering effect may cause weight gain, reduce sexual enjoyment, and lower a person's drive to stay fit.[4]

Managing cholesterol and blood pressure have helped reduce the rate of heart attacks and strokes, but they don't do enough. That's because we're focusing on the wrong issue.

What is the 30-Day Heart Tune-Up? It's all about shrinking arterial plaque, improving circulation, and strengthening your heartbeat. I recommend neither an extreme vegan diet, which few people, despite their best intentions, can maintain for more than a week or two, nor deprivation (let's be realistic!), nor expensive medications that merely treat the symptoms rather than the cause, although I agree that some medications, when indicated, do help you make the transition to optimal heart health. So how can you accomplish this goal in such a short time? In a nutshell, here are your tools:

1. Incorporate five easy-to-remember categories of heart-healing foods into your diet.
2. Engage in exercise that strengthens your heart and arteries.
3. Learn how to better manage your stress.
4. Follow a customized, heart-friendly supplement plan.

If you've had trouble dieting or sticking to extreme diets to get healthy, take heart. Eating well and becoming fit are much more important. Don't look at this program as a weight-loss diet although, if you are overweight, you likely will lose weight if you stay on it. *The truth is that you can make your heart younger and stronger whether or not you lose weight.*

I have worked with thousands of patients who have used my program to revitalize their heart by at least ten years. Jeff, a 62-year-old executive of a major company, was diagnosed with advanced plaque growth and was on the verge of a cardiovascular event when he first came to see me. Rather than make any lifestyle changes, he originally opted to begin a well-known statin—a cholesterol-lowering medication. He took it for one year, yet still managed to increase his arterial plaque by 5% (typical plaque growth is 1% to 1.5% a year), and he developed several worrisome findings on his heart evaluation, including a newly abnormal stress test, despite his medication. He was aggravating his heart disease and increasing his risk for a heart attack, stroke, and death. Frightened by the accelerated aging of his heart, Jeff decided to follow my program. Over the following year, not only did he shrink his plaque by 8%, but he lowered his cholesterol level and blood pressure to normal and lost 25 pounds. By the second year, his cardiac evaluation results showed not even a hint of heart damage or risk of heart attack. As his arterial plaque continues to shrink, he'll soon have normal arteries for a man his age.

My medical center regularly consults with patients like Jeff to help them prevent and reverse their heart disease. And as a bonus, our patients rejuvenate their lives by having their blood pressure, cholesterol, and blood sugar levels lowered and their weight reduced in ways that the standard blood pressure and cholesterol protocols never could accomplish. For tens of millions of Americans who are at advanced risk for a cardiovascular disease, the 30-Day Heart Tune-Up offers new hope. What's more, these same healthy-heart recommendations have been proven to make the average American trimmer, fitter, and mentally sharper.[5]

## WHY DO WE NEED THE 30-DAY HEART TUNE-UP?

Sadly, many physicians have given up hope that their patients will make the meaningful changes that I recommend. Cardiologists and primary care physicians have complained to me, "My patients never listen." My response is, "Of course they won't listen if they only have a ten-minute office visit and are not provided with tools or hope for success." The saddest result of patients' despair is the suffering that could have been avoided, the lives that could have been saved.

In addition to thinking about yourself, think of your family. According to a prominent article in the *New England Journal of Medicine*,[6] for the first time in recorded history, our children's generation is expected to have a shorter life span than their parents' generation. Despite improvements in health care, drugs, and genetic therapies, technology cannot overcome the fact that our lifestyle is killing us—and our children. So when you think about adopting heart-healthy habits, it won't only help you, it will benefit your children and other loved ones, too!

With my program, I aim to reverse the misguided and out-dated thinking that has hampered our efforts to prevent heart disease. I will help you take control of your heart health, to extend your life, and to enhance your enjoyment of it. With the 30-Day Heart Tune-Up, I'm giving you the rationale, the tools, and the hope.

## THE TRUE RISKS AND BENEFITS OF HEART PROCEDURES

As I explained earlier, many Americans will undergo an invasive cardiac procedure, such as the insertion of a stent, instead of opting to change their lifestyles. Heart catheterization is usually presented to people as an easy, "not to worry about" procedure. Yet in rare cases, it can be very dangerous. Consider the angioplasty used to open a narrowed artery. A cardiologist inserts a catheter, a narrow, flexible tube, equipped with various tools, into an artery in your groin and passes it via the blood vessel through the pelvis, the abdomen, and chest, until it finally reaches the arteries of the heart. The doctor then injects dye, takes pictures, and, depending upon the degree and location of the blockages, may dilate (expand) a few of the arterial narrowings and keep the dilations open with a wire mesh tube called a stent.

Sounds complicated, right? If you are having a heart attack, this procedure can truly be life-saving. It is critical to reopen a blocked heart artery as quickly as possible, because the lack of oxygen to heart tissue can cause massive heart cell death. So clearly the sooner you have the blockage opened, the better!

Yet in my opinion, as well as in those of a growing number of physicians, heart procedures are often performed on patients when there is not a true emergency. In randomized clinical studies reviewing elective (nonemergency) procedures, compared with standard medical care, researchers and cardiologists themselves have stated that 50% to 79% of the heart procedures were performed when they would have shown no benefit or only a very limited benefit.[7]

Rare but serious complications can occur with these elective procedures. How rare depends upon the setting. In an emergency room situation, the procedure benefit is likely well worth the risk. But in an elective community setting, where patients just want to know their heart status and their cardiologist agrees, I would say the risk might be greater than the benefit. The total risk for all heart catheterization procedures combined averages 6 serious events per 1,000 procedures. Strokes are the most common adverse events; heart attacks and deaths also occur.

Consider that most of the time patients who need this type of procedure have arteries lined with plaque. Some of the plaque may have formed lesions, as described above. If one bursts during a procedure, it might release tiny pieces of calcified plaque (like broken china), that could float through your arteries to your brain and other organs. Rupturing a plaque lesion may also cause blood clots to form. The combination of tiny clots and plaque hit the brain with a meteor shower effect. Strokes and other complications following heart catheterization are a rarity, but they are devastating.

Now consider heart bypass surgery, during which a surgeon creates a new blood vessel to go around a blocked artery in the heart—a much more invasive procedure. Not only is the chest typically opened by sawing through the sternum and/or ribs to access the heart, but the heart arteries are manipulated much more than during an arterial catheterization procedure. This too has the potential to shower the brain with tiny fragments of plaque and clots, although the incidence is rare. Studies have shown a nearly 20% decrease in cognitive function long term after bypass surgery in up to 40% of patients,[8] although, over time, the degree of cognitive decline has diminished with better surgical techniques.

When should one have cardiac bypass surgery? If you have advanced heart disease and can no longer exercise because of chest pain from narrowed arteries, then your condition will likely worsen. At this point, the benefits of open-heart surgery might outweigh the risks. Yet too often this type of procedure is performed on people who could have completely reversed their symptoms with the lifestyle changes and medications I suggest in *The 30-Day Heart Tune-Up*. The bottom line is that you need to have all the information so you can make an educated decision before having these types of invasive procedures.

## FOR ME THIS IS PERSONAL

*My approach to healing embraces holistic, functional, and integrative medicine to empower my patients to optimize their health and manage the aging process.* I have had broad professional experience in helping patients lower their risk of heart attack and stroke by encouraging them to change their lifestyle. I have been inspired by my own personal experiences to guide as many people as I can—that's the purpose of this book—but I believe a deeper impulse stems from very painful family experiences I've witnessed firsthand. I've watched loved ones have their lives destroyed by cardiovascular disease. My mother-in-law, Joy, and my stepfather, Chuck, suffered more from cardiac procedures than they did from cardiac disease itself. I have vowed to help others avoid similar tragedy. Let me share their stories with you.

I met Joy 27 years ago. As time passed, her health was powerfully impacted by the lifestyle choices she made, which in fact, made the difference between life and death. Back then in the 1980s, I was engaged to a delightful young woman, who is now my wife Nicole. Her mother, Joy, was witty and smart, and she and I had an instant rapport. I enjoyed her personality greatly, and we shared many happy moments together.

Shortly after I met Joy, she developed shoulder discomfort and shortness of breath, typical angina symptoms for women, whenever she walked briskly. Because of these new symptoms, her other son-in-law, Bob, also a physician, referred her to a cardiologist for a treadmill stress test to have her heart checked. Because of abnormal findings, she was admitted to the hospital and was immediately scheduled for coronary artery bypass surgery at the young age of 54. Our concern turned to relief when she survived the surgery, but her medical status at follow-up visits was troubling, revealing persistently high cholesterol and high blood pressure. Joy was still in danger of reclogging her arteries. Further, she noticed substantial memory loss after this surgery, for reasons that I did not fully understand at the time.

Like many patients after bypass surgery, Joy mistakenly believed that the procedure, combined with a few medications, had made her good as new, and so she initially ignored my advice to institute lifestyle changes that would improve her overall health. I waited patiently as she struggled to accept her grave risk and frailty. No advice was forthcoming from her surgeon or cardiologist. Finally, when she asked me for help, I designed a diet and exercise program to help her reverse the plaque in her arteries and control her blood pressure and cholesterol levels.

My program was incredibly successful for her. Joy's cholesterol plummeted 170 points, and her ratio of total cholesterol to high-density lipoproteins (HDL) dropped from 8 to 2.5—an excellent finding. (I will explain this in greater detail in Chapter 2.) To Joy's delight, her vitality improved so dramatically that she felt as well as she had in her youth. All of these wonderful results occurred because Joy's new lifestyle reduced the plaque that was clogging her arteries and met her nutritional needs, which gave her renewed energy. The changes she made extended her life and vitality by 20 years, giving Joy time to revel in her grandchildren and time for them to have the incredible pleasure of knowing her.

But, over time, I found myself wishing I'd met Joy sooner so that we could have prevented some of her heart problems before they'd occurred. Sadly, by the time Joy had bypass surgery, her heart valves had already stretched and been damaged. And, like 20% to 40% of those having this type of surgery, she suffered an immediate and permanent drop in brain function as a result of the coronary bypass surgery. Despite these issues, Joy's angina symptoms disappeared for nearly 20 years, as she thrived by following my food and fitness program.

However, 18 years after her bypass surgery, Joy's heart valve finally gave way, causing heart failure. She underwent yet another cardiac surgery and had an even greater loss in memory and cognitive function. That loss, combined with her family history of Alzheimer's disease, resulted in continued decline in mental function until she could no longer care for herself. Joy encouraged me to share her story with others so they could be spared the suffering she is enduring during her final years.

I met Chuck when I was finishing high school; my parents had divorced years earlier. Chuck was the director for Washington State Parks at the time, involved in dozens of national organizations, yet he always took time for every event and holiday in my life. I remember telling my mom, "You should marry this guy. He's great!" They did get married, and he went on to become a regional National Parks director, taught parks administration at the university level, and looked forward to a wonderful retirement consisting of endless community activities. Years went by, and he became a fantastic grandfather to my two young boys.

Chuck had never mentioned any health issues—he told me his

doctor gave him an annual clean bill of health—meaning perhaps that he didn't need me looking into his medical history. But out of the blue, shortly after he'd retired, Chuck developed chest pressure and was admitted to the hospital. His symptoms resolved in the hospital, yet the emergency room cardiologist took him to the catheterization lab to "take a look" with an angiogram. During the procedure, a section of plaque in Chuck's artery was unintentionally dislodged, which caused a massive stroke, destroying much of the right side of his brain. Chuck left the hospital legally blind, with severe memory loss, and was unable to shave or dress himself. The wonderful retirement he had dreamed of, indeed the rest of his life, was suddenly ruined. He, and my mother, who cared for him, suffered greatly for seven years until he died.

The last time I saw him, I sat at the edge of his bed and cried as I said goodbye. This is the most painful thing I can ever remember doing. Chuck's parting words echo in my mind today: "Don't let what happened to me happen to others."

In retrospect, I know that Chuck's nightmare medical experience could have been prevented. I found out later that his cholesterol had been in the high 200 range, but his doctor said his HDL was good, so he was protected. (I will explain this more fully in Chapter 2.) Nobody had thought to measure his plaque growth or the function of his arteries, or to give him an advanced cholesterol profile assessing low-density lipoprotein (LDL) cholesterol size and type of HDL cholesterol. These more definitive tests would have clarified his true risk for a future heart attack or stroke. However, had Chuck taken proper action and responsibility for himself, it likely would have precluded his health problems and the need for an angiogram. It was so tragic!

These painful experiences with Joy and Chuck propelled me to intensely investigate what I could do to help people avoid such devastating outcomes. I wish I had known then what I offer my patients now: the ability to determine the age of their heart and arteries and their true risk for a heart attack or stroke, plus an easy-to-follow program that can rejuvenate their hearts. I want to prevent my patients and now you, my readers, from ever needing an invasive cardiac procedure. And so I've developed the 30-Day Heart Tune-Up, which has helped thousands of patients reverse arterial plaque growth and regain their lives.

## THE FUNCTION OF FUNCTIONAL MEDICINE

I am an advocate of functional medicine. Traditional health care requires a doctor to label a patient with a diagnosis and then develop a treatment plan for that disorder. Let's take hypertension as a good example. During a screening, a traditional doctor would observe your high blood pressure and then would diagnose you with hypertension. But during that typical 10- to 15-minute visit, there wouldn't be enough time to address your diet, fitness level, weight control, and nutrition. The result? Most likely, your doctor would provide some very brief lifestyle advice, but without enough information to bring your blood pressure back to normal. You would return some weeks later, after having made some minimal changes that were inadequate to correct the blood pressure problem fully. Likely you'd be treated with a drug, which unfortunately, doesn't reverse the underlying problem, although this stopgap measure will slow your demise.

In contrast, as a functional medicine physician, I would strive to enhance your cardiovascular system through a broad and holistic range of options, which must involve the weblike interactions among your diet, activity level, weight, environmental toxins, hormones, stress, and biochemical factors such as blood sugar control and inflammation levels. My aim, and that of functional medicine, is to lower your blood pressure from elevated, to normal, to optimal with a lifestyle plan that matches your unique needs. Instead of a diagnosis of hypertension, I would likely call this something like: "not enough exercise, not enough fruits and vegetables in the diet, high emotional stress, and excessive body fat." The plan wouldn't be to treat the blood pressure problem with a drug, but rather to view the whole matrix of health issues, optimize a new lifestyle plan with customized tools designed for your success, and correct the underlying cause of the high blood pressure once and for all. The result would be a personalized plan that achieves normal blood pressure without medication.

Dr. Mehmet Oz, who has endorsed my work, recently mentioned on his TV program that if a member of his family went to see a doctor, he would want one who specializes in functional medicine. I have used functional medicine in my clinical practice for 20 years, and it is the foundation of my 30-Day Heart Tune-Up.

## THE 30-DAY HEART TUNE-UP IN ACTION

As a board- and fellow-certified physician in family medicine and a nutritionist, health researcher, author, and trained chef, I speak each year at dozens of physician and scientific conferences, as well as at meetings organized by the American Heart Association. While doing background research for my first book, *Ten Years Younger*, I participated in a five-part series on the Discovery Channel. Over the past 15 years, I have helped thousands of patients trim down, get fit, improve their libido, and tap into unsuspected energy sources. As the president of the Masley Optimal Health Center in St. Petersburg, Florida, and the medical director of the Ten Years Younger Program, I've won acclaim for helping hundreds of patients reverse type 2 diabetes and eliminate the symptoms of cardiovascular disease. Let me share one patient's story. Her name is Judy.

At 50, Judy was a partner in a company headquartered in the Tampa Bay region of Florida. Over the years, her business had grown from several stores to a national chain. Her husband worked for a local law firm, and her young adult children were living mostly financially independent lives, with occasional visits home for the holidays. Not only was Judy successful, she was charming and had a radiant smile.

Yet Judy's health on the inside was anything but radiant. Fortunately for her, Peter, the company's chief executive officer, had come to me six months earlier for an optimal health assessment of his own. Based on my analysis and coaching, Peter had lost 30 pounds, was able to come off his cholesterol and diabetic medications, and now felt fantastic. Judy was clearly impressed with his progress and scheduled an appointment to see me as well.

During our discussion, Judy revealed that she was working 50 hours a week. No less than 70 e-mails found their way into her smart phone daily. She aimed to exercise three days a week, but in reality managed to do so only once a week, and that single weekend workout was getting shorter and lighter. Her eating habits had never been healthy, but the recent increase in business dinners, which included schmoozing over cheesy appetizers, artery-clogging entrees, rich desserts, and too much alcohol, were adding to her problems.

Judy's previous physician had put her on cholesterol, blood pressure, and heartburn medication, but when the prescriptions ran out, she didn't bother to refill them. She complained that the drugs made her tired, and even worse, they further suppressed her already waning sex drive; the latter was taken personally by her husband. During her evaluation in our office, Judy wasn't surprised that her blood pressure, cholesterol level, and weight had all jumped several points since her previous doctor's checkup, nor that during her nutrition consultation with me, I determined that she failed to meet her nutrient needs, despite the fact that she consumed far more calories than she should for her weight. She was surprised, though, that her body fat percentage had reached 35% of her total weight, which meant she was slipping toward obesity, although in fact, she admitted that few of her stylish suits fit her anymore. We used a computer to test her cognitive skills, and they turned out to be only average—not in the top percentile, as she had expected. She was annoyed that her push-up and sit-up scores were below average for a woman her age, and she was clearly concerned that her blood sugar level was prediabetic, especially since her grandmother had died from diabetes after a leg amputation.

Judy's full attention was captured, however, during the treadmill stress test. Her blood pressure shot up to 220/118, prompting us to stop the test just before reaching her maximum exertion, to avoid risking a stroke. She reached only the 20th percentile for aerobic fitness for her age. The final and most significant motivation to change her life came during an ultrasound test that measures plaque in the carotid artery, the artery that runs along the side of the neck and carries blood from the heart to the brain. Not only did she have the plaque of a woman 15 years her senior, but we could see irregularities growing along the artery wall—essentially plaque lesions ready to burst and devastate her heart and brain.

As the evidence accrued, Judy became frightened by her results. She was at high risk for a heart attack or stroke. To wrap up her consultation, we then talked for more than an hour about her condition. Then, with a smile, I shared the good news that she could reverse this whole process; clear her arteries of plaque and restore their function; reestablish her fitness, libido, and mental sharpness; and revitalize her life. Faced with this clear, comprehensive assessment, she was more than ready! And so she began the 30-Day Heart Tune-Up, following similar step-by-step instructions to those I will be detailing for you in this book.

We coached and encouraged Judy's progress with weekly phone calls the first month, and then with an office visit every three months. At the 30-day point, her results were impressive. Judy lost 6 pounds (all from fat), her blood pressure dropped 10 points, her bad LDL (low-density lipoprotein) cholesterol level decreased 31 points (I'll speak about the kinds of LDL cholesterol soon in Chapter 2), and her heartburn was gone. Equally important, she reported that her fitness level, energy, quality of sleep, and libido had improved dramatically. Her husband was delighted.

At the one-year mark, Judy returned for a follow-up comprehensive evaluation. She had lost 35 pounds of fat (about the volume of 7 footballs!) and added 10 pounds of muscle to her frame. Her body fat percentage was now an excellent 22%. Her blood pressure and cholesterol were beautifully controlled without medications. Her mental sharpness had increased dramatically, and her sex life had returned to normal. During this consult, she completed a full treadmill test, reaching the 90th percentile for aerobic fitness for women her age, with excellent blood pressure. The plaque growth in her carotid artery had dropped an incredible 10% in just one year, and the irregularities on the artery walls were now mostly gone. Plus, she looked and felt fantastic! Trimmer, sexier, livelier, joyful, and revitalized!

How did Judy change her life? The simple truth is that she adopted my program without hesitation. Instead of drug side effects, she enjoyed my prescription for vitality foods, tasty recipes, a customized supplement regimen, age-busting workouts, and moments of peace and calm. Three years later, Judy still feels fantastic, and her plaque continues to shrink as well.

Jeff and Judy are among the thousands of patients in my care who have reversed the rapid aging of their cardiovascular system. The best news of all is that you too can revitalize your heart and your life. *The 30-Day Heart Tune-Up* contains all the information you need to turn back the clock and add healthy, productive, pleasurable years to your life. You have the power to dissolve plaque from your arteries, reverse heart disease, and enjoy a heart ten years younger than when you started.

In the following chapters, you'll learn more about the real age of your heart and blood vessels, your cardiac risk factors, how to incorporate the five simple heart-healing food groups into your diet, how to strengthen your heart with exercise, how to manage stress and find inner peace, and how to develop a targeted supplement program that will speed your rejuvenation program. You will discover why international studies have concluded that we can prevent 90% of heart disease today.[9] You'll also learn about the sexual benefits of following the 30-Day Heart Tune-Up. As a bonus, you'll find 60 fantastic recipes to support your new eating style—everything you'll need to develop a younger, stronger heart.

Our hearts are everything to us emotionally and physically—the essence of our lives, the source of our love. We sing about our hearts, we praise and honor them. Indeed, we cherish our hearts in poetry and song, but in reality we don't provide the attention and care our hearts deserve. In this book, I am offering you a set of innovative strategies for your heart. These recommendations will make you feel fitter, trimmer, mentally sharper, sexier, and stronger, day by day and week by week. As you embark on this program, make sure to use your physician as a resource and include him or her as a partner in your progress. The great news is that there is a reasonable way for you to reverse your heart problems, regardless of your size, shape, gender, or age, that doesn't require costly medications, surgery, or tests. A way that gets at the real heart of the problem.

Your first step is to get rid of the myths that may have cluttered your thinking and to develop a real understanding of what your risks for heart disease are today.

## Chapter Two

# Truths and Myths about Cardiovascular Risk Factors

Cardiovascular risk factors accurately predict your chance for a heart attack or a stroke 80% of the time For the 20% of people who have a heart attack without any warning, risk factors are not very good predictors.

However, I'm simply unwilling to dismiss the fact that 20% of people are at risk without knowing it. So in my clinic, I look at the functional health of the cardiovascular tree to identify those people whose classic risk factors are not setting off an alarm. I look at arterial age in men over 40 and women over 50, using carotid IMT testing, which assesses the thickness and measures other qualities of plaque—something I'll cover in much more detail in Chapter 3. I also check aerobic fitness markers to ensure we don't overlook someone who is, in fact, at very high risk for a cardiovascular event. As you will see, I go beyond standard measures and focus more on lifestyle-related factors, because I have discovered that, as scientific research refines our knowledge, some of the commonly accepted risks are actually misleading or don't tell the whole story.

# MYTHS ABOUT YOUR RISK OF HEART DISEASE

There are far too many myths about your risk of developing heart disease. *None* are true, as you will discover in this chapter. The following myths are those I've heard most often from my patients:

- High cholesterol is the leading cause of heart disease.
- If your HDL is normal or if your total cholesterol/HDL ratio is good, you are always protected from heart disease.
- The amount of cholesterol in your food determines your blood cholesterol level.
- Moderate egg consumption causes your cholesterol level to jump.
- Eating shrimp also increases your cholesterol levels.
- LDL cholesterol is your enemy and should be as low as possible.
- A high body mass index or BMI (a formula based on dividing your weight by your height, as explained in Appendix I, "Body Mass Index Chart," page 353) is a major risk factor for heart disease.
- Once you start medications for high blood pressure or high cholesterol, you will need to take them the rest of your life.
- Your family history determines if you are at high or low risk for cardiovascular disease.
- If you take a statin cholesterol-lowering medication, you're protected and you can eat whatever you want.

It's easy to be convinced that these myths are true because they're so prevalent in our society. So to understand your *real* risk of experiencing a cardiovascular event, let's start with the basics. There are five classic cardiovascular risk factors that have been used for decades to predict your future chances for a heart attack or stroke. In addition, we must also consider a few recently identified risk factors. For some individuals, these are even more significant than the original five, yet sadly, as a result of time constraints in medicine today, they may be left unmentioned in your consultation with your doctor.

# FIRST LET'S LOOK AT THE CLASSIC CARDIOVASCULAR RISK FACTORS

## Classic Risk Factor #1: High Cholesterol

We have become so accustomed to thinking of cholesterol as dangerous that most of us have lost sight of the fact that we need it. This fatty substance makes your cell walls flexible, and it constitutes the building blocks for hormones, such as testosterone, and nutrients, such as vitamin D. It also helps cover your nerve cells with a myelin sheath—think of this sheath as the rubber that coats electrical wires to prevent short circuits. Cholesterol also plays a key role in digesting fats, as it is converted into bile acids that your gallbladder secretes.

Keep in mind that there are many forms of cholesterol, and some are more beneficial than others. Indeed, some forms of cholesterol contribute to arterial plaque growth, while others help prevent that very problem. So, in truth, it doesn't make much sense to lump the different kinds together with a measure of your "total cholesterol."

Some scientists consider LDL cholesterol to be bad for you (think L for "lousy"). In fact, it is the target of many cholesterol-lowering drugs. Yet LDL is actually a bubble of cholesterol containing fat and protein. It carries fat-soluble nutrients like vitamin E, which don't dissolve in your blood, from your intestines to the rest of your body. So LDL cholesterol is the delivery truck when you eat nutrient-rich foods. It isn't bad for you unless you eat harmful foods that create abnormal levels of LDL cholesterol—which I will explain below.

The fact is, not all cholesterol is created equal. There are three general types in your body, which blood test results will usually report:

- **LDL(Low-Density Lipoprotein)**, the largest choles-terol component, is a bubble of fat and protein that, with a healthy diet, carries nutrients from your intestinal tract to your cells. If you fill your LDL with bad fat that has been modified from eating too much sugar and trans fats (such as shortening or other fats used in fast food or packaged foods), it can transform from a nutrient-carrying bubble to dangerous plaque, lining your arteries, just as trash blocks traffic in an alley. Most of us keep an eye on high levels of LDL because they are a much stronger risk factor for a heart attack than total cholesterol levels. A normal LDL level is less than 100 mg/dL (milligrams per deciliter) of blood. The average LDL level for people in the United States is around 130 mg/dL; a high LDL level is 160 mg/dL, and an LDL over 190 mg/dL is very high and can be dangerous.
- **Triglycerides** are small beads of fat that hitch a ride through your bloodstream in LDL. The higher your tri-glyceride levels, the greater your risk for plaque buildup. When your blood sugar is elevated, you typically have high triglyceride levels. Your minimal goal should be a blood level less than 150 mg/dL. Better yet would be a reading of 90 mg/dL or less.
- **HDL (High-Density Lipoprotein)** or "healthy cho-lesterol," as I like to think of it, is the trash collector that cruises your blood vessels, picking up all the "bad LDL" and triglyceride garbage in your bloodstream as it works to clean your arteries. Ideally, in most cases, you need more HDL. The minimal goal for men is an HDL over 40 mg/dL blood, and for women, over 50 mg/dL. Any scores above 55 mg/dL for men and above 65 mg/dL for women are great!

Instead of just LDL and HDL numbers, many medical providers prefer to look at your ratio of total cholesterol (TC) to HDL, basically a comparison of total garbage to garbage trucks. This is like trying to estimate if your streets and alleys are open enough for traffic to pass through. A normal TC/HDL ratio is less than 3.5, and 3 or lower is excellent. However the average in the United States is 4.5. If your ratio is more than 5, you are probably growing arterial plaque quickly. For example, if you have a total cholesterol level of 240 mg/dL and an HDL level of 40 mg/dL, your ratio is 6.0, and over time you may be in danger of a cardiovascular event. In my published study identifying cardiovascular biomarkers that predict arterial plaque scores, the TC/HDL ratio was the only cholesterol marker that was predictive—total and LDL cholesterol didn't help predict plaque growth.[1]

However, as you'll see from my discussion below of *abnormal* cholesterol, these numbers do not tell the full story. Obviously a person with a cholesterol level of 300 mg/dL should not ignore these test results. But the picture is actually a bit more complicated. A relatively good cholesterol score of 180 mg/dL in the presence of other abnormal factors can be much more dangerous than a cholesterol level of 240 mg/dL with otherwise normal cholesterol features.

---

### *Truths to Replace Old Cholesterol Myths*

- You don't need to be on cholesterol medications forever! Even people who have taken them for years can change their diet and exercise, shrink their arterial plaque, and may be able to stop further arterial plaque growth without any medication.
- Most cholesterol doesn't come from your diet. Your liver makes it while you sleep. Eating saturated fat (found in fatty dairy products and meats) does more to increase cholesterol production than can be caused by simply eating foods high in cholesterol.

- Not all saturated fat is the same. All forms increase your cholesterol levels, yet some, such as fat from dark chocolate, increase large, fluffy LDL cholesterol, which is less likely to cause plaque to grow, compared with butter, cheeses, and fatty meats.
- Some foods that are high in cholesterol don't raise cholesterol levels at all. For instance, eggs have been falsely labeled as unhealthy. Moderate egg consumption doesn't raise cholesterol levels. Even better, organic, free-range chickens fed flaxseed produce eggs with much less saturated fat and much more healthy fats. (However, skip the bacon and syrup-drenched pancakes on the side.)
- Shrimp is higher in cholesterol than many other foods, yet studies show it seems to have a form that doesn't cause human cholesterol to increase. Eating shrimp is safe, as far as cholesterol goes.
- If you take a statin cholesterol medication, you are only partly protected! You may not eat whatever you want. Statins tell your liver to make less cholesterol when you're sleeping. But they can't stop bad food choices from coating your arteries with slime and plaque. Think about a glass filled with whole milk. Empty it, and you see a film inside. This is what happens to your arteries when you eat unhealthy food.
- In restaurants, people order prime rib, slather butter on their dinner rolls, load their baked potato with sour cream, indulge in ice cream for dessert, and then pop an extra statin pill, thinking it will take care of the cholesterol problem. This just makes me cringe! Statins have no effect whatsoever on the food you have eaten. They can lower your LDL production, which makes your profile look good in theory, but your arterial plaque is still growing with this type of lifestyle. As I'll discuss in Chapter 7, I believe the greatest benefit from statin medications isn't that they lower cholesterol, but rather that they decrease artery inflammation and blood stickiness—and these actions reduce the risk of having a heart attack or stroke. Notice that statin commercials state correctly, "This medication, when combined with a healthy lifestyle, can reduce the risk of heart disease." *Healthy lifestyle* is the operative phrase here. Drugs alone have not been shown to shrink plaque.

## Classic Risk Factor #2: Diabetes

Diabetes isn't just about elevated blood sugar levels, but happens because of a much more profound issue—namely, that your body can no longer *regulate* blood sugar levels. This means that multiple hormonal systems are out of balance. The resulting sugar-coated proteins cause every organ in your body to age more quickly, leading to an increased risk not only for heart disease and strokes, but also for cancer, Alzheimer's disease, amputations, blindness, and kidney failure. Sugar impacts your cholesterol profile. If your blood sugar levels are elevated, your liver produces small-sized LDL, which is more likely to cause the growth of arterial plaque, as well as small-sized HDL, which does not clean your arteries effectively.

The best test to monitor people with type 2 diabetes is the HgbA1C level (or hemoglobin A1C). This essentially measures the degree to which your blood proteins are sugar-coated. The more sugar that is caramelized on your proteins, the faster the proteins burn and the quicker you age. A normal HgbA1C level is less than 5.7%. Levels over 7% are considered uncontrolled and unhealthy, and anything over 8% is just plain terrible. Most doctors use drugs to lower a very high level to 6.5% or 7%. Using my 30-Day Heart Tune-Up, I have helped hundreds of patients drop their HgbA1C level from a dangerous 9% or 10% to less than 5.7% without any medications at all. The key is adopting a lifestyle that matches your own genetic makeup.[2] Typically, you will need to add much more daily activity and get rid of all the refined carbs in your diet to succeed.

Before full-blown type 2 diabetes develops (this was called "adult onset diabetes" in the past, but now even adolescents develop obesity-related diabetes), blood sugar and insulin levels rise. This is commonly called prediabetes, which I'll discuss in more detail in the metabolic syndrome section on page 38.

## Classic Risk Factor # 3: High Blood Pressure

High blood pressure is important in that it's more accurate in predicting cardiovascular disease than all other risk factors. The reason is simple—blood pressure is not merely a risk factor; it is also a direct marker of cardiovascular function.

Blood pressure is typically recorded as two numbers, written as a ratio like this: 118/78 mm Hg (millimeters of mercury). The top number is the systolic blood pressure, which is also the higher of the two numbers, measuring the pressure in the arteries when the heart beats (when the heart muscle contracts). The bottom number is the diastolic blood pressure, which is also the lower of the two numbers, measuring the pressure in the arteries between heartbeats (when the heart muscle is resting between beats and refilling with blood). Your blood pressure rises with each heartbeat and falls when your heart relaxes between beats. While BP can change from minute to minute with changes in position, exercise, stress, or sleep, it should normally be less than 120/80 mm Hg (less than 120 systolic *and* less than 80 diastolic) for an adult age 20 or over.

Generally speaking, if the systolic number is high that is a sign that your arteries are stiff and your blood pressure jumps with each beat. If the diastolic number is high, that suggests that the heart is stiff and your blood pressure doesn't drop normally.

If you have high blood pressure, you're probably growing arterial plaque as well. Elevated blood pressure—more than 120/80 without medication—means your arteries are sick and are not functioning properly. Poor diet and low fitness are the most common reasons for having high blood pressure. Eating refined carbs and sugar causes proteins in your blood to become sugar-coated, and these in turn irritate (inflame) the lining of your arteries. When deprived of nutrients from vegetables, beans, fruits, and nuts, your arteries lack the ability to dilate, so instead they constrict, which leads to a rise in your blood pressure.

Your arteries, which carry oxygen and nutrients to your tissues and remove waste, are simply muscular tubes. Just as your biceps will turn flabby if you don't lift weights, your blood vessels will weaken and grow stiff without exercise. With time, elevated blood pressure causes the arteries to constrict. Hardened arteries generate abnormal blood flow or turbulence within their walls, and this accelerates arterial plaque growth.

Hypertension occurs once your blood pressure is greater than 140/90 mm Hg, and this leads to a strong likelihood of advanced arterial thickening. If the 140/90 level persists during the course of a few doctor's consultations, the standard treatment is to start a blood pressure medication. Yet drugs don't fix the underlying problem—and so your arterial plaque typically keeps growing while you take drugs. The truth is that having high blood pressure means that your lifestyle is not in sync with your genetic needs.

Let me share three examples of lifestyle choices that cause hypertension. First, if you're inactive or not aerobically fit, your arterial walls will become weak and stiff because you are not exercising them enough. Second, if your diet does not include a daily portion of leafy green vegetables, you will lack vitamin K. Without it, your arteries will also become calcified and stiff. Third, if you don't eat enough of all kinds of fruits and vegetables, you will not get sufficient potassium—a mineral essential for your blood vessels to dilate and keep blood pressure normal. All of these lifestyle factors contribute to your risks for cardiovascular disease.

Salt consumption is another lifestyle risk factor that can create a spike in blood pressure. However, we have recently discovered with genetic testing that this doesn't hold true for everyone. We now know that one third of us experience a big jump in blood pressure with high salt intake, another third of us have a fairly mild increase, and in the remaining third, there is hardly any relationship between salt intake and blood pressure. However, aside from genetics, another marker ties high blood pressure with salt intake. If your blood sugar levels are elevated, you are much more likely to have a spike in blood pressure with the increased use of salt.

Most people can reduce their blood pressure to a normal level if they are empowered to make lifestyle changes. I explain how to do this in Part II of *The 30-Day Heart Tune-Up*. I have treated many patients who were on four or more medications for uncontrolled high blood pressure. These drugs caused numerous unpleasant side effects, including fatigue, weight gain, depression, sexual dysfunction, and a drop in libido. After some coaching, most were able to return their blood pressure to normal levels and stop their medications, but substantial changes in their former lifestyle routines were also required.

In my research on cardiovascular biomarkers that predict arterial plaque scores, systolic blood pressure (the top number) was by far the most powerful predictor for arterial plaque formation.[3] So make sure to keep your blood pressure nicely controlled at less than 120/80 mm Hg.

### Classic Risk Factor #4: Tobacco Use

Tobacco use ages people in hundreds of ways. The 300 toxins in tobacco impair the function of your arteries, causing them to constrict and grow extra arterial plaque. In addition to the well-known problems it causes related to lung disease and cancer, tobacco use raises blood pressure and blood sugar levels and accelerates arterial plaque growth by damaging cholesterol within the lining of your arteries. Even one passive exposure (for example, being in a smoky bingo hall for 20 to 30 minutes once a week) will increase your risk of a heart attack by 20% for up to seven days. The damage caused by passive exposure to tobacco is one of the primary reasons why smoking is now prohibited in public.

If you use tobacco, the single most important step to take for your overall health is to stop.

## Classic Risk Factor #5: Family History

Your family history represents the wild card in your risk for arterial plaque growth. It may have a very strong impact on your cardiovascular health, or it may have no effect at all. In other words, you can't rely on it to predict how you will fare! If either of your parents had a heart attack or stroke, you may or may not be at risk. If your parents lived into their eighties without any cardiovascular issues, you can still have a heart attack by age 50, if you have other risk factors. Most often, your family history impacts your risk if you have had the same lifestyle as your parents, but this is often not the case today, as lifestyles (diet and activity) have changed dramatically—often for the worse—from past generations to the present generation. Most of us no longer walk to our place of work or perform manual labor—for some, even getting up to change the TV channel can seem too arduous a task. And in previous generations, many of our stay-at-home mothers used to cook healthful meals from farm fresh, unprocessed foods—a nearly unheard of activity nowadays.

Consider Frank. His 70-something-year-old parents were very health-conscious. They hiked, bicycled, gardened, or went to the gym daily. They seldom touched a sweet or an unhealthy fat and cooked most of their meals at home from fresh produce they bought at the farmer's market. They were trim and fit and were active in their communities. They had been this way their entire lives.

Frank rebelled! At 46, he refused to exercise, took breakfast and lunch at the local fast-food emporium, never met a dessert he didn't like, and consequently became nearly 50 pounds overweight. At our first meeting, I identified all the classic cardiovascular risk factors, except smoking. His treadmill stress test was slightly abnormal, but his arterial plaque was typical for a person 20 years older. In fact, he was on the verge of a heart attack, so there was no point in Frank's counting on his family history to protect him.

Family history is a double-edged sword. Consider Mary. She felt she was doomed to live a shortened, disabled, and painful life, because every family member on her dad's side had suffered from cardiovascular disease, heart attacks, and strokes, resulting in bypass surgery and stents by age 50. No relative had lived past 62. Mary ate fairly well, but not ideally, since she hated all green vegetables. She was trim and fit, but by the time she reached 50, she too had been hospitalized for chest pain (angina). A heart catheterization revealed that many of her coronary arteries were blocked. Although her blood sugar, blood pressure, and even her advanced cholesterol profile levels were all normal, when I measured the age of her arteries with ultrasound, I found them to be consistent with those of a 70-year-old woman. Mary's doctors had put her on a statin medication, but she kept complaining of chest pain. The only solution they offered was bypass surgery.

After meeting her, I discovered that Mary had a common genetic defect in her vitamin B metabolism. Since she ate very few greens, her vitamin K intake was extremely low. Considering this information, we optimized Mary's eating plan by including the heart-friendly foods you'll learn about in Chapter 4. I also gave her special supplements, designed to counteract her genetic and lifestyle deficiencies and—amazing! Her angina disappeared. Her arterial plaque is now gradually shrinking. Mary didn't need heart surgery after all. Her family's history with cardiovascular disease was not to become her destiny!

How was this possible? Well, some of our genes are fixed, such as those that determine some forms of early onset breast cancer (genes known as BRCA-1 and BRCA-2 breast cancer genes). In this situation, young women have a high risk for breast and ovarian cancer whatever their lifestyle may be. However, most of our genes are not fixed. Rather, they can express many different outcomes, depending upon the lifestyle you choose. Fortunately for people with a family history of cardiovascular disease or type

2 diabetes, most of the causes of the disease are multifactorial. The outcome can be modified by the choices you make.

If you have always had the same lifestyle as your parents, a rarity today, then your family history is apt to closely predict your health outcomes. But if your lifestyle is different than those of prior generations, the expression of your genes will be different than that of your parents. And as we have seen from Frank and Mary's experiences, this change can be either detrimental or beneficial.

The bottom line is that if your parents had type 2 diabetes and heart disease, then yes, you are at increased risk for those diseases. Yet you also have the ability to minimize that risk by pursuing a lifestyle that matches your genetic design, likely a lifestyle that follows my 30-Day Heart Tune-Up.

## NEW RISK FACTORS THAT MAY BE UNFAMILIAR TO YOU

Many of us are already aware of the cardiovascular risk factors I've listed above. However, I'm asking you to take into account some factors that may be unfamiliar to you. Why? There are two primary reasons. First of all, our scientific knowledge has been growing by leaps and bounds, especially in the last 20 years. For instance, we have discovered that inflammation plays a critical role in arterial plaque growth and therefore increases the risk of heart attacks and strokes. We have also learned that there are many different types of LDL cholesterol, and that some forms cause much more plaque to grow than others. In addition, some genetic patterns may cause heart disease, even when other classic risk factors are "normal."

As important as these scientific breakthroughs have been, however, I believe the second reason is more significant. Our lifestyle has changed dramatically over the last 50 years. Risk factors that were not in existence 20 or 30 years ago are problems now. Let's take the case of the teenagers today who are obese at the age of

16 or 17. They're not old enough to buy a beer, but they may have arterial plaque of a 40-year-old.

For more than 85,000 years, we humans were hunter-gatherers. We spent most of our days outside walking, running, and carrying heavy loads. Our diets consisted exclusively of lean protein, vegetables, nuts, fruits, beans, plus a few whole grains (not many) and an abundance of herbs and spices. Now we typically sit at a desk 50 or more hours a week. After work, we come home tired and either flop down in front of the TV or play on the computer. Highly processed foods predominate at mealtime. This change in how we communicate with our genes has altered our genetic expression from living healthy to living a life that results in abnormal cholesterol, prediabetes, and inflammation. Our modern sedentary lives and our eating habits are killing us. So, for the sake of your heart, let's look at some of these newer risk factors.

### New Risk Factor #1: Metabolic Syndrome and High Blood Sugar

We used to believe that high cholesterol was the #1 risk factor for cardiovascular disease. But we must look at the whole picture. Having metabolic syndrome, appropriately called "diabesity" by Mark Hyman, MD, in his excellent book, *The Blood Sugar Solution*, and also known as prediabetes and Syndrome X, is a greater risk factor than having high cholesterol. In fact, it is now the #1 cause of cardiovascular disease.

Metabolic syndrome is a *huge* problem nationwide. More than 30% of adults in the United States (which translates to nearly 50% of baby boomers) have this condition. The bad news is that metabolic syndrome can kill you before you ever develop diabetes. Because it changes your cholesterol profile, increases inflammation, and raises your blood pressure levels in ways that are similar to those of diabetes, it too can cause a heart attack or stroke.

## Do You Have Metabolic Syndrome?

The answer may be yes. National standards for metabolic syndrome require you to have 3 of the first 5 of the following features. I diagnose my patients with metabolic syndrome if they have 3 of any of the following 6 criteria:

1. Expanding waistline (more than 40 inches in men and more than 35 inches in women. (Guys: your pants size is typically 3 inches less than your waistline)

2. High fasting blood sugar (more than 100 mg/dL)

3. High triglycerides (more than 150 mg/dL)

4. High blood pressure (blood pressure more than 130/85 mm Hg)

5. Low HDL cholesterol (HDL less than 40 mg/dL in men and less than 50 mg/dL in women)

6. Inflammation, as measured by a high-sensitivity C-reactive protein (hs-CRP) blood test. (See New Risk Factor #5, page 46.) Any hs-CRP level over 1.0 mg/L (milligrams/liter), and especially over 3.0 mg/L, should be considered one of the signs of metabolic syndrome. Apart from high blood pressure, especially in women, this may be the most dangerous feature of all.

High fasting blood sugar levels (#2 in the "Do You Have Metabolic Syndrome?" box, above) mean that your body has lost the ability to regulate blood sugar properly. If your levels are high, your proteins and tissues are being sugar-coated, making your tissues burn and age much more quickly than they would otherwise. I have successfully helped hundreds of my own patients reverse this condition. In fact, I published a study with the Florida Academy of Family Physicians showing that metabolic syndrome can be completely reversed with lifestyle changes in as little as two weeks.[4]

However, most people are surprised to learn that they had metabolic syndrome for 5 to 10 years "before" they developed high blood sugar levels. The problem is that their lifestyle is killing them, without their knowing it. The first signs of metabolic syndrome are usually not elevated blood sugar levels, but the factors I listed in the "Do You Have Metabolic Syndrome?" box (page 39). If anyone measured these people, they would see that their insulin levels were elevated and working overtime to keep their blood sugar controlled.

I am delighted to share that the 30-Day Heart Tune-Up is designed to reverse metabolic syndrome and bring you back to a state of vitality and optimal health.

### New Risk Factor #2: Abnormal Cholesterol

The basic cholesterol numbers (and even the TC/HDL ratio) I've already discussed don't predict nearly 20% of heart attacks and strokes—this 20% of the population has normal levels, but cardiovascular events occur anyway. It happens rarely too that some people with very high cholesterol levels do not get any cardiovascular disease. Why? It is because overall heart health is not determined by cholesterol numbers alone. Not just the levels, but the type of HDL and LDL cholesterol circulating in the blood makes a big difference.[5] Yes, there are different types. That's where advanced lipid profiles come in. This new blood test can be very useful in explaining why some people have too much arterial plaque even with normal cholesterol numbers. In fact, it would be especially important to check your advanced lipid profile if you have accelerated plaque growth.

Consider my patient Will. His cholesterol numbers were all very satisfactory, as were his blood pressure and blood sugar. He was a trim nonsmoker, and even his diet was decent. He came to me because everyone on both sides of his family had suffered from heart disease, and understandably, he wanted to avoid their fate. I checked the thickness of the plaque in his arteries with the carotid IMT test, and given his excellent cholesterol numbers, I was astonished to find that the deposits were equivalent to those of a person 15 years older than Will's stated age. So I looked to the advanced lipid profile for an answer. And there it was: We found that although Will's HDL level was high (which is good), he had the wrong type. His brother Gene had the same findings. Did this explain why his whole family had heart disease? Happily, this was probably the case. Why did I consider this good news? Because I knew we could take some action to correct the situation for both men—and we did.

We now know there are different forms of LDL and HDL, which are either more or less harmful or protective. Fortunately for Will and Gene, the latest research has shown that size and density of LDL and HDL cholesterol (as determined by an advanced lipid profile) and not just the levels, matter greatly. And it is exactly these factors that can be improved upon with lifestyle changes.

- LDL cholesterol can be small and dense or big and fluffy. The latter is packed with nutrients and carries fat-soluble vitamins and antioxidants to your cells. The smaller LDL bubbles are the ones to worry about, because they cause much more plaque to grow. Lack of physical activity and a diet high in refined carbohydrates (carbs) and low in healthy fats shrinks your LDL. This small LDL grows much more plaque. Big, buoyant, fluffy LDL does not.
- HDL cholesterol also comes in mainly two sizes. HDL2 is big and is effective in hauling away the garbage in the arteries. HDL3, smaller HDL, is not. So, like Will and Gene, you may have an excellent HDL score, but this may not be protective. By the way, ineffective HDL3 increases with alcohol consumption.
- Lp(a) cholesterol, or lipoprotein (a) cholesterol, is an abnormal type of cholesterol (it is very small) that has the potential

to cause much more plaque to grow than one would predict based on other classic risk factors. Sadly, you can't affect Lp(a) levels to any great degree with lifestyle changes. Yet, if you do everything else right (as outlined in this book) and if the rest of your advanced lipid profile looks good, you can overcome an abnormal Lp(a) level and either stop plaque from growing or have it reverse its growth over time. If you discover that you have an abnormally high Lp(a) level, living a very healthy lifestyle will help to protect you.

So the bottom line for you is: *While traditional total LDL and HDL cholesterol markers are accurate 80% of the time, you can't rely upon them fully! If you feel you are at high risk or have a worrisome family history of cardiovascular disease, then consider having your physician check your advanced lipid profile.*

---

### Ideal Goals in an Advanced Lipid Profile

- Lots of effective type HDL2 cholesterol
- Big fluffy (buoyant) LDL cholesterol
- Normal Lp(a) cholesterol

---

Be sure to control excessive alcohol, because it tends to elevate dysfunctional HDL cholesterol. Far too often, I have met patients like John, who, at age 50, had a cholesterol level of 240 mg/dL (which is high) and an HDL level of 70 mg/dL (which should be very protective). Because his ratio of total cholesterol to HDL (240 divided by 70) of 3.4 was good, his previous physician told him he didn't have to worry about cholesterol. However, during my evaluation, we determined that he had the arterial plaque of a 65-year-old—15 years of extra plaque for his age, and close to the range where a heart attack or stroke would occur. Upon taking his advanced lipid profile, I realized he had small, dense LDL (susceptible to accelerated plaque growth), and his HDL2 was very low, as he had mostly ineffective HDL3, which was not protecting him after all.

Ideally, I would have met John sooner, but the good news is that this type of abnormal cholesterol profile can be corrected with lifestyle changes. Often people like John, who drink more than two servings of alcohol daily, have a good cholesterol ratio, but the wrong type of HDL, so they may keep growing plaque without realizing it. As we discussed John's living habits, alcohol use emerged as the obvious culprit here. By adding daily exercise and increasing his consumption of healthy fats, his HDL2 levels can increase. But be aware that the traditional recommendation to be active for 20 minutes for 3 or 4 days a week has little if any impact on HDL2 levels. On the other hand, these levels increase nicely once you start exercising at least 30 minutes, five days a week.

### New Risk Factor #3: Obesity and Excessive Body Fat

Obesity appears to be an obvious risk. Extra body fat raises cholesterol, blood pressure, and blood sugar levels. In addition, fat cells produce inflammatory compounds that make your blood stickier, increasing your risk for a blood clot or stroke and accelerating arterial plaque growth. Yet the advantage of being highly fit can offset some of the risk associated with being overweight.

The standard definition of obesity is a body mass index (BMI) greater than 30 for men and women. Nearly one third of all adults in the United States are obese, and this fraction of the population is increasing nationwide. (You will find a tool to calculate your BMI, the "Body Mass Index Chart," in the Appendices, page 353.) A normal BMI would be less than 24, while 24 to 30 is considered overweight.

As your fat increases above your target BMI, your risk of major health problems skyrockets not linearly, but exponentially. I do have a few reservations when it comes to relying on your BMI, however. The major limitation with this measure is that it can't differentiate between muscle and fat mass. Adding your fat mass to your lean-muscle mass and then using the grand total (your weight) to decide your health status makes as little sense as combining your HDL and LDL cholesterol for a single "total" cholesterol number. The BMI can be misleading, because many people with a normal score are in fact "obese." That's because their muscle mass is low and their body fat is high. And in rare instances, some people with extra muscle are falsely labeled obese, since the BMI scale doesn't give them any credit for highly beneficial muscle mass.

A much better method I rely on is measuring your actual body fat. You'll find a tool for body fat goals and calculations in Appendix II, "Dr. Masley's Recommended Body Fat Percentage Rates," page 355. However, you'll need a special scale (such as a bioelectrical impedance scale) or other high-tech equipment (DEXA scanner or water immersion tank) to get an accurate result. Although the bioelectrical impedance scale has a fancy name, it is available at many stores that sell housewares. I have two of these: a highly accurate $2,500 model at the office that I use for my patients and for research, and an $89 model at home—both are manufactured by a company called Tanita. The cheaper scale works nearly as well as the expensive one, when readings are averaged over time. A less precise but commonly used way to calculate body fat percentages is a skin thickness test. If you don't have access to any of these measures, you can ask your doctor or a trainer at the gym to help you. Or you'll have to rely on BMI, which only requires that you know your height and weight.

Before you feel stressed about your weight goals, please note that the best results from my research on plaque growth show that several other factors play a more important role than weight. In particular, from a heart perspective, being fit markedly reduces any risk from being overweight. And if you eat more fiber, your heart risk drops even further, regardless of your weight. In fact, new research published in the *European Heart Journal* confirms that people who are overweight but physically fit can be at similar risk for heart disease or cancer as those of normal weight.[6] In this study, researchers looked at data from more than 43,000 people in the United States, more than a third of whom were obese. Of these, half were assessed as healthy after a physical examination and lab tests. This group of people didn't suffer from diabetes, high cholesterol, or high blood pressure. However, they exercised much more than the other, less healthy obese people in the study. The key is being fit, and the result of being fit in this study was having no sign of high blood pressure, abnormal cholesterol, or elevated blood sugar.

Take heart! If you follow my program, your heart will be younger and stronger, whether or not you lose weight. I'll also bet you'll achieve a healthier weight as a happy side benefit.

### New Risk Factor #4: Inactivity

The public health definition of "inactivity" is doing less than 30 minutes of moderately aerobic movement a day. You may think that you're exercising when you take a walk every day or so, but if you're not walking briskly and getting your heart rate up for more than 30 minutes, this doesn't count! It's like driving your car at 10 mph in fourth gear. The engine will sputter and stall. And no diet can substitute for inactivity! The human body was designed to move. Ideally, you should be moderately to vigorously active for one to several hours every day.

Activity is the best treatment for weight loss, elevated blood pressure, and high blood sugar levels. It even helps prevent and reverse depression and anxiety. Perhaps the strongest predictor of arterial plaque growth in our research at the Masley Optimal Health Center is aerobic fitness—if your aerobic fitness is good to excellent, very likely you will have less plaque than expected for your age.

However, while the definition of being "active" might be moderate activity 30 minutes a day, studies have shown that that is not enough for long-term weight control in women. *In fact moderate activity for 150 minutes a week over decades is associated with weight gain. Most women require 60 minutes every day for good weight control.*[7] This is yet another reason to get fit. You'll be able to rev yourself up in less time.

The key components of successful exercise are a true aerobic workout (keeping your heart rate appropriately elevated for at least 20 to 30 minutes most days), strength training to build muscle mass, and doing a stretch at the end. We'll review how to optimize your workout in Chapter 5.

### New Risk Factor #5: Inflammation

In Latin, inflammation (*inflammo*) means "to ignite." When your tissues are inflamed, they do feel afire—red, hot, and sore. Inflammation is the vascular tissues' biological response to a harmful assault such as an infection or injury. The classic signs of inflammation include pain, heat, redness, swelling, and loss of function.

In the short term, inflammation is the body's way to protect itself. If inflammation is prolonged, then unfortunately it causes accelerated aging. If your joints are chronically inflamed, you get arthritis. If your lungs are inflamed, you develop asthma. If your brain is inflamed—Alzheimer's. And if your arteries are chronically inflamed, your blood pressure is elevated, and you have accelerated arterial plaque growth.

The liver produces a compound called C-reactive protein (CRP) when the tissues in our bodies become inflamed. CRP levels give an indication of how much inflammation exists in your body. The more inflammation, the higher your CRP level, and the greater your risk for a cardiac event. High-sensitivity CRP levels are so precise that in some women they may be more accurate than cholesterol levels in determining the risk of a future cardiovascular event.[8] You want a high-sensitivity CRP (called hs-CRP or cardio CRP) reading to be no higher than 1.0 mg/L (milligrams per liter). A score of 3.0 mg/L poses a high cardiac risk.

---

### Caution! Don't Measure Your CRP When Ill

When you are acutely ill (with a cold or stomach flu) or have had a soft tissue injury (including any surgery), your inflammation levels will appropriately increase tenfold. Therefore, don't measure your hs-CRP levels if you have been sick, injured, or have had a medical procedure during the last month. Ask your doctor to check your hs-CRP levels when you are in your normal state of health.

---

## A HEART TUNE-UP CHECKUP

The startling news is that if you have two or more of the classic risk factors that I've just outlined, your lifetime risk is 500% higher (600% for men and 400% for women) for a cardiovascular event than if you have none of them. And as you now know, even if you have none of the classic risk factors, you could still be in danger. So take the following quiz to help you understand your own situation.

Many of you may have used a heart attack risk factor assessment tool in your doctor's office, similar to the questions in the "Gauging Your Risk" box on page 48, to assess your 10-year risk for cardiovascular disease. I do want to emphasize one caution in using the 10-year risk calculating tools. The misleading fact remains that the majority of adults who are considered to be low risk with these tools over one decade are actually high risk across their life span. So don't be lulled into living with these risk factors long-term.[9] Fixing these risk factors makes a big difference and has been associated with 14 extra years of life free of cardiovascular disease.[10]

# *Gauging Your Risk*

Is your heart aging prematurely? Here's a quick way to find out. You may have to ask your doctor to order a few tests so that you can answer some of these questions fully. Chances are, if you're an average American who is not living a fit lifestyle, you're going to answer yes to at least 3 or 4 questions. Unfortunately, that means you're at higher risk for cardiovascular disease than if you said no. Whatever the result, this could be a very good quiz to review with your doctor once all of the results are in. The good news is that the 30-Day Heart Tune-Up will give you the tools to correct most of these risks.

1. Is your LDL cholesterol too high (more than 100 mg/dL)? Or do you take a cholesterol-lowering medication?

2. Is your healthy HDL cholesterol too low (less than 40 mg/dL for men and less than 50 mg/dL for women)?

3. Do you have an abnormal advanced cholesterol profile with small-sized LDL, the wrong type of HDL, or a high level of Lp(a)?

4. Is your blood pressure elevated without medication (more than 120/80 mm Hg)? Or do you have to take blood pressure medication?

5. Is your blood sugar level elevated? (Elevated means more than or equal to 100 mg/dL; optimal is under 90 mg/dL.) Or do you take diabetic medication?

6. Is your waistline expanding (more than 35 inches for women; for men, larger than a 37-inch pants size, which is a 40-inch waistline)?

7. Are you overweight (body mass index greater than 24, especially a body fat percentage of more than 24 for men and 27 for women)?

8. Is your high-sensitivity C-reactive protein (hs-CRP) level (an indicator of inflammation) higher than 1.0 mg/L? A reading of 3.0 mg/L or more poses a high cardiac risk.

9. Do you use any form of tobacco products?

10. Do you exercise less than 5 days a week? More important, take the fitness tests discussed in Chapters 3 and 5 to clarify whether you are as fit as you should be for your age.

11. Do you eat fatty meats and dairy products more than twice a week?

12. Do you eat one or more servings of refined carbs daily?

13. Do you eat less than five cups of fruits and vegetables daily?

14. Do you have a family history of cardiovascular disease?

15. Do you eat trans fats (hydrogenated fats) from processed food or restaurant food?

Now that you have a basic idea of your risk factors for cardiovascular disease, the next step is to clarify your capacity to start the program by determining the true age of your heart.

## Chapter Three

# How Young Is Your Heart?

From my research, I have found that measuring the virtual age of a person's cardiovascular system is much more important than measuring the patient's other cardiac risk factors. It gives us an excellent assessment of heart function. Your aerobic fitness is also a better predictor of your arterial plaque age than laboratory blood tests are. Besides, many people find doing a fitness test more fun (or at least less painful) than having their blood drawn!

To understand your heart's age, let's first look at the anatomy of the whole cardiovascular system, which includes your heart, which pumps blood, the arteries that carry the blood to your tissues, and the veins that return the blood to your heart. Blood brings oxygen from your lungs and nutrients from your intestinal tract to your cells. It also transports toxic waste out of your cells to be processed by your kidneys and liver. Your brain, heart tissue, kidneys, intestines, muscles—indeed, every cell in your body depends upon this constant circulation.

If you stop blood flow to a part of your heart muscle, even for as little as 20 minutes, a portion of your heart dies, resulting in what we call a heart attack. Similarly, if you stop blood flow to a part of your brain, you have a stroke. Too often, people with cardiovascular disease experience a devastating heart attack or stroke as their first symptom. They were totally unaware they had any disease, and as a consequence they now have a permanent injury. The "luckier" people have been diagnosed because of symptoms they have developed, such as angina—pressure in the chest upon exertion. Or their condition is discovered during medical screening with, for example, a treadmill stress test, even though no "event" has yet been identified. But by the time symptoms actually appear, the blood flow in the arteries around the heart is already blocked by at least 70%.

The truth is that you may be in danger of having a heart attack without ever being aware of it. That was the case with Mike, a 52-year-old vice president of marketing. A father of four children and a volunteer swim coach, Mike had a loving family. His wife was a full-time homemaker, hustling from one child's event to another. All of the kids were involved in music and sports, and they all excelled at school. The family ate dinner together every evening that Mike was not traveling, even if they had to wait for him to return home after a long day at work.

Mike's job had always been stressful, but it became nearly unbearable during the recent recession. I saw him that summer for a consultation. He was not complaining about any worrisome heart symptoms, but it soon became clear to me that he was on the verge of cardiovascular breakdown.

Since his previous visit with me, Mike had gained 25 pounds. His cholesterol had increased 60 points, his HDL (good) cholesterol had dropped, his blood sugar had jumped to near-diabetic levels, and his blood pressure was also high. Not only had he developed metabolic syndrome, but his arterial plaque growth had increased 15%. On an ultrasound, I could see telltale plaque lesions growing at the branch points in the carotid artery. His stress treadmill test was abnormal as well, which suggested blocked arteries in his heart. Mike's lifestyle was an issue too. Apart from a decent homemade family dinner, he had been eating junk food for breakfast and lunch, hadn't exercised in two years, and looked totally stressed out.

I felt badly for Mike. But perhaps more important, it was clear to me that in the two years I hadn't seen him, Mike's heart and cardiovascular system had aged faster than his actual years. He was in grave danger.

## HOW YOUR CARDIOVASCULAR SYSTEM AGES

The goal for my patients, and now for you, is to keep your arteries unclogged long enough for you to live to 100 without the risk of a heart attack or stroke. Healthy arteries remain dilated, optimizing blood flow and preventing arterial wall plaque formation. They are lined with a protective film called a glycocalyx, which helps prevent inflammation and injury to the artery wall.

Each meal you consume has the potential to cause a fine layer of plaque to grow in your arteries. Let us first consider what happens after a healthy meal. LDL cholesterol bubbles carry nutrients from your intestines to your cells, and this stimulates the lining of your arteries to release healthy compounds that keep them wide open and prevent clots from forming (see Figure 3.1a). Your arteries dilate when they receive these healing nutrients.

In contrast, after an unhealthy meal, your LDL cholesterol becomes filled with bad fat. As soon as your body senses this, white blood cells are sent to attack the LDL cholesterol. The damaged, unhealthy LDL particles stick to the lining of your arteries and cause arterial inflammation. It's the inflammation that makes your arteries constrict, blocking blood flow. You actually lose 20% of your circulation for at least six hours after a meal high in unhealthy fats (see Figure 3.1b). You are at elevated risk for a cardiovascular event during this time. If you consider hot dogs, prime rib, or whipped cream–filled Napoleons a treat and eat them only on rare occasions, the film is likely to dissolve and the artery functions eventually return to normal.

But if bacon cheeseburgers and fries are regular lunch items, the fat is converted within the lining of your artery wall into plaque. This is similar to the pus within a pimple on your skin.

Figure 3.1a

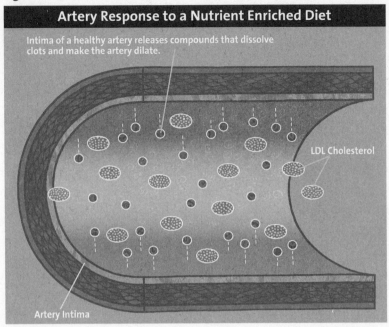

**Artery Response to a Nutrient Enriched Diet**

Intima of a healthy artery releases compounds that dissolve clots and make the artery dilate.

LDL Cholesterol

Artery Intima

Figure 3.1b

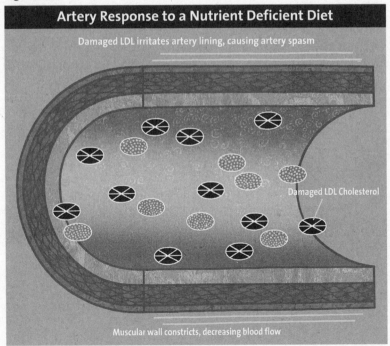

**Artery Response to a Nutrient Deficient Diet**

Damaged LDL irritates artery lining, causing artery spasm

Damaged LDL Cholesterol

Muscular wall constricts, decreasing blood flow

If you eat too much sugar, this accelerates the conversion of fat into pustule-like plaque. If you smoke, much more plaque forms. If you are overweight, your fat cells produce inflammatory compounds that grow yet more arterial plaque. If your blood pressure is elevated (above 120/80 mm Hg), it creates turbulence in your arteries, causing inflammation and vasoconstriction, which are damaging to the arteries and promote even more plaque growth.

The protective lining, the glycocalyx, is also eventually lost, and inflamed compounds leak from the bloodstream through the artery wall into the lining of the artery. Figure 3.2a shows gradual plaque growth in arteries.

As we age, arterial plaque continues to grow and thicken; eventually it becomes harder and harder, much like cement. Newly formed plaque can pop and cause tremendous damage, while the

Figure 3.2a

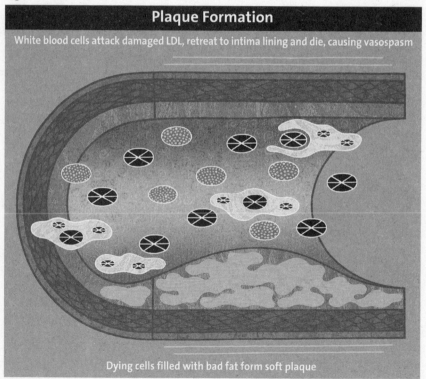

## Plaque Formation

White blood cells attack damaged LDL, retreat to intima lining and die, causing vasospasm

Dying cells filled with bad fat form soft plaque

older, more calcified plaques gradually restrict blood flow. The older plaque causes symptoms, but it seldom triggers life-threatening events. However, as shown in Figure 3.2b, when a small arterial plaque lesion ruptures, releasing inflammatory compounds into the artery, it causes a massive clot to form, which blocks blood flow in the artery and triggers a cardiovascular event.[1]

## MEASURING THE AGE AND FUNCTION OF YOUR CARDIOVASCULAR SYSTEM

How do we gauge plaque growth? It is simple, safe, and easy using high-tech ultrasound equipment similar to what monitors the growth of a fetus in the womb. I use this new carotid intimal medial thickness testing (carotid IMT testing) to precisely calculate arte-

Figure 3.2b

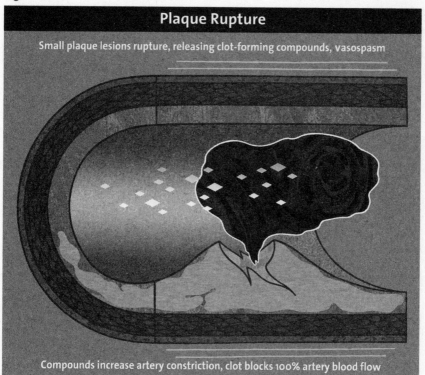

**Plaque Rupture**

Small plaque lesions rupture, releasing clot-forming compounds, vasospasm

Compounds increase artery constriction, clot blocks 100% artery blood flow

## Should I Be Taking a Daily Dose of Baby Aspirin?

A small dose of aspirin is effective in decreasing heart attacks and strokes, especially for men. When a plaque pustule ruptures, it starts forming a blood clot. Aspirin blocks this clotting mechanism. Even a baby aspirin (which is only 81 mg per tablet) is enough to save a life. Keep in mind, however, that aspirin is a double-edged sword. It has benefits and risks. People at low risk for cardiovascular problems are more likely to suffer serious or life-threatening bleeding when taking aspirin than to benefit from it. On the other hand, people with elevated cardiovascular risk factors have more benefit than risk. Because heart attacks in women have more to do with artery spasm and less with clotting than heart attacks in men do, women don't benefit as much as men do from taking aspirin. Talk to your doctor to clarify whether you are a candidate for daily aspirin therapy.

rial plaque growth and to reliably estimate my patients' arterial age.

The carotid arteries are the large ones that carry blood from the heart to the brain. The thickness of the plaque growth within the artery can be measured without radiation or needle sticks, just by a touch of gentle pressure on the neck. Research studies have shown that more than 90% of the time, the carotid arteries, the coronary arteries, and even the arteries in your legs all grow plaque at the same rate.[2] Therefore, the thickness of plaque in the carotid artery reflects plaque growth everywhere in the body, including the arteries that feed the heart. Several studies have also shown that carotid IMT is an excellent and safe predictor of risk for future cardiovascular events.[3]

## TAKING A CAROTID INTIMAL MEDIAL THICKNESS (CAROTID IMT) TEST

The carotid arteries are much easier to get to than the arteries in your heart. To receive a carotid IMT test in my office, my patient simply lies comfortably on an exam table. I apply warm ultrasound gel on his neck over the artery. I gently pass a measuring device from the ultrasound machine over the skin and take pictures of the carotid arteries, which are just beneath the surface. Typically I'll take 12 or more pictures from the right and left carotid arteries, with different views and angles. The whole process usually takes 10 to 12 minutes. At this point, the patient's job is done. I transfer the images to my computer, enlarge them on my screen, and use extremely fancy software to measure the artery lining thickness. These measurements are accurate to hundredths of millimeters.

Multiple studies published in major medical journals have already calculated average carotid artery plaque thickness in thousands of men and women.[4] So once I've calculated my patient's score, I can use these figures to project the average age of his arteries. A 50-year-old man, for instance, might have the plaque of a 40-, 50-, or 60-year-old...or someone older, and might never know it (unless he was tested).

We then monitor the artery age over time (checking every year or two) to clarify whether my patient's plaque is growing, staying the same, or if he follows the 30-Day Heart Tune-Up long-term, actually shrinking.

The Prevention Group of the American Heart Association considers carotid IMT testing to be an excellent way to assess future cardiovascular disease risk.[5] The group recommends it as a safe and dependable tool. Several studies have confirmed their recommendations. If performed regularly over years, repeated carotid IMT scans can project the age at which one will become high risk for a heart attack or stroke and, most important, can give us time to recommend the appropriate therapy to prevent and reverse this aging process.

Because of its safety and efficiency when compared to heart catheterization, IMT testing should be the new gold standard for cardiovascular plaque testing. However, this is not yet the case. Despite its usefulness, 95% of doctors are not ordering this screening test for their patients. You can rest assured that this is a situation I aim to change.

**Figure 3.3**

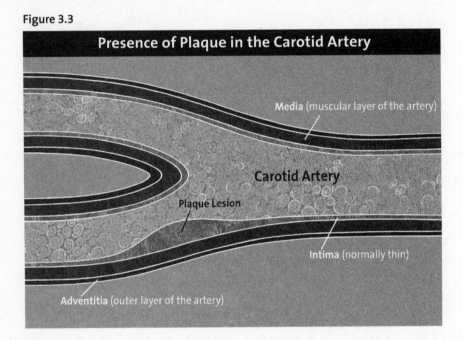

## Presence of Plaque in the Carotid Artery

Media (muscular layer of the artery)

Carotid Artery

Plaque Lesion

Intima (normally thin)

Adventitia (outer layer of the artery)

## *But What If I Have Already Had a Carotid Test?*

It is possible that your doctor tested your carotid artery. But don't be confused by the results from current testing. The standard carotid ultrasound test performed in 95% of hospitals and medical clinics around the country does not measure plaque thickness the way a carotid IMT test would. Rather, this Doppler flow study determines whether the blood flow in your arteries is blocked. A 70% or greater blockage is usually called "significant" and may result in a recommendation for carotid artery surgery. Any lower percentage might be called "no significant obstruction," even though someone with advanced plaque growth and on the verge of a heart attack or stroke might fall into this category. "No significant obstruction" in this case means you are not yet a candidate for surgery, but it says nothing about the age of your arteries, the thickness of the accumulated plaque, or whether those dangerous plaque lesions on the artery wall have formed. So the question should be: Did you have a carotid artery test that measured the thickness of your arterial wall and estimated your arterial age?

Aside from its accuracy, another benefit of IMT testing is that it doesn't require cardiac catheterization, which, as you know from my stepfather Chuck's tragic experience, can cause a stroke in very rare occasions. For more than 10 years, I have used non-invasive IMT testing to monitor my patients' arterial plaque growth. And, as they follow my 30-Day Heart Tune-Up, I've seen many whose arterial plaque load has actually shrunk by up to 10% a year, with and without the use of cholesterol medications. I demonstrated this in a recent study, in which I investigated 400 subjects who had had serial carotid IMT exams once a year for an average of three years, although some patients were actually tested over a 6-year period. Nearly 100 of them (in particular, those who followed my 30-Day Heart Tune-Up recommendations) had a significant decrease in their IMT scores. In fact, many had arteries that were truly 10 years younger![6]

Just be aware that IMT testing must be done under a doctor's supervision. I recommend that carotid IMT scores should be checked at least once in your lifetime for the following reasons. First, it's important for you and your doctor to know your score if action must be taken, and if your score is high, you might want to repeat it yearly over time. Second, I've also found this score to be a powerful motivator for making lifestyle changes—it's much more effective than knowing your values for cholesterol and blood sugar levels. In fact, published studies report that people are much more willing to change their diet and exercise routine after discussing their artery plaque score than they are upon knowing their traditional risk factors.[7]

If you don't have a carotid IMT medical center near you that does these measurements, photos can be taken from regular ultrasound machines, copied as digital images, and sent for analysis to medical centers that measure plaque thickness.

## Should I Have a CT Scan of the Heart?

A chest computed tomography (CT) scan is an imaging method that uses X-rays to create a detailed picture of the heart and its blood vessels. The results are measured as a calcium score of the heart arteries. The higher the calcium score, the more calcified plaque exists. Cardiac CT scanning helps to predict the risk for a future heart attack or stroke.

If you have had a heart scan and your score is high, that means you are at elevated risk for a heart attack or stroke,[8] so clearly you should take action and follow the 30-Day Heart Tune-Up program. However, there are two reasons that you shouldn't repeat a heart CT scan yearly to see if your plaque has grown, shrunk, or stayed the same, the way you can with carotid IMT testing. First, new, soft plaque growth doesn't show on CT scanning. CT only shows the calcification of old plaque, formed years ago. Second, CT scanning causes substantial radiation exposures that increases your risk for cancer—I believe the risk associated with yearly CT scanning is just too great!

I had the experience of testing my patients with both a CT heart scan and a carotid IMT for a few years. With time, I discovered that the CT heart scan had several disadvantages when compared with carotid IMT testing:

- The heart scans did not provide any "extra" useful information. I have never had an abnormal heart scan and a normal carotid IMT. Plus, sometimes they missed critical information. If a patient has advanced plaque growth that is still soft and hasn't calcified, this won't show up on a CT scan. The patient will be at risk but will believe that his or her blood vessels are in good shape.
- The scan costs patients twice as much as the carotid IMT.
- It adds a dose of radiation exposure that increases the lifetime risk for developing cancer.

The bottom line from my experience is that the CT heart scan provided no more information than I was acquiring from carotid IMT testing, but CT heart scans had the problems I've just noted, so I stopped ordering the scans and have been relying on carotid IMT testing instead.

## OTHER WAYS TO PREDICT YOUR PLAQUE SCORE

My research has successfully shown that even if you've never had the IMT test performed, or if it's not available to you, other means are available to help you predict your carotid IMT plaque score and estimate the age of your cardiovascular system. The best predictors are:

1. aerobic fitness
2. fiber intake
3. how many times a week you eat fish
4. systolic blood pressure, which is not just a risk factor but a measure of artery function
5. your total cholesterol/HDL ratio (not to be confused with a simple cholesterol test)
6. body fat. But guess what? While elevated body fat is a risk factor for growing arterial plaque, if you take care of the predictors listed above, your weight will take care of itself!

In fact, if you are unable to schedule a carotid IMT study with your doctor, there are straightforward measurements you can take on your own at home with a friend or with an exercise physiologist or trainer at the gym that will help you measure your fitness and your heart's function:

- your blood vessel function as determined by your blood pressure response to exercise
- your aerobic fitness—metabolic equivalency (MET) level achieved—measured while on a standard gym treadmill, elliptical machine, stationary bicycle, or during a simple 3-minute step test
- your heart resilience after exercising as shown by your 1-minute heart rate recovery

Let's look at these more closely.

## THE IMPORTANCE OF BLOOD PRESSURE

The most common measure of cardiovascular health is blood pressure, the degree of pressure within your arteries. In fact, if you compare blood pressure with all of the other classic risk factors—high cholesterol, obesity, smoking, and diabetes—it is the strongest predictor of future risk for a heart attack and stroke.

When high blood pressure persists over time, doctors call it hypertension. This doesn't mean you have a disease that is attacking your heart and that you need a prescription medication. Rather, hypertension is a sign that your arteries aren't functioning well. With time, they will get sicker as they grow more and more plaque. There are drugs that lower blood pressure, but the high blood pressure is the sign that warns us that something is wrong in our arteries and heart. Even while you are taking blood pressure medication, plaque typically continues to grow within the arteries.

As we all know, blood pressure can be an imprecise measure of heart age, as it changes from moment to moment—typically it can increase rapidly if you become excited, upset, or frightened. Nevertheless, it is very easy to measure, and most grocery stores, fire stations, and pharmacies have the equipment for this. You can even buy a blood pressure measuring device yourself.

Since blood pressure can vary from day to day and even from hour to hour, it is important to assess it when you are calm and relaxed. Use the lowest reading from several observations. Your blood pressure basically tells you whether your cardiovascular system is:

- young and fit
- aging and stressed
- elderly and sick

You can have your blood pressure measured during exercise in most gyms with the assistance of an exercise physiologist, or at a medical office during stress exercise testing.

The blood pressure at rest of a young and fit vascular tree is below 120/80 mm Hg. A reading of 110/70 is healthy and good. During vigorous exercise, the top (systolic) number climbs from 120 to 150 and up to 160 or 170 as the heart pumps harder. The bottom (diastolic) number drops as your arteries dilate, usually it drops from 10 to 20 points, and may drop 40 points or more in highly trained athletes. So at peak exercise, a fit person might have a blood pressure of 170/40, and this is considered normal.

In comparison, an aging and stressed vascular tree has a blood pressure at rest of between 120/80 and 140/90, which is called an "elevated blood pressure." In this case, during vigorous exercise, the top systolic number climbs as the heart pumps harder from 120 to 150 and may go as high as 180 to 200. The bottom (diastolic) number will stay the same, or it may climb 5 to 9 points with strenuous activity. So when exercising, a person with an aging and stressed vascular system will have blood pressure that jumps to 190/85. Elevated blood pressure is a sign that your arteries are growing sick and likely forming plaque.

An elderly and sick vascular tree has a blood pressure (without medication) that is more than 140/90. During vigorous exercise, the top (systolic) number climbs as the heart pumps harder, from 120 to 150, and often goes above 180, sometimes over 200. The bottom (diastolic) number will increase by at least 10 points, which is an abnormal response. Basically, the arteries constrict, which is not a desirable result of physiological stress. So with vigorous exercise, the blood pressure of a person with a sick or elderly vascular tree might reach 200/105. An elderly vascular tree probably has been neglected for years.

Your blood pressure test is a simple, inexpensive way to assess your cardiovascular risk. If you are a healthy individual, an exercise physiologist at the gym can check your blood pressure, as outlined above, while you exercise. If you have multiple risk factors for heart disease and your physician requests a stress test to have your heart checked, be sure to tell the technician or your doctor in advance that you want to see the numbers to clarify how your blood pressure responds to exercise. You'll also want to know your 1-minute heart rate recovery number, which I will discuss shortly.

## STOP COUNTING CALORIES AND BECOME A METS FAN

A second way to determine the function of your heart is to measure your METs. And no, I am not referring to the New York baseball team, even though you pronounce the word the same way! METs is a term that health professionals use to describe how much energy you spend while performing a particular activity, as in METabolic equivalency level, or energy-burning rate, compared to the resting metabolic rate. The usual measurement for your overall exertion level is called your "MET level achieved." One MET of energy designates how much energy (oxygen) you burn when lying completely still in bed. The more physical activity you do, the higher your MET level. For instance, a person doing gardening or housework (depending on how strenuous it is) will burn between 1.5 and 4 METs; a construction worker on the job will burn between 4.0 and 8.5 METs. Running 3.4 miles per hour on a treadmill set at an elevation of 14% should yield an 8 to 8.3 METs level in the first minute.

| MET Levels for Various Jobs and Activities | | | |
|---|---|---|---|
| Occupation | METs | Activities | METs |
| Receptionist | 1.0–2.0 | Walking with a suitcase | 7 |
| Housekeeper | 1.5–4.0 | Cleaning floors | 4 |
| Farm worker | 3.5–7.5 | Cooking | 3 |
| Construction worker | 4.0–8.5 | Gardening | 4 |
| Miner | 4.0–9.0 | Pushing a power mower | 5 |
| Mail carrier | 2.5–5.0 | Sexual intercourse | 5 |
| Medical professional | 1.5–3.5 | Running on a treadmill | 5–18 |

Physicians worldwide use the MET scale on a standardized treadmill test to gauge cardiovascular function. The most common standardized test used in the United States is called the Bruce Protocol Treadmill Stress Test. During a stress test, the treadmill speed and incline are increased every three minutes. Even if you're not taking a stress test, the number of METs achieved at the end of each minute you complete will appear as a reading on most treadmill or cardiovascular exercise machines. Ideally, this test should be done with a physician, but with your doctor's permission, you can also determine your MET score with the help of a skilled exercise physiologist or trainer at the gym.

After a heart attack, many of the people referred to my cardiology colleagues are very unfit. They are unable to achieve even 4 METs of exertion. Identifying this level of poor fitness is very important, because it clarifies that at least for the moment, they may be unable to perform even basic activities of daily living (cleaning, gardening, etc.) without straining their hearts.

Most healthy people should "comfortably" achieve a total of at least 10 to 12 METs on a standard treadmill fitness test that lasts anywhere from 12 to 18 minutes. Many of my robust 80-year-olds still reach at least 10 to 12 METs, and with time and training you should be able to attain this level too. For a middle-aged person, 12 METs is a decent level of fitness, and 15 METs is very good. My more athletic participants from their thirties through their seventies may reach 15 to 18 METs, which is excellent. From my research,[9] we now know that those who reached 15 METs seldom have an elevated carotid IMT score—more on this in Chapter 5.

Doing well on a MET assessment has important implications for your life! For every single MET increase in fitness, your risk of a heart attack, stroke, or sudden death drops by 12.5%. So forget about burning calories; if you can increase your fitness level by 2 METs (from 8 to 10, or from 10 to 12) you will decrease your risk of a cardiovascular event by 25%! You will find instructions on how to perform your own METs test in Chapter 5.

## HEART RATE RECOVERY AFTER EXERCISE ASSESSES THE RESILIENCE OF YOUR HEARTBEAT

An equally good predictor of your heart's fitness and ability to accommodate varying levels of physical exertion is to track how quickly your heart rate drops after one minute of peak exercise. At maximum exercise, your heart can race as high as 200 beats per minute. When you stop, the quicker your heart rate drops, the better. In published studies using treadmill testing at the Cleveland Clinic on tens of thousands of patients, poor heart rate recovery was the strongest predictor of future heart attacks and cardiac death.[10] In fact, in several other studies across the country, the one- or two-minute heart rate recovery was judged to be the best tool to predict the risk of future cardiovascular events in people with or without heart disease between the ages of 30 and 80.[11] One minute after stopping at your peak exertion level, your heart rate should drop by at least 25 beats, and dropping more than 30 beats is very good. Some athletes will have a 40–60 point drop in heart rate at one minute. If your heart rate drops less than 20 beats at one minute I call that concerning. If it drops less than 12 beats, that may be alarming.

If you have found that you have any of the risk factors listed in Chapter 2, you need to begin this kind of exercise testing with your physician. With your doctor's permission, a second and excellent option is to work out at the gym with an exercise physiologist or trainer; a fantastic investment in your health would be to perform an annual fitness test in a gym. Obviously, if you're young, healthy, and fit without cardiac risk factors, you might choose to do this testing on your own. A good rule of thumb: the more significant medical problems you have, the more important that you undergo testing with a physician or an exercise physiologist.

Of course, the mentally tough and hardheaded might choose to push it quite a bit, strain themselves, and get to the point of dizziness and collapse when taking the treadmill test. Clearly, that's going too far! You run the risk of fainting, having a head injury, or pulling a tendon. You could face months of rehab. *Absolutely don't overdo it.* Total exhaustion would be running until you can't run anymore. The example I often give patients while in the early stages of the treadmill test is as follows: "Imagine that a lion has been chasing you. Exhausted, you give up, stop, look the beast in the eye, and say, 'Okay. Eat me!' That's verging on collapse, and we won't go that far! We're going to stop when you can no longer speak two short sentences." You should observe the same guidelines too!

Also be aware that if you're taking blood pressure medicine or other medications that modify your heart rate, your response may vary from my usual recommendations.

Having clarified the risks, let's repeat that there's a huge benefit to pressing on with exercise and defining your real maximal heart rate. This fitness test will help you make the best use of your exercise program and will provide the most benefit within a reasonable time. In Chapter 5, you'll find instructions on how to do this.

## THE 3-MINUTE STEP TEST

If you don't have access to a gym, the easiest assessment of your aerobic fitness that you can take is a 3-minute step test. You can get a couple of important results from this simple test. The Queens College Step test is one of many variations. A similar test is the YMCA 3-minute step test. They both provide a measure of your cardiorespiratory or endurance fitness.

But we're not talking about running up and down the stairs in your house. The "step" is a 16.25-inch-high box. You'll also need a stopwatch, a metronome (optional), and heart rate monitor (optional, but recommended). You'll find instructions on how to do this test in Chapter 5.

## SHOWING RESULTS

Remember Mike? He was the marketing VP who had lost his good health during the recent recession. We made a METs fan out of him, and it saved his heart and his life! After seeing his abnormal stress test, lab work, and carotid IMT results, he committed himself to making a change. Mike cleaned up his diet, adding nearly all of our heart-friendly foods. He did a complete oil change with his revised fat intake, but perhaps most important, he decided to work out five days every week—and he stuck to it. Our heart rate exercise recommendations led to positive results. One year later, Mike's MET level score had jumped from 10 to 15, lowering his predicted risk for a cardiovascular event by 62.5%. His blood pressure response to exercise changed as well. His prior peak had been 190/100, but only one year later it had been lowered to 170/70. Not surprisingly, Mike's heart rate recovery improved too. Initially he showed a worrisome 15-beat drop one minute after peak exercise. But this improved to a 30-beat drop once he regained his fitness.

After seeing these changes in his conditioning and cardiovascular function, I knew that Mike's carotid IMT scores must have also improved. In fact, his plaque had shrunk by nearly 10% in just one year. That gave all of us reason to celebrate.

The truth is that I have seen many patients make improvements just as Mike has. With a little encouragement, you can have fantastic results, too!

## PREPARING YOURSELF FOR YOUR HEART TUNE-UP

I know that you're eager to begin the 30-Day Heart Tune-Up, and I will be behind you when you take the leap. However, now that you've decided to take your heart's fitness into your own hands, it will be wise to create a baseline with your physician. If you are healthy and you know that you are relatively fit, that you have normal cholesterol, blood pressure, blood sugar levels, inflammation markers, and body composition, you don't smoke, nor do you have a worrisome family history, then you are ready to get started.

However, if you don't know your risk factors, or if you've been a couch potato for years and are unhealthy or unfit, you should seek your doctor's permission to begin this program. Start by having a checkup. Uncontrolled diabetes, high cholesterol, and hypertension could create a dangerous situation, so all of your medical conditions must be taken into account. You just want to be sure you can proceed safely. If you are tested properly, you will know where you stand and what you are capable of handling.

Here is how I suggest you approach your physician:

1. First, call and schedule an appointment with your doctor. Tell the receptionist you want to make a "wellness" appointment to confirm you are safe to start an exercise program. If your regular follow-up exam is overdue, depending upon your physician, it might be advisable to also schedule a second appointment to get caught up on all your appropriate health screening.

2. At your visit, tell your physician that you want to take charge of your health by adding regular exercise, by eating healthy foods, and by managing your stress. Explain that you hope your doctor can confirm that it is safe for you to start. Tell him or her that you are following my 30-Day Heart Tune-Up. I have presented lectures on this subject to tens of thousands of physicians over the last 10 years, so your doctor might already be aware of my program. If not, I suggest you provide your doctor with this book, or refer your doctor to my website, www.hearttuneup.com, so he or she can see the type of program you are following. If you have uncontrolled health problems such as diabetes, high cholesterol, or hypertension, your doctor may recommend a stress test—there is a ton of information you can gain from this. But please don't let anyone rush you into an invasive procedure such as a heart catheterization without getting at least a second opinion from another physician. Make sure that you have read this entire book and discussed what you have discovered with your own physician.

3. The key safety issues to resolve during your physician's assessment are to clarify that your heart, lungs, and joints are ready for exercise.

4. If you are not up-to-date on your laboratory testing, I hope your doctor will order the tests I'm about to suggest, plus measure your body fat, blood pressure, and resting heart rate. But if this doesn't occur for whatever reason, then I will suggest you ask for the following tests (if you have had these tests in the last year, you don't need to repeat them unless your physician believes otherwise):

   a. fasting lipid profile; if you have several cardiac risk factors or a family history of heart disease, ask for an advanced lipid profile

   b. fasting blood sugar; optimal is under 90 mg/dL and normal is under 100 mg/dL; include a hemoglobin A1C and a fasting insulin level, if you have elevated blood sugar

   c. hs-CRP (high-sensitivity C-reactive protein) test; a measure of inflammation; normal is less than 1.0 mg/dL

   d. TSH (thyroid-stimulating hormone) level; a measure of thyroid function; normal should be less than 3.0 mIU/L (milli-international units per liter). If you have symptoms of low thyroid hormone levels, such as low energy, constipation, cold intolerance, and/or weight gain, request a full thyroid panel, which includes free T3, free T4, reverse T4, and thyroid antibodies.

   e. hemoglobin (or complete blood count) to check for anemia

Ask for a carotid IMT study to measure your plaque growth. For the most part, insurance companies are not yet covering carotid IMT testing, despite the fact that it is now considered a state-of-the-art diagnostic tool. (However, there are exceptions, as the state of Texas has proposed a bill stating that if a physician orders it, insurers are required to pay for a onetime IMT carotid scan.) There are, as you have seen, many benefits to the carotid IMT test. If this test isn't covered by your medical insurance, let your doctor know you are willing to pay for it out of pocket. Depending upon the equipment and who performs the study, prices for a carotid IMT study vary from $150 to $450—less than you might pay for a new iPad upgrade. Isn't it worth spending those dollars for a test that could literally save your life? But don't be surprised if your doctor hasn't heard of carotid IMT testing, or if your physician mistakes it for Doppler carotid artery testing. This is a common misunderstanding. There are also many other useful tests your physician might consider, so listen to what studies he or she may suggest.

## WHO PAYS FOR THIS TYPE OF CARDIOVASCULAR TESTING?

This brings up a subject close to *my* heart. Medical insurance coverage varies dramatically. Typically, it covers only the very basic cardiovascular risk factor measures (blood sugar, cholesterol profile, and blood pressure), or if you have already had a heart attack or stroke or suspicious symptoms, more advanced testing such as standard carotid ultrasound studies and treadmill.

Unfortunately, many people may not be able to afford to pay for tests measuring how they're aging, which would include a carotid IMT and stress treadmill testing. Yet for most all of us, following the 30-Day Heart Tune-Up long-term has the potential to save a fortune in future medical expenses, and very likely will lessen the need for these tests in the first place. So whether or not you participate in the fancy testing, you'll still benefit enormously by following the program itself.

The truth is that our current medical system has little concern for measuring aging factors or optimizing health screenings for fitness or nutrition. Medical insurance only reimburses for treating diseases once they've already occurred. Think about it this way: If you've had a stroke, it's like being involved in a serious car wreck—your insurance will cover your medical costs related to the stroke. But if you want new brakes, they will not cover this preventive measure even if the brakes would have averted the accident in the first place.

After 25 years of helping people optimize their aging process, my beliefs about insurance coverage have changed. For instance, I discovered that people get much better test results if they take more responsibility for their own health. Measuring cardiac fitness, arterial age, and nutritional status are steps we should take to enhance our health and aging process without asking others to pay for them.

During my college years, I spent a semester studying in Washington, D.C., which included a stint with a historian at the Smithsonian Institution. My research project was related to medicine practiced by Native American healers in the fifteenth and sixteenth centuries. One of the take-home messages that I now recall, more than 30 years later, is that the medicine men always charged for their treatments. Powerful medicine and teachings always required a higher charge than simple ones. The "payment" was an essential part of the cure—somehow, without adequate payment, the therapy wouldn't work. Over the years, I've worked in many medical settings and have spent extended time doing volunteer work as well. When I compare the results my patients have achieved, clearly those who paid out of pocket for the services they received have had far better results.

If we are to improve the aging process and stop the #1 killer in America today, it might mean we must all have some "skin in the game." This may empower us to achieve the results we all deserve but few achieve. Admittedly, advanced, preventive cardiovascular screening is expensive. A carotid IMT study can cost between

$150 and $450; an advanced lipid profile may cost $100 to $250; and a stress treadmill test with VO$_2$ max testing (a measure of oxygen consumed by the body) may cost from $300 to $600. Yet for many, this can be a onetime expense. Either your tests look good, and your doctor doesn't have to keep ordering them, or if the results are bad, your insurance may actually cover this type of testing in the future to help keep you out of the hospital.

## WHAT THE TUNE-UP WILL DO FOR YOUR HEART

The simple assessments I've outlined above should give you an estimate of your heart's age and your cardiac fitness level. I'll show you how to do these tests in Chapter 5. You may be surprised to learn that your heart and blood vessels are not as young as the rest of you and that you may be at risk for a cardiovascular event. If so, this is the moment to take action—before you get into trouble and have an episode that could damage your heart, your brain, and your life.

So today, right now, I can offer you a medically sound plan designed to markedly reduce your cardiovascular risk without surgery, drugs, or frequent and expensive trips to the doctor. I can offer you a scientifically proven program that can reduce the plaque in your arteries—the main culprit behind heart attacks and strokes. I can offer to make your heart younger and stronger and at the same time make you feel healthier, more vigorous, trimmer, mentally sharper, and sexier than you have in over a decade. I promise with this tune-up you'll begin to see results in as little as 30 days. I strongly hope *you* will follow this plan!

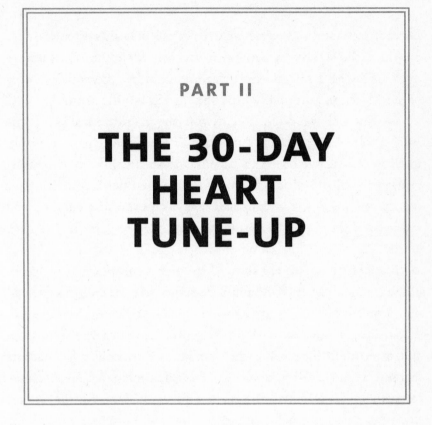

**PART II**

# THE 30-DAY HEART TUNE-UP

Sometimes it takes a catastrophe to get somebody's attention. Let me share the story of a patient in my clinic who chose to ignore my 30-Day Heart Tune-Up recommendations, the consequences of her inaction, and finally how she turned her life around.

Silvia is a 55-year-old executive with a communications company. I liked her as soon as I met her. She was cheerful, charming, intelligent, and we shared a passion for tennis. Like that of most businesspeople, her life was stressful. She used her 50- to 60-hour workweek and weekly plane travel as excuses to skip exercise and order from the dessert menu (as a misguided reward for her hard work).

Silvia's first assessment showed the arterial plaque of a 69-year-old woman, and her blood pressure response to exercise suggested sick arteries that were growing plaque. Her fasting blood sugar was modestly elevated, 110 mg/dL (something her prior physician called normal). The rest of her classic cardiovascular risk factors seemed fine, including a "normal" HDL cholesterol level. However, an advanced lipid profile showed she had very little HDL2, the super garbage truck that cleans our arteries, which very likely caused her advanced arterial plaque growth.

We discussed adding daily aerobic activity, drinking less alcohol, adding fish oil, and cutting way back on sweets and refined carbs in her diet, which, when combined in a comprehensive treatment plan, can raise HDL2 nicely. Although we'd spent a good deal of time together, Silvia was not ready to make any changes at that time. Sadly, she disregarded my recommendations.

Six months later, during an intense business meeting, Silvia developed heavy chest pain, felt nauseated, and became sweaty. She didn't let her colleagues know, but when the meeting was over, the pain worsened. She called 911 and was admitted to the hospital with a heart attack. Several hours later, while in the intensive care unit, her heart stopped. She had suffered what's known as "sudden death." The emergency room staff shocked her heart twice, and she was successfully resuscitated. She left the hospital four days later, but not before cardiologists placed a defibrillator device in her chest that would shock her if her heart stopped again. She was also given several medications to help prevent dangerous heart rhythms from recurring and to prevent blood clots from forming in her heart. The side effects of some of these drugs, which she would need to take for the rest of her life because of the injury to her heart, can include depression, low energy, wheezing, and sexual dysfunction.

Not surprisingly, after this terrible incident, Silvia returned to me with motivation. Today, following the 30-Day Heart Tune-Up, her blood sugar and cholesterol are nicely controlled, and she has lost weight. She also works out every day. We should be able to prevent her from having another life-threatening event, but the heart attack has left her with a permanent scar on her heart, which increases her future risk for sudden death. As a result, she will now live with a defibrillator, extra medications, and a good bit of anxiety.

We were able to restore Silvia to an active life. But the key is to make changes *before* serious, irreversible problems occur, not after! For those who need it, the 30-Day Heart Tune-Up is also designed to help reverse much of the arterial damage already done.

What's the Tune-Up all about? It is about shrinking arterial plaque, improving circulation, and strengthening your heartbeat. You will be using four important tools:

- heart-healing foods
- exercise that strengthens your heart and arteries
- stress management
- a customized heart-friendly supplement plan

Plus, you need to commit to adopting this plan and sticking with it!

Each of these tools will be clearly explained to you in the following chapters—why they're important and how to incorporate them into your life. As an extra, added benefit, many of my patients have found that, along with a healthier heart, their sex lives have improved markedly as a result of the 30-Day Heart Tune-Up plan. So in Chapter 8, I'll explain how the program will add zest to your life in more ways than one!

Living this healthy lifestyle will be valuable to you in many ways. You'll feel younger, happier, stronger, and sharper mentally. You'll have more stamina and energy. You'll improve your immune system and feel less achy. And, you'll be fitter and trimmer than you have been in years.

But the purpose of this book is not just to improve your quality of life—although it most certainly will. I have in mind a higher purpose that will benefit all of us as Americans. We can attribute a big part of the national rise in health care expenses to paying for the treatment of cardiovascular disease. Indeed, heart disease is bankrupting us on a national level. It is taking hundreds of billions of dollars from our budget, when that same money could go toward preventive health care, education, and our own pocketbooks.

The sad truth is that heart disease likely will affect someone you love dearly—or possibly even yourself—during your lifetime. If nothing else motivates you to change your lifestyle—this should.

Finally, the 30-Day Heart Tune-Up has been based on my life's work. I've devoted every hour of every day striving to make my patients' lives and hearts better without their having to resort to surgery or other invasive procedures. This has become a calling for me—one that I believe will improve the quality of life for all of us. After all, the losses we suffer due to cardiovascular disease are great—personal pain, decreased income, reduced productivity, physical suffering, and even premature death. So much of this anguish is unnecessary. Instead of your muddling through as a helpless, hopeless victim of heart disease, with the 30-Day Heart Tune-Up you will have all the tools you need to attack and defeat this scourge. It is possible to reverse cardiovascular disease, and certainly to prevent it. This book will help you take charge of your own well-being, starting right now!

## Chapter Four

# Eat Right for Your Heart

How many times have you heard of or read about the "basic food groups"? Government-issued healthy eating guidelines first named four food groups, then changed it to seven—now it's five, to be eaten in varying proportions. They issued educational pie charts and food pyramids and illustrated plates. Adding to the confusion has been an endless variety of diets that have been promoted by so-called health experts and idolized by our national media: Ornish? Pritikin? Atkins? South Beach? Paleo? Grapefruit? Cabbage soup? Liquid? Starvation? The choices are as confounding as they are dizzying, since experts swear by their own methods.

I believe it's time for a little common sense when it comes to food and your heart. And I certainly don't want to add to the confusion. So let's set aside the government's recommendations and fad diets and think clearly about which foods will help you take better care of your heart—the foods that will actually lower your harmful cholesterol and raise the beneficial cholesterol, reduce arterial plaque and inflammation, prevent clots from forming, and open your arteries, thereby diminishing your risk for a cardiovascular event. I propose an eating plan that you will be able to adopt for the long run so that it becomes a normal part of your life, not a crash diet that is the topic of cocktail party conversation, but results in you giving up, famished and frustrated, to binge on fast food or dig out the Ben & Jerry's from the back of your freezer. Relapses such as these are more injurious to your heart health than having maintained your former lifestyle choices, because overindulging in toxic food accelerates arterial plaque growth and undermines your motivation to maintain a healthy lifestyle. So I truly don't want you to fall into that trap!

## HOW I DEVELOPED THE 30-DAY HEART TUNE-UP EATING PLAN

Over the years, I have had extensive experience working with people who have type 2 diabetes and heart disease. In the 1990s, I tried to bring the Dean Ornish Program to a 500,000-member cooperative clinic in Olympia, Washington (the Group Health Cooperative). I wanted to offer something more than just drugs and surgery to our patients, and I spent nearly one year fighting to initiate a lifestyle program that had been proven to reverse heart disease. The difficulty following the Ornish Program was that it was ultra-low-fat, vegetarian, and required daily meditation. Fewer than 5% of our high-risk cardiac patients would even consider it. So instead, I created my own program, which I shared with groups of patients, and they had excellent success in changing their lifestyle and improving their outcomes.[1]

Years later, when I was the medical director for the Pritikin Longevity Center in Florida, people would arrive with advanced diabetes or heart disease. Often they were on multiple medications and had poor blood sugar control. After two or three weeks, their blood sugar levels had improved to the point that they were normal, so we were able to wean them off most of their medications. Often their angina disappeared. We were thrilled that we had transformed their lives!

Why were these Pritikin patients so successful? They exercised an hour or two every day, their stress levels had dropped substantially, and there were no junk foods or refined carbs to be had. But the fact is, they were not home in their usual surroundings. Instead, they lived in a controlled environment at the Pritikin Center, where their diets were tightly monitored. They ate only whole, unprocessed foods. It was a very high-fiber, high-carb regimen with little protein or fat.

But the story, rosy as it seems, doesn't end there. As time went on and patients cycled through the center, I saw that they couldn't stick with the program once they returned to their homes and families. Nearly all of my patients had setbacks. Not only that, but despite the improvements in blood sugar, the HDL cholesterol levels of many of my patients dropped (as you now know, this is a bad thing) because their diets lacked adequate healthy protein and fats.

When I left Pritikin, I saw ways to improve on their program. I resumed using my own original high-fiber, low–refined carb diet, based upon my previously proven results. It provided the same blood sugar–lowering benefits, but now my patients were able to stick with it long-term. The difference was that I added healthy fat and protein sources, which made their food much more palatable, nutritious, and fun to eat! My approach has been confirmed by the recent Mediterranean Diet Study for Cardiovascular Disease, which has also shown that adding olive oil and nuts to your diet is heart-healthier than following a moderate-fat heart-healthy diet alone.[2] Now my patients can stay on my eating plan at home and even follow it in restaurants for years to come.

The heart-healthy diet I'm about to recommend has been thoroughly researched and is the best and easiest way for you to begin your journey toward a younger, stronger heart. Not only that, there are only five components for you to remember:

1. adequate fiber
2. healthy fats
3. lean protein

4. beneficial beverages
5. fabulous flavors

None of my recommendations and the 60 recipes I've created (see Chapter 10) are exotic or outlandish! You'll recognize all of the foods. You'll eat none in excess. And I can guarantee you won't be bored! How can you be, when you'll choose from among entrees such as grilled salmon, almond-crusted white fish, shrimp, crab, mussels, oysters, and lobster? Herb-seasoned chicken or turkey breast, pork tenderloin, bison steaks, and other game meats will share your plate with fresh, colorful vegetables and wild rice or quinoa. There will be berries in abundance and peaches, apples, and cherries, plus tomatoes, green salads, and artichokes. Almonds, pistachios, pecans, walnuts, and avocados— yes, these have fats in them, but they're healthy fats, the kind your body needs, and fiber too! You'll enjoy rich and flavorful minestrone soup, or spicy garlic-shrimp tostadas laden with fresh tomato salsa, black beans, and red cabbage.

Eggs—the organic, free-range, omega-3 variety—are definitely on the menu! I know they cost a little more, but they're so worth it when you consider the alternatives. So how about an omelet with sautéed artichoke hearts, spinach, and green onions for Sunday brunch?

And there's even room for dessert: strawberries dipped in dark chocolate! Or fresh blueberries, nuts, and dark chocolate chips sprinkled on Greek yogurt. For a treat, how about a dark chocolate raspberry orange soufflé, or pear, peach, and blueberry crumble? To drink? Iced or hot green or black tea, cocoa, blueberry smoothies, purified water, and even coffee, merlot, cabernet, or pinot noir, in moderation.

You will feel satisfied and full—not deprived or hungry! And if you are overweight, weight loss will be a happy side benefit of your following the 30-Day Heart Tune-Up eating plan. Sound fantastic? Too good to be true? Not at all.

## WHY THIS DIET WORKS

Food is not only a source of calories and nutrients; it provides information that regulates your gene expression. Your genes tell your cells to either self-destruct or thrive. In fact, one third of your genes respond to what you eat. Given the right food information, your genes stimulate your cells to manufacture enzymes that can lower cholesterol, open your arteries, and prevent blood clots from forming. The 30-Day Heart Tune-Up eating plan is designed to empower you to select foods that will tell your genes to make your heart and your whole cardiovascular system more functional and essentially younger at a cellular level.

It is time to adopt a heart-friendly diet that includes heart-healing foods. These are specific foods you should *add* to your diet to revitalize your heart and circulation. Adding is my theme, and it's essential. Not only is adding food more beneficial, it is easier and much more fun than depriving yourself of foods you love. Strict programs such as the Pritikin Plan and Dean Ornish's regimen dictate what you can't eat. Yes, both programs offer healthy food ideas and good exercise tips. But the truth is, while many of us may start these diets with good intentions, I have seen that most Americans won't stay on them. In fact from my experience, more than 90% of people will *not* accept these austere recommendations over the long haul. Most give up within a few weeks and return to where they started—discouraged, defeated, and less willing to try again.

In contrast, I have published scientific research in *Alternative Therapies in Health and Medicine* and the *Journal of Family Practice* proving that at least 70% of the people who have started the 30-Day Heart Tune-Up eating plan follow my recommendations for up to two years.[3] And in my clinic, my patients have been thriving on it for nearly a decade.

# A WORD OF CAUTION BEFORE WE BEGIN

I strongly believe in the value of adding certain foods to your diet, as you'll see. But the one thing I don't want you to add is a toxin. Yes, that's right, toxic food! Most food-related heart disease comes from eating the two most common toxins found in the American diet—both of which lead to the metabolic syndrome. The first toxin is too much inflammation-inducing sugar and the second is artery-clogging trans fat (also called hydrogenated fat).

You know what sugar is; we see it all the time. But trans fat/ hydrogenated fat is less well understood and usually hidden in the food supply. Trans fat does not exist in the natural world in any significant amount. It is manufactured by the food industry to prolong the shelf life of processed foods in order to boost profits. This substance was created for us to eat, despite the fact that bio-chemically it has more in common with liquid plastic than with food. Scientists combine regular oil with harmful metals and then pump hydrogen into the mixture. This creates a stiff fat. Studies show that trans fats increase your risk for cancer, diabetes, and heart disease. A common name for trans fat is margarine, but I prefer to call it embalming fluid, as chemically they have much in common. Trans fat is found in many processed foods and is commonly used in restaurants, too.

Eating sugar and trans fat is like putting dirt in your car's gas tank. Obviously the engine won't run well with dirty gas, so nobody would stop at the gas station and sprinkle dirt into their tank. Yet many people will walk inside the gas station shop to buy chips, candy, cookies, soda—foods that are full of sugar and trans fats. They are literally poisoning themselves. This drives me crazy. Why do Americans worry more about gas for their cars than the fuel they provide for themselves?

Why are sugar and trans fats so dangerous? In the past, the #1 cause of heart disease appeared to be related to high choles-terol levels. We were active, didn't eat a great deal of processed sugar-rich foods, and people who developed heart disease ate far too many fatty cuts of meats such as burgers and prime rib; and ate rich dairy products, in particular cheese, 2% and whole milk, whipped cream, and butter. Today, there is actually much less cholesterol-raising saturated fat in our diets. In fact, if you recall from my discussion in Chapter 2, the leading cause of heart disease is now related to having metabolic syndrome. So let's deal with our national overuse of sugar.

## THE SUGAR CONUNDRUM

Over the last ten thousand years, we have developed a natural affinity for sugar, a useful source of energy for ancient tribes that often faced famine. The brain rewards us for eating sugar with a blast of chemicals that make sweets extremely satisfying. The problem is, we no longer endure famines. So we don't need sugar, but our brain does not have a shut-off switch that would help us just say no to sweets.

The first step to achieve control over your sweet tooth is to broaden your understanding of the word "sugar." I propose that we redefine sugar as any harmful carb that causes a spike, rather than a gradual rise, in blood sugar levels. These bad carbs are found in white bread, white rice, white flour tortillas, white flour pasta, sports drinks, processed fruit juices and fruit drinks, table sugar, cookies and chips, and sodas. Please remember that "enriched flour" is really just white flour without fiber. If you search their ingredient lists, you will see that popular cereals use these types of harmful carbs too.

Harmful carbs are usually easy to find in cookies, chips, and sodas. But many bad carbs are hidden in foods we eat where it is much harder to detect them. For instance, natural or organic "whole-grain" cereals will also cause a jump in your blood sugar levels if the grain has been ground into flour. Most people are unaware that a bowl of white rice, a bowl of white flour, and a bowl of whole-grain flour all result in nearly the same abnormal spike in blood sugar levels. In fact, a sudden spike also comes from eating whole-grain breads (such as whole wheat), and whole-grain corn tortillas too.

---

## Hidden Toxic Sugar

The food industry is required to list all the ingredients on food labels, but their marketing departments don't want sugar to be listed first (as the principal ingredient), so they hide it. To do this, they will often add three, four, or even five sources of sugar to a package so that "sugar" doesn't show up first on the ingredient list.

The next time you look at a food label, search for the following sources of sugar:

- sugar, glucose
- corn syrup, cornstarch
- any fruit juice
- cane products
- honey, fructose
- any syrup
- potato starch
- any flour that isn't whole-grain flour

---

The bottom line is that if a grain has been processed into flour, it acts like a refined carb on your blood sugar control. So if you have any signs of metabolic syndrome (elevated blood pressure, blood sugar, and triglycerides; increasing waistline; low HDL; and inflammation), you should avoid everyday use of products that contain flour.

Let me explain why even whole wheat flour causes the same jump in blood sugar levels as granulated sugar. The flour particles are ground so finely that they are absorbed across the intestinal wall into the bloodstream as quickly as sugar molecules. In both cases, your blood sugar level surges. This spike causes inflammation, which we now know is detrimental to your arteries. Not only are you inflamed, but the same spike also stimulates your pancreas to produce insulin—a hormone that quickly returns blood sugar levels to normal. The higher your sugar spikes, the faster insulin will counteract it to make your levels plummet. Your body senses this drop intensely, because it triggers hunger and cravings. Suddenly you feel famished and exhausted so you grab another snack—repeating the process over and over again until it becomes a vicious cycle.

---

### Would You Like Some Chopsticks with That Bowl of Sugar?

Why is it so bad to eat refined grains such as white rice? Well, in truth, there's no difference between a bowl of white rice and a bowl of sugar! White rice turns into sugar in your body and ruins your metabolism, so they have exactly the same effect. Whole wheat has far more nutrients than white flour, but once ground, the calories dissolve into your bloodstream just like table sugar. So my advice is to treat any moderate serving of flour like an occasional treat, especially if you have metabolic syndrome.

---

Not only is your energy low, but these recurrent blood sugar surges act as a double whammy on your cholesterol profiles. This is because when the sugar spikes, your liver converts it into a harmful form of triglyceride, and at the same time, it stops making the beneficial HDL cholesterol.

The final consequence of eating flour and/or sugar periodically through the day is that in addition to feeling exhausted, it will give you all the signs of metabolic syndrome: high blood sugar levels, an expanding waistline, high triglyceride levels and low HDL levels, and high inflammation—all of which inflame your arteries and cause arterial plaque growth. So it should be no surprise that this eating pattern increases your blood pressure as well as your risks for a cardiovascular event.

## PARTIAL EXCEPTIONS TO THE FLOUR RULE: OAT FLOUR, PUMPERNICKEL BREAD, AND PASTA

For people with signs of metabolic syndrome (most Americans) who need to avoid or limit whole-grain flour consumption, there are some mini-exceptions to the no-flour rule. Let's review them one at a time.

If you need a small amount of flour for a recipe, whole grain *oat* flour is a better choice than whole wheat. Oats have more soluble fiber, which lowers both blood sugar levels and cholesterol levels. When used in small portions, oat flour will limit blood sugar spiking and will lower bad cholesterol too.

Some pumpernickel bread includes a substantial quantity of whole grains (actual pieces of grain) along with the flour, so it is a moderate exception to the bread rule. If you are going to eat bread, better to eat one with some whole grains, rather than one that is 100% flour.

Another partial exception to this no-flour rule is pasta. This is because the flour in pasta is so densely packed that it isn't absorbed nearly as quickly by the intestines and therefore doesn't cause the same leap in blood sugar levels that occurs with bread and cereals. But even with pasta, you clearly need to watch your portion size. Italians traditionally serve it as a first course, on a small salad plate. Typically, you enjoy a few bites of delicious pasta with a heavenly sauce. Then go on to your protein and vegetable course. In contrast, we Americans tend to stuff ourselves with pasta by the platter. To prevent your sugar levels from spiking when eating cooked pasta, don't eat more than ½ cup to 1 cup of it at any meal. And select a product that is fiber and protein enriched, such as Barilla PLUS. It uses lentil, chickpea, flaxseed, and oat flour and has much more protein and fiber than regular pasta. From a culinary perspective, it is a huge improvement over whole wheat pasta, as it has a really nice texture and good flavor.

## BUT WHAT ABOUT THE NUTRIENTS IN WHOLE-GRAIN FLOUR?

White flour is clearly worse than whole-grain flour as it lacks fiber and other whole-grain nutrients. So from a nutrient perspective, whole-grain bread is much better than white bread, whole-grain corn tortillas are much better than white flour tortillas, and brown rice is much better than white rice. If you are active and have normal blood sugar and cholesterol profiles, then you can likely have whole-grain flour products in moderation.

The problem is that far too many Americans have metabolic syndrome, and for them eating sugar, and even whole-grain flour, puts them into a downward spiral toward inflammation, weight gain, and growth of arterial plaque.

---

### What If I Feel I'm Healthy? Am I Permitted to Have a Little Sugar?

If you have trouble controlling your weight or have one to two signs of metabolic syndrome, then generally you should consider refined carbs and flour to act like toxins. However, if you're active, and all of your metabolic syndrome markers are normal, then certainly you can enjoy an occasional treat. For an average person, *occasional* may imply once or twice a week. If you are highly active (you work out vigorously daily) you may tolerate even more treats.

Fortunately, by following the 30-Day Heart Tune-Up, you can avert a health crisis and indulge in foods you love in moderation. You will notice in the Chapter 10 recipe section that some of the dessert recipes contain small amounts of maple syrup or sugar. Your challenge is to put this program in motion so you can enjoy these recipes on special occasions.

---

Now that you understand the perils of sugar and other harmful carbs, let's have a look at all of the wonderful foods you can and should eat.

## THE FIVE HEART-FRIENDLY FOOD GROUPS TO EAT EACH AND EVERY DAY

The goal of the 30-Day Heart Tune-Up Eating Plan is for you to enjoy meals that dilate your arteries, reduce inflammation, prevent clotting, and promote circulation. The five heart-healthy food groups—adequate fiber, healthy fats, lean protein, beneficial beverages, and fabulous flavors—are easily available essentials you should eat daily for heart health and vitality. In Part III, "The Eating Plan," I will expand this list to more than 60 wonderful and easy-to-prepare recipes that will help you find creative and delicious ways to include these foods regularly in your diet. But for now, let's look at the five heart-healthy food groups in more detail.

### Adequate Fiber

I have listed fiber first because it is clearly the most critical! Fiber used to be called roughage. It's the woody part of the plant, which is partially digested by people. Although scientists have divided fiber into two categories (soluble and nonsoluble) based on how it behaves in laboratory settings, the bottom line is that all fiber is good for you. Sources of soluble fiber (beans, nuts, oats, vegetables, and fruits) are especially effective at lowering cholesterol levels, because they block cholesterol's absorption from the gut into your bloodstream. They also lower blood sugar levels by slowing the release of sugars from your stomach to your intestines. Several companies sell fiber supplements (such as ground flaxseeds, chia seeds, psyllium, and other mixtures that contain fiber from fruits, oat bran, and seaweed) that can be added conveniently to a protein smoothie, 1 tablespoon every day. Some fiber sources help protect the glycocalyx and the lining of your arteries. See Chapter 7 for details on fiber supplements.

Fiber does much more than just lower blood sugar and cholesterol levels. Fiber-rich foods contain thousands of anti-aging nutrients, many of which we probably haven't even discovered yet. In particular, plant pigments slow aging and oxidation. The blue in blueberry, red in tomato, green in kale, orange in butternut squash protect every cell in your body from aging. They protect your heart's ability to pump and produce energy, and they decrease artery stiffening that occurs with aging,[4] lower blood pressure,[5] and prevent the cells lining your arteries from growing plaque.

Sadly, in the United States, the average person eats only 12 grams (about 0.4 ounce) of fiber a day, but I recommend that you eat from 30 to 50 grams (1 to 1.8 ounces). That may be much more than you're consuming right now, so it's wise to take it easy and increase your fiber intake slowly, by 5 to 10 grams a week. Eating too much fiber too quickly (say, zealously jumping from less than 10 grams a day to more than 40 grams a day) could cause abdominal bloating and perhaps even cramping. At the end of this section, you'll find a table to help you increase your current fiber intake, "How to Increase Fiber Gradually Over 30 Days." You can use this table to easily reach 40 grams per day over a 30-day period. Perhaps 40 grams seems like a lot, but here's how to get enough fiber into your system to make a difference.

## VEGETABLES AND FRUITS

All vegetables and fruits in their whole, unprocessed form are packed with valuable anti-aging nutrients. And any vegetable that holds it shape after cooking—green beans, cauliflower, artichokes, fennel, asparagus, red peppers, carrots, broccoli—will also have plenty of healthful fiber. *There are 3 to 5 grams of fiber in a*

*1-cup serving, so if you eat 5 cups of vegetables and fruits a day, you'll score 20 grams of fiber.* Figure 4.1 shows you the benefit to your cardiovascular system of eating more vegetables and fruits. Enjoying at least 4 or 5 cups of these daily will reduce your risk of a heart attack and stroke by 35% all by itself, without having any negative side effects. No drug is this beneficial! And every study that has ever researched vegetable and fruit intake shows that eating more of them will not only reduce some cancer risks, but also will result in weight loss. Diets that tell you to stop eating vegetables and fruits have got it all wrong!

Even though salad doesn't have a lot of fiber, it still has many heart-healthy benefits. Each cup of leafy green vegetables (kale, romaine, arugula, spinach, cabbage) added to your diet cuts your risk of a cardiovascular event by 25%. So even two cups daily of leafy green vegetables—a plate of salad—should reduce your risk by nearly half. That's a lot of benefit with a very small change in diet.

Figure 4.1

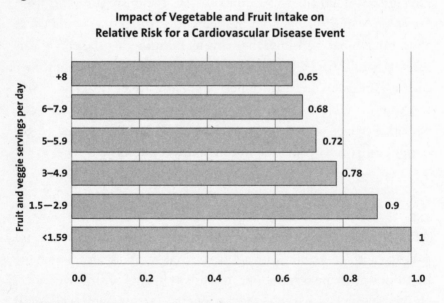

**Impact of Vegetable and Fruit Intake on Relative Risk for a Cardiovascular Disease Event**

*(Compiled from data published in Hung HC, Joshipura KJ, Jiang R, et al. Fruit and vegetable intake and risk of major chronic disease.* J Natl Cancer Inst *2004;96:1577–84.)*

## Fruit Juice Peril

You may be tempted to fill your fruit and vegetable quota with juices. This is a mistake! Stay away from fruit juices, as they're basically all sugar and no fiber. It's far better to eat an orange or an unpeeled apple than to drink orange juice or apple juice. Vegetable juices have more nutrients and less sugar than fruit juices, but they also lack the fiber your heart needs to stay healthy.

Greens are also rich in calcium, fiber, vitamin K, magnesium, potassium, and folic acid, as well as a host of cancer-preventing plant pigments. Eating at least two cups of leafy greens daily will help your arteries to dilate and will block inflammation— stopping arterial plaque growth. I'll give you some great recipes to enjoy them. However, bear in mind that there are some limitations with salads. Lettuce and fresh spinach are mostly water, so they collapse down to a much smaller amount when cooked. That's why salads, though excellent sources of nutrients and plant pigments, shouldn't be your main source of fiber. It's best to rely on beans and other vegetables instead.

### CRUSADE FOR CRUCIFEROUS VEGETABLES

Every day, toxins in the environment assault your body. These are poisonous foreign chemicals (heavy metals, industrial chemicals, pesticides, drugs, and various other pollutants) that enter through your skin, lungs, and especially your intestines. Your body also produces toxins (free radicals) when you metabolize hormones and drugs and burn calories for energy. These accumulate in your tissues and can lower energy, reduce calorie burning, and stiffen your arteries too.

Fiber-rich cruciferous vegetables—cabbage, bok choy, broccoli, kale, cauliflower, and Brussels sprouts—are high in enzymes that remove these toxic compounds from your body. Eating one cup of these vegetables daily will help to control your blood pressure as well. They're also great sources of vitamin C, magnesium, potassium, and calcium. And they contain compounds that fight cancer and help restore normal hormone balance for women and men alike. You can eat these vegetables raw, steamed, or lightly sautéed, but be careful not to overcook them or they'll lose their valuable properties.

## BERRIES ARE BEAUTIFUL

Blueberries, blackberries, strawberries, cranberries, raspberries, bilberries, and cherries are among the brightly colored fruits and vegetables that have so many antioxidant benefits. They're also a great source of fiber. Toss them on your oatmeal or mix them with your nonfat yogurt for breakfast. Sprinkle them on your salad. Take them for a snack. In particular, berries improve artery function and protect your brain from aging. Aim to have at least ½ cup to 1 cup of berries every day.

## BEANS ARE A WONDER-FOOD

Beans are fiber superstars, and we don't eat nearly enough of them! *In fact, beans have more fiber than any other commonly eaten food: 10 to 14 grams of fiber per cup. If you add a half cup daily at first, you'll score 6 grams of fiber.* Over 30 days, you can build to 1 cup and score 12 grams of fiber. This is important because ½ to 1 cup of beans a day reduces your LDL cholesterol by 5% as it increases your healthy HDL cholesterol by 2% to 3%. Beans also help you to feel full, and their very high fiber content can control blood sugar levels. The antioxidant compounds in beans lower bad cholesterol levels, help block inflammation, and they protect your arterial lining beautifully. It's not surprising, then, that eating 1 cup of beans daily has been shown to reduce your risk of cardiovascular events.[6]

The musical fruit? You fill up with gas if you eat beans only once in a while, but studies have shown that if you eat beans every day for a month, gas production drops. It is better to eat them in small daily quantities (begin with ¼ cup, then build toward ½ cup daily) and gradually increase portions over time. The "How to Increase Fiber Gradually Over 30 Days" chart at the end of this section will help you.

It's easy to enjoy beans as a side dish or add them to soups, salads, and rice and pasta dishes. One half cup of hummus dip with baby carrots makes a great snack. There are dozens of different types of beans. If you're too busy to cook them, canned beans will make your life easier. Just rinse them well, since they are packed with extra salt and sugar. Aim to eat beans regularly, because if you limit yourself to the rare double helping of chili, watch out!

## Whole Grains Hold You

There are about 4 grams of fiber per cup in most whole grains. If you add 2 cups of whole grains to your diet daily, you'll score 8 grams of fiber—*but because of their impact on blood sugar, be sure to avoid having more than 1 cup of grains at any one time.* The fiber in whole grains helps your intestinal function, and sources like steel-cut oatmeal are great for lowering cholesterol. The fiber in whole grains means you'll feel satisfied after a meal, even though you've eaten fewer calories as you follow the 30-Day Heart Tune-Up eating plan. If you are one of the 20% of people who should follow a gluten-free diet, fear not. There are plenty of grains available that are gluten-free, like brown rice or wild rice, quinoa, millet, corn, and oats.

Many diets restrict the intake of grains in particular because of patients' blood sugar (glycemic) response to them. The key to success is enjoying them as whole grain—not as flour—and in small portions. By "small portions," I mean a serving of no more than

½ cup to 1 cup of any cooked grain at any meal. The easy-to-prepare grains with the highest nutrient content include quinoa, oats, wild rice, and brown rice. Your plate should have twice as many vegetables as grains and they should be complemented with some form of lean protein.

## NUTS ARE GREAT FOR FIBER

People think of nuts as a source of healthy fats, yet they also are loaded with fiber. *There are 3 grams of fiber per 1 ounce serving (about a handful). If you add one handful of almonds, pecans, walnuts, or pistachio nuts a day, you'll score 3 grams of fiber.* I'll share more about the properties of nuts in the "Healthy Fats" section of this chapter (page 99).

## FIBER SUPPLEMENTS CAN HELP YOU REACH YOUR GOALS

Most people may find it difficult to reach 30 to 50 grams of fiber a day, so supplements can help. Ground flaxseed and other seeds (e.g., chia seeds) are excellent sources of fiber. *Add 1 tablespoon daily—a reasonable goal—to score 2 grams of fiber.* Flaxseed oil, on the other hand, lacks fiber and goes rancid quickly. It can become packed with free radicals so it is a poor choice. Make sure your flaxseed is ground. Ground flaxseed lowers LDL cholesterol and improves blood sugar control,[7] but whole flaxseed passes through your intestinal tract like birdseed, without being absorbed. If you can't find ground flaxseed in the market, use an old coffee mill or mini-chop to grind it. Freshly ground flaxseed has a pleasant nutty flavor. I keep it in an airtight container in the refrigerator, so it's handy to sprinkle on my oatmeal, smoothies, and salads. The great news about chia seeds (yes, as in chia pets) is that you don't even have to grind them.

## PSYLLIUM FIBER

Psyllium fiber is an easily purchased product. It is 70% soluble fiber, and it has cholesterol-lowering and blood sugar–lowering properties. It's an easy fiber to add to drinks. The powder is generally gluten-free, although you should read labels carefully as some psyllium wafers contain gluten.

## FIBER POWDERS

There are a variety of supplements you can choose. See Chapter 7 for details.

| How to Increase Fiber Gradually Over 30 Days | | | |
|---|---|---|---|
| Food Source | Fiber when you start the Heart Tune-Up (in grams)* | Fiber after 2 weeks on the Heart Tune-Up (in grams) | Fiber after 30 days on the Heart Tune-Up (in grams) |
| Vegetables and fruits (3–5 cups) | 12 | 16 | 20 |
| Beans (¼ to 1 cup) | 3 | 6 | 12 |
| Whole grains (2 to 3 cups/day) | 8 | 8 | 12 |
| Nuts (1 ounce) | 3 | 3 | 3 |
| Flax or chia seeds (1 Tbsp) | | 2 | 2 |
| Fiber supplements (1 scoop) | | | 4 |
| Total fiber intake: | 26 | 35 | 40+ |
| *1 gram = .035 ounce (weight) | | | |

## Healthy Fats: Time for an Oil Change?

Not all fats are created equal. Many of us have been told to avoid foods high in cholesterol in order to prevent heart disease. But cutting out saturated fats found in rich dairy products (cheese, butter, and high-fat milk, so-called low-fat 2% milk, whole milk yogurt) and meats (red meat, sausage, and bacon) is much more effective in lowering dangerous LDL than watching how much cholesterol you eat. Excessive saturated fat raises your cholesterol and speeds the formation of plaque, especially in people with metabolic syndrome and diabetes. But worst of all, this kind of fat actually stimulates your liver to create cholesterol—and your liver can produce up to 4,000 to 5,000 mg of cholesterol daily! This kind of fat has a huge impact on your LDL level—much more than simply eating an extra 100 mg of cholesterol has.

However, it is fair to say that there are controversies regarding how bad saturated fat is for you. First, saturated fat intake can modestly improve your HDL cholesterol, so it's not all bad. Second, some saturated fats are worse than others. For example, saturated fats found in fatty meats and full-fat dairy products are worse than those that come from coconut. Also, nonorganic fatty meats and dairy products often contain hormones, pesticides, and dioxins, which have cancer-causing properties. In contrast, dark chocolate mostly has a form of saturated fat called stearic acid, which acts like olive oil biochemically and is likely good for you. And, if you follow the recommendations in this book to add my heart-rejuvenating foods, you can still enjoy some saturated fat in moderation. The key is avoiding excess.

The "Saturated Fat Content of Various Foods" table on page 101, will help you estimate how much saturated fat you typically eat daily. It provides a list of foods, with their calories and saturated fat content per serving. My goal would be for you to stay in the moderate range, not more than 12 to 20 grams of saturated fat daily. (You don't have to count dark chocolate!) If you have known heart disease, then good sense would dictate that you limit yourself to less than 15 grams daily.

# Saturated Fat Content of Various Foods

| Seafood | Calories per Serving | Saturated Fat (grams) |
|---|---|---|
| Catfish (6 oz) | 115 | 1.5 |
| Cod (6 oz) | 218 | 0.3 |
| Mahi mahi (6 oz) | 218 | 0.5 |
| Salmon (farmed, Atlantic, 6 oz) | 400 | 5.0 |
| Salmon (wild, Atl, 6 oz) | 360 | 2.4 |
| Salmon (wild, Coho, 6 oz) | 278 | 2.0 |
| Shrimp (6 oz) | 200 | 0.5 |
| Sole (6 oz) | 155 | 0.5 |
| Tuna, bluefin (6 oz) | 360 | 3.2 |
| Tuna fish sandwich (1) | 533 | 4.0 |

| Poultry | Calories | Saturated Fat (grams) |
|---|---|---|
| Chicken breast, fried (6 oz) | 319 | 3.0 |
| Chicken breast, baked (6 oz) | 230 | 2.0 |
| Chicken leg, fried (6 oz) | 208 | 3.5 |
| Turkey breast, baked (6 oz) | 200 | 2.0 |
| Turkey leg, baked (6 oz) | 270 | 2.2 |

| Meat | Calories | Saturated Fat (grams) |
|---|---|---|
| Bacon (4 strips) | 140 | 4.0 |
| Hamburger (6 oz) | 490 | 14.0 |
| Cheeseburger, large | 580 | 20.0 |
| Hamburger, lean (6 oz) | 467 | 12.5 |
| Hot dog | 140 | 6.0 |
| Pork chop (6 oz) | 280 | 6.0 |
| Steak, sirloin (6 oz) | 360 | 7.0 |
| Steak, prime rib (6 oz) | 692 | 24.0 |

| Fast Food | Calories | Saturated Fat (grams) |
|---|---|---|
| Chicken nuggets (1 serving) | 430 | 5.0 |
| Pizza, Sicilian (2 slices) | 590 | 13.2 |
| Sandwich, roast beef | 473 | 9.0 |
| Taco, beef (2) | 520 | 12.0 |
| Taco, chicken (2) | 410 | 8.0 |

| Appetizers | Calories | Saturated Fat (grams) |
|---|---|---|
| Chicken wings (6 oz) | 607 | 10.0 |
| Nachos (7 chips) | 570 | 13.0 |
| Onion rings (1 serving) | 450 | 8.0 |

| Dairy | Calories | Saturated Fat (grams) |
|---|---|---|
| Egg, regular | 75 | 1.6 |
| Egg, omega-3-enriched | 75 | 1.0 |
| Butter (1 Tbsp) | 100 | 7.0 |
| Cheddar cheese (1 oz) | 112 | 6.0 |
| Whole milk (1 cup) | 149 | 5.0 |
| 2% milk (1 cup) | 137 | 3.0 |
| 1% milk (1 cup) | 118 | 1.8 |
| Nonfat milk (1 cup) | 86 | 0.3 |
| Half and half (2 Tbsp) | 40 | 2.0 |
| Yogurt, whole milk (1 cup) | 160 | 4.5 |
| Yogurt, low-fat, 2% (1 cup) | 145 | 3.0 |
| Yogurt, nonfat (1 cup) | 120 | 0.1 |

| Spreads | Calories | Saturated Fat (grams) |
|---|---|---|
| Almond butter (1 Tbsp) | 95 | 1.0 |
| Mayonnaise (1 Tbsp) | 100 | 2.0 |
| Peanut butter (1 Tbsp) | 100 | 1.5 |

| Oils and Nuts | Calories | Saturated Fat (grams) |
|---|---|---|
| Almond oil (1 Tbsp) | 120 | 1.15 |
| Olive oil (1 Tbsp) | 120 | 2.0 |
| Almonds (1 oz) | 170 | 1.1 |
| Cashews (1 oz) | 163 | 2.6 |
| Peanuts (1 oz) | 166 | 2.0 |

*continues*

## Saturated Fat Content of Various Foods (continued)

| Snacks | Calories | Saturated Fat (grams) |
|---|---|---|
| Corn chips (1.5-oz bag) | 240 | 2.5 |
| Potato chips (1.5-oz bag) | 230 | 4.0 |
| Popcorn, air-popped (1 oz = 3 cups) | 110 | 0.2 |
| Popcorn, oil-popped (1 oz) | 142 | 7.9 |
| Tortilla chips (1.5-oz bag) | 260 | 2.0 |
| Tortilla chips, baked (1.5-oz bag) | 165 | 0.1 to 0.7 |

| Breakfast | Calories | Saturated Fat (grams) |
|---|---|---|
| Cinnabon (1) | 700 | 14.0 |
| Croissant (1) | 350 | 11.0 |
| Scone, cinnamon (1) | 530 | 13.0 |
| Oatmeal with nuts & berries | 362 | 0.8 |
| Veggie omelet | 145 | 1.9 |

| Dressings | Calories | Saturated Fat (grams) |
|---|---|---|
| Vinaigrette (oil & vinegar) | 125 | 2.0 |
| Ranch | 120 | 2.5 |
| Blue cheese | 120 | 3.0 |
| Thousand Island | 116 | 2.0 |

| Desserts | Calories | Saturated Fat (grams) |
|---|---|---|
| Chocolate chip cookie (1) | 250 | 8.0 |
| Donut, (1) glazed | 491 | 7.0 |
| Ice cream (1 cup) | 520 | 18.0 |
| Ice cream, nonfat (1 cup) | 200 | 0.5 |
| M&M's (2-oz bag) | 270 | 8.0 |

Much worse than the harm caused by saturated fat, however, is that caused by trans fats or hydrogenated fats (found in shortening, margarine, and many processed foods and packaged baked goods, as well as in many fried fast foods).

## The Trouble with Trans Fats

Trans fats are doubly dangerous. They raise your LDL cholesterol while simultaneously dropping your healthy HDL levels. They cause your blood sugar levels to rise and your cell walls to stiffen. Eating these nasty fats boosts your risk of heart attacks and cancer and heightens your chances for developing diabetes. In many ways, eating trans fat is like having liquid plastic or embalming fluid injected into your veins with an IV while you are still alive. This is why I have traveled the country for the last 15 years warning tens of thousands of physicians and millions of people regarding the dangers of this substance. Always read the labels of packaged foods. If it lists "partially hydrogenated" anything, skip that item altogether. In a restaurant, ask if they use hydrogenated fats, such as hydrogenated soybean oil or a restaurant product called "phase vegetable oil," in the foods they serve. If they do, request that they cook your food in olive oil. If they won't honor your concern, it may be time for you to find another restaurant. Fortunately, many restaurants are starting to avoid these nasty fats.

That's the bad news about fats. To make the point, look at Figure 4.2. It shows how very damaging replacing even a tiny amount of carbohydrate with trans fat is for your heart. In Figure 4.2, you can see that a 2% increase in trans fats (as in typical French fries cooked in shortening, cookies, pie crust, chips, and crackers) will increase your risk of heart disease by 62%. In contrast, adding 5% more calories from saturated fat or cholesterol instead of carbohydrates will have a smaller adverse effect on the heart (the difference was not clinically significant). Fortunately, adding 5% more healthy fats (polyunsaturated, such as from nuts) is clearly very good for you, as they reduce the risk of coronary heart disease by 35%. And a 5% increase in monounsaturated fat (as in olive oil or avocado) will decrease your risk of heart disease by 16%.

So we see there are good fats, which are beneficial to your health. This is especially true for foods high in long-chain omega-3 fats. They are some of your most effective heart-healthy allies. Excellent sources of long-chain omega-3 fats come from cold waters and include salmon, trout, sole, sardines, herring, mussels, oysters, and seaweed. These foods decrease clotting within blood vessels, inflammation, and abnormal heart rhythms.

Healthy plant sources of omega-3 fatty acids (also called medium-chain omega-3 fats or alpha-linoleic acid) are soybeans and soybean oil, organic expeller-pressed canola oil, leafy green vegetables, flaxseeds and chia seeds, tofu, and many nuts. These plant-based omega-3 fats lower cholesterol. However, unlike seafood and seaweed sources of omega-3 fats, they don't have the

Figure 4.2

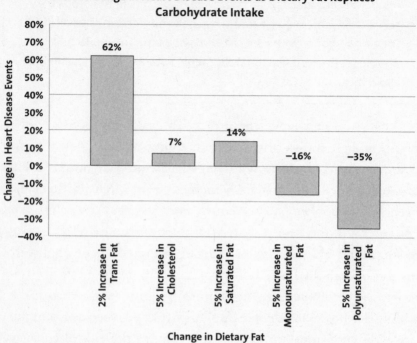

**Percent Change in Heart Disease Events as Dietary Fat Replaces Carbohydrate Intake**

*(Source: Adapted from data published in Hu et al. Dietary Fat Intake and the Risk of Coronary Heart Disease in Women. N Engl J Med 1997;337:1491–99.)*

ability to reduce clotting, heart rhythm irregularities, or inflammation. It is really false marketing to say that these plants have true omega-3 benefit because all the advantages noted in clinical trials come largely from seafood.

You've already read about the benefits of leafy green vegetables and flaxseeds. Here's how to incorporate some of these other foods rich in healthy fats into your eating plan.

### FISHING FOR FISH

Eating fish several times a week can reduce irregular heartbeat, blood stickiness, and triglycerides. This means it actually lowers death rates. The omega-3 fats in seafood can also decrease inflammation. Aim to eat cold-water, small-mouth fish (like salmon, sole, and trout) at least three times a week. (On pages 109–110 I explain why small-mouth fish are the best for you.) In addition to helping your cardiovascular system, these small-mouth fish are also low in mercury. You can safely enjoy cold-water shellfish (shrimp, lobster, clams, mussels) 1 or 2 times a week as well. The benefits are twofold. Not only are you getting the fish oil your body needs, but you're potentially replacing an unhealthy entrée high in saturated fat with one that's good for you. To support the benefit of seafood, please consider that in my study that analyzed how biomarkers predict arterial plaque growth, fish consumption was more beneficial than fish oil alone, when we measured carotid IMT scores. However, if you don't enjoy these types of fish, and you eat mostly warm-water fish or lean fish, then their active ingredients can also be taken as fish oil supplements. The two active compounds in fish oil are called EPA (eicosapentaenoic acid) and DHA (docosahexaenoic acid), special long-chain omega-3 fats. But choose your supplements carefully, since many brands of fish oil contain very little of these active ingredients. Studies have shown that taking 600 to 1,200 mg of EPA and DHA daily will lower the inflammation marker hs-CRP by up to 40%. In Chapter 7, you will discover how you can add high-quality omega-3-rich fish oil supplements to your 30-Day Heart Tune-Up.

## Go Nuts Over Nuts

Many people shun nuts because they believe them to be too fatty, but this is a mistake. Nuts are another miracle food, because they decrease your risk of cardiovascular disease.[8] They are packed with protein, anti-aging compounds, and fiber. They make you feel full, so you're less likely to reach for an unhealthy snack. And they contain mostly healthy fats. Most recently, research published in the *New England Journal of Medicine* showed that adding extra olive oil and nuts (2 handfuls daily of pecans, pistachios, almonds, walnuts, or hazelnuts) to your diet was better at reducing rates of cardiovascular events (especially strokes) than following the traditional American Heart Association–recommended moderate fat diet.[9] Further, these same nuts have been shown in randomized clinical trials to lower cholesterol levels when you eat 1 to 2 ounces a day.[10] Research published in the *American Journal of Clinical Nutrition* found that people who ate 1 to 2 ounces (1 to 2 handfuls) of almonds daily lost more weight than those who ate other complex carbohydrates, so nuts appear to benefit both your heart and your waistline.[11] Every study published to date has shown that eating nuts regularly decreases your risk of heart attacks, strokes, and death.

---

## What About Peanuts?

You may have noticed that peanuts are not on my list of recommended nuts. This was purposeful. First, peanuts are actually a bean (a legume) and not a nut. But more important, peanuts do not have the same heart-healthy benefits as tree nuts like almonds, pistachios, walnuts, and pecans. Besides that, they're sometimes contaminated with an aflatoxin from mold, and they're a common cause of food intolerances and allergies. So I intentionally avoided them.

If, like some people, you crave peanut butter, be sure it's organic, sugar-free, and without hydrogenated fats or trans fats. As an alternative to peanut butter, try almond butter—I like the texture much better.

---

What about salted nuts? Happily, they don't have much sodium. My recommendation of 1 to 2 ounces may contain 125 to 150 mg of salt. Depending upon your health status, your total daily sodium intake should be around 1,500 to 2,500 mg. So, yes, there is room to enjoy salted nuts in your diet, especially when you consider that a cup of commercial soup may contain over 1,000 mg of sodium by itself. If you prefer unsalted nuts, then even better, as this will allow you to have more salt with other foods! And, as I explained in the previous chapter, not everyone experiences a spike in blood pressure from salt.

Keep in mind, though, that nuts are high in calories. I could easily eat a whole can at one sitting watching a sports event and then go eat dinner, but that is way too many calories. Aim for 1 to 2 ounces (1 to 2 handfuls) daily—not more—unless you are trying to gain weight. By the way, nuts are a great source of healthy calories for children who don't get enough.

## Enjoy Avocados

Avocados also are perceived as fatty, but like nuts, they are excellent for your cardiovascular system. Avocados are high in mono-unsaturated fats, which are associated with lower cholesterol levels. These fats also protect your cholesterol from being oxidized into artery plaque.

## The Right Kind of Cooking Oil

When choosing among oils you'll use for cooking, baking, and salad dressing, I'd stick mostly with olive oil and nut oils (almond oil is my favorite nut oil, and walnut oil is a good choice, too). Extra virgin olive oil will smoke with high heat, so virgin olive oil is better for hot skillet cooking. Olive oil and avocado oil are rich in monounsaturated fats, which optimize your heart health. Avocado oil is also good for high heat cooking as it doesn't smoke easily and is packed with very healthy fat. Occasionally, you can use modest amounts of coconut or sesame oil for their flavoring. Coconut oil can tolerate high-heat cooking; sesame oil is more delicate so I add it after the cooking is completed. (I'll expand upon the benefits of coconut oil in Chapter 9.) Finally, I'd save butter as a treat, only for special occasions. And hydrogenated fats, such as margarine and shortening, should never cross your tongue.

## Eggs!

If you eat eggs, consider buying organic, free-range, omega-3-enriched eggs commonly sold in grocery stores; the hens have usually been fed flaxseed. Though more expensive than ordinary eggs, they have half the saturated fat and a healthy dose (225 to 300 mg) of omega-3 fats per egg. Healthy egg yolks are loaded with beneficial nutrients.

### Lean, Not Mean, Proteins

Mean proteins—in the sense that they're bad for your heart—include fatty dairy products and fatty red meats, such as hamburger and sausage. These are loaded with saturated fat and, unless they are organically raised, may be high in pesticides and other toxins. And don't be fooled. "Low-fat" or 2% milk gets 35% of its calories from fat! Stick with nonfat milk and skim milk, or consider almond milk, soy milk, or coconut milk as alternatives.

On the other hand, seafood, chicken and turkey breast, free-range game meats, beans, soy, and nonfat dairy products are excellent lean protein sources. Eating more lean protein helps you feel fuller on fewer calories. If you want to control your weight, you can enjoy 20% to 30% of your calories from healthy, lean protein sources. You could start and end the day (breakfast and dessert) with a protein shake. It helps you build muscle mass after working out with weights and raises your basal metabolic rate so that you burn calories as well.

The following are ways to add lean protein to your life:

1. **Select free-range, grass-fed, organic protein whenever you can.** Beef, poultry, and pork that have been fed grains produce fats that increase your inflammation and sicken your heart. Free-range and grass-fed land animal protein sources are much healthier and have more beneficial long-chain omega-3 fats. Fatty meats and dairy products also contain most of the dioxins (the most common and potent carcinogens in the human diet) that Americans eat. The best way to reduce your exposure to hormones and pesticides is by selecting free-range, grass-fed, organic animal protein whenever possible. See my food sources and links list in the "Helpful Resources" section, page 364, for organic meals.

2. **Seafood.** Fish and shellfish are rich in protein and low in saturated fat. As noted, cold-water fish and shellfish are high in valuable omega-3 fats; warm-water fish (such as tilapia and catfish) are a good source of protein but don't add omega-3s to your diet. Aim for at least 2 to 3 servings of fish and/or shellfish per week.

If you are vegetarian, then be sure to enjoy some form of seaweed every day. Seaweed from cold water has the same beneficial fats as fish, but fish have them in much higher concentrations. So you'll need to eat seaweed in abundance—at least one half cup of fresh (not dried) seaweed salad daily or two sheets of nori. One caveat: you should not eat kelp in these quantities as it is high in iodine and excessive dosing is associated with thyroid problems.

*Caution!* If you eat fish more than once a week, be aware that some fish are high in mercury. In particular big-mouth fish are high on the food chain, so they have much higher mercury levels than small-mouth fish. That is why a medium-sized snapper with a big mouth likely has more than 10 times the mercury content of a wild salmon, and a big ahi tuna or grouper might have 100 times the mercury content of the same-sized wild salmon. Salmon may be big, but they have small mouths and can eat mostly little shrimp and herring. Fish that are high in mercury include tuna, grouper, snapper, bass, swordfish, and shark. Don't eat these big-mouth fish more than 1 or 2 times a month without asking your doctor to check your mercury level. For pregnant women, these high-mercury choices are totally off limits. (See "Long-Chain Omega 3-Oils (Fish Oils)," page 199, in Chapter 7, for details.)

3. **Use protein powders.** It is easy to add protein powder to a smoothie. These come in the form of whey protein, soy protein, and pea and rice blends. Scoop the powder into your blender or VitaMix, add some frozen berries; a cup of brewed green tea; almond milk, soy milk, nonfat milk, or plain yogurt; and blend. For extra fiber, add a scoop of fiber powder or a tablespoon of flax-seed or chia. Blend the ingredients, rinse the blender, and you have a great meal or snack in less than one minute from start to finish.

A protein-fiber smoothie in the morning revs up your metabolism and helps you burn calories. The added fiber will suppress your hunger for hours. It's a great trick for successful weight control. Aim for 20 to 30 grams of protein per smoothie.

4. **Enjoy beans daily.** Beans and legumes are good sources of protein; typically 25% to 35% of their calories come from protein. They are packed with fiber, nutrients, and anti-aging compounds. Eating beans prevents your blood sugar levels from rising and provides you with an even source of energy for hours. Have a bean dip like hummus or black beans with veggies. The classic dinner plate might be a mixture of protein, vegetables, and grains; a great new dinner plate would substitute beans as a side dish to complement your veggies and protein.

5. **Appreciate the joys of organic soy.** Today you can enjoy soy every day without even touching tofu! In the market, you'll find a variety of soy products, including calcium-fortified soy milk. These products lower cholesterol and blood sugar lev-

els, improve artery function, and are packed with cancer-fighting compounds. Edamame (fresh soybeans out of the pod) make a terrific snack, and they're so easy to prepare—just pop them into the microwave or boil in water for a few minutes. Of course, that's not to say that tofu is off the menu. In Part III, I'll provide you with some delicious recipes that put zing into a food usually considered very bland.

You may want to experiment with different brands and types of soy products, because you may like some more than others. For instance, when I decided to give soy milk a chance, I bought six brands at once, poured myself a glass of each, and taste-tested them until I found the one I liked best. Although none tasted like milk, a few brands were quite palatable. Then I poured my favorite into my cereal, coffee, tea, and cocoa. Although chocolate soy milk has 10 more calories than plain, it can make a great light dessert. The challenge with soy is finding organic products.

If you look on the Internet, you'll find that soy foods are embroiled in a great deal of controversy. The biggest real issue is that somewhere between 5% and 15% of people are soy intolerant. They get gassy and bloated. Some even have systemic intolerance symptoms. As I'll discuss in Chapter 9, where I cover the elimination diet, if you have a history of unexplained gastrointestinal problems, fatigue, joint aches, brain fog, etc., you should try an elimination diet. If giving up soy improves your symptoms, then by all means avoid all soy products.

That having been said, if you use soy, it is critical to choose organic soy. I prefer sources that have not been processed and are served as whole food, rather than soy products that have been processed with a variety of preservatives. Commercial products may contain high levels of pesticides, or they could come from genetically modified (GM) crops (as an example, a GM plant can be genetically programmed to make its own toxic chemicals to repel pests so that pesticide spraying isn't needed). Choosing organic soy helps avoid this. Ironically, some people avoid eating soy and corn products because of their GM content. Instead they substitute lots of meat and poultry, which have been fed GM corn and soy. And all the pernicious chemicals from the grains and soy have accumulated in the meat at much higher concentrations than you would ever find in even commercially grown soy products. The bottom line: look for free-range, grass-fed protein and organic soy instead.

Finally, despite all the soy controversy and recent rumors that soy intake is low in Japan, Japan's National Nutrition Survey and the Food and Agriculture Organization (FAO) of the United Nations confirm that the longest-lived population on the planet, the Japanese, continue to eat soy products in abundance as they have done for a millennium.

6. **Plain nonfat yogurt is the healthiest dairy food!** It's loaded with lactobacilli that protect you from harmful bacteria. It's also a good source of lean protein and calcium. Eating yogurt improves intestinal function and lowers inflammation levels, so it is a heart-healthy choice. It's also low in saturated fat, so unlike fatty dairy products, nonfat yogurt will not raise your bad cholesterol levels. Try yogurt in dips and sauces in place of sour cream or mayonnaise. I like to add a dollop to a bowl of spicy lentil or black bean soup—it cools the heat while adding lean protein and calcium. Mix it with lemon juice, mustard, or tamari sauce for a great veggie dip. Add it to curries at the last minute. Just don't cook it or it will curdle. Some people are dairy protein intolerant and should even avoid yogurt. Intolerance to lactose (a sugar found in milk and ice cream) is the most common food intolerance on the planet. Yogurt does not contain lactose. On the other hand, if you are intolerant of milk *protein*, then likely you need to avoid yogurt too. See the elimination diet section for details, in Chapter 9.

## Nonfat Fruit Yogurts?

You may be tempted to snack on nonfat fruit yogurts. After all, they have no fat. But they may have sugar! Lots of it. Also beware of nonfat "sugar-free" yogurts. These have artificial sweeteners that leave your body hungry, so you'll crave more food later! Ideally, it's best to enjoy your plain nonfat yogurt with a half cup of berries, other fresh fruit, a teaspoon of ground flaxseed, and/ or a sprinkling of sliced almonds. Now, if it was a nonfat yogurt sweetened with just one teaspoon of a natural sugar (like honey or organic cane sugar), and it came with the benefits of 6 to 8 ounces of yogurt...that is a close one—you would have to decide.

## Beneficial Beverages

Our bodies are 80% water. We all need fluid to survive—6 to 8 cups a day would be ideal. But we need to drink the right kinds of liquids. Don't tack on extra calories by drinking soda, for instance. A 12-ounce can of regular cola typically has 140 calories. If you drink only one a day for a whole year, unbelievable as it may seem, you've added an extra 51,100 calories—or 14 pounds of body fat weight. That is nearly 3 to 4 footballs of extra fat mass added to your frame in one year. If you normally drink soda daily, switch to iced tea, seltzer, or bubbly water, and you should lose 14 pounds of fat over the next year. Diet sodas can be deceptive—just like "sugar-free" fruit yogurt. The sweeteners stimulate hunger, so you're not taking in any calories for the moment, but you'll end up eating more later. Coffee and alcohol need to be taken in moderation because they're diuretics—they don't actually hydrate you. As for drinks that help your heart, why not try the following?

1. **Make my tea green.** You can have 1 to 2 cups of coffee daily (without sugar and cream, although a skim-milk or soy latte would be fine), but tea is better for you. Yes, you read about

coffee being rich in many healthy compounds and that it is associated with lower rates of cognitive decline. But also remember, in excess it will stiffen arteries and raise blood pressure and cholesterol levels. In contrast, green tea is all good. Drinking 3 to 4 cups of green tea daily is associated with a marked drop in heart attack and stroke rates. Green tea is so powerful that its benefits are similar to those of cholesterol-lowering drugs. It has a pleasant, although slightly bitter flavor that you can learn to enjoy. Make a weak cup at first to appreciate the subtle flavor. If it still seems bitter, dilute it even more. Over time, you may learn to enjoy stronger green tea.

2. **Limit caffeine.** Be sure to limit your total caffeine to no more than 2 to 4 servings daily; 2 cups of tea or 1 cup of regular coffee (½ cup of Starbucks coffee) makes one caffeine serving, 60 mg of caffeine. I have good news for tea drinkers, as tea consumption decreases your risk for heart attacks and strokes, and green tea is the best, so aim for 3 to 4 cups of tea daily.

3. **Fiber- and protein-rich drinks.** As I've mentioned, a smoothie made with a combination of berries, peaches, or other fruits; ground flaxseed or chia seeds; and almond milk, coconut milk, soy milk, or nonfat yogurt provides many benefits—fiber, lean protein, and omega-3 acids—and can satisfy your hunger while helping you quickly achieve a few of your heart-healthy goals in one fell swoop. I've sometimes even added green tea and protein powder to my smoothies to boost their nutritional effectiveness.

4. **Red wine in moderation is divine.** Although red wine may seem like an indulgence, one daily 5-ounce glass helps keep your cardiovascular system young. It reduces your plaque buildup, the risk of clotting, and overall oxidation, and it decreases death rates, too![12] The key for health is stopping at one glass, and definitely not drinking more than two. Four a day? Who are we

kidding? Red wine is preferred, as it is the richest source of anti-oxidants and resveratrol (a plant compound thought to have many health benefits) of all the alcohol choices, but if you avoid red wine, I'd suggest white wine over beer, and beer over hard liquor. Of all the alcoholic choices, hard liquor is the most irritating to your liver and the poorest choice. Yet, at one serving daily, all can be a good choice. If you don't drink alcohol, you may have a good reason not to, so you need not start now. The heart-healthy pigments in red wine are also found in unsweetened pomegranate juice, beets, or in any smoothie prepared with a mixture of colorful berries. You can also take a supplement of resveratrol, which typically contains 50 to 100 times what is found in one glass of red wine.

5. **Dream of dark chocolate.** A cup of unsweetened cocoa decreases clotting and the oxidation of LDL into plaque.[13] Cocoa also helps dilate your arteries—improving their function, your blood pressure, and lowering the risk of clotting.[14] Cocoa is rich in magnesium, fiber, and is packed with anti-aging and stress-relieving compounds. I find a cup of hot cocoa (made with skim, almond, or soy milk) to be a great dessert and surprisingly satisfying. Caution: Although unsweetened cocoa lowers blood pressure, the improvement disappears if you add sugar. Soy milk tends to be sweeter than other kinds of milk, so if you find cocoa without sugar to be too bitter, it can be a good choice. If you are soy intolerant, a natural sweetener like stevia may work for you.


## Fabulous Flavors

I've just outlined a diet I know you can not only live with, but also live longer with! Still, I'd like to add more enjoyment to your life. The following foods not only make your meals tastier, but they're also terrific for your cardiovascular system. I'm throwing them in as a bonus for you. Okay, some of you may think that garlic, spices, and herbs aren't technically a food group, and I'll admit it is a stretch, but these ingredients are essential for food flavor and for your health. Yet who is going to argue with dark chocolate—it is so healthful and delicious. If not for my Fabulous Flavor group, it should have a food group of its own.

1. **I sing the praises of fresh garlic.** One clove of fresh garlic lowers total cholesterol by about 7% to 9%, raises HDL slightly, decreases clotting, lowers blood pressure, and boosts your immune function.[15] That's an awful lot of benefit from such a small item. Allicin is the chemical that gives garlic its aroma as well as its cholesterol-lowering punch. (That means you should stay away from deodorized garlic pills, because they do nothing to reduce cholesterol.) To maximize allicin in the foods you eat, use a garlic press or smash the cloves with the flat side of a chef's knife. You want the juices to meld a bit. I suggest 1 to 2 cloves for each person daily. Throw it into your salad dressing, stir-fry dishes, soups, and rice dishes. Most meals benefit from garlic, be they American, Mexican, Chinese, Indian, French, Spanish, Greek, or Italian cuisine.

Do be careful, though. If you brown the garlic, it will become bitter. Aside from affecting the taste, overcooking also ruins garlic's medicinal properties. So throw it into the pan when you're almost done cooking. This will preserve garlic's rich flavor while also boosting its heart-healthy benefits.

2. **Herbs and spices.** Thyme, rosemary, oregano, parsley, sage, basil, cumin seed, mint, chili, chives, turmeric, dill, and cilantro. We are biochemically attracted to herbs in the same way that bees are captivated by flowers. Why? Because by weight, they're the most potent heart-healthy foods you can find. Add at least 1 teaspoon of dried or 1 to 2 tablespoons of fresh herbs daily to your diet. (The recipes in Chapter 10 will make this easy for you to do.)

Also, don't be gingerly with your ginger. It adds zest to meals, especially Indian curries, Asian stir-fries, teas, desserts, and marmalades. Not only does it improve the flavor of food, but like garlic, ginger helps decrease blood stickiness, which prevents unwanted clots. Ginger eaten regularly acts as an anti-inflammatory that relieves joint pain and arthritis without increasing the risk of stomach ulcers. In fact, people use ginger to treat ulcers!

Turmeric is another wonderful spice, typically found in Indian curries, which has very powerful anti-inflammatory products. If you don't enjoy curry spice, turmeric has so many wonderful benefits that you might consider taking a turmeric extract called curcumin daily. I'll discuss this supplement in Chapter 7.

Don't forget chili. It adds a whole extra dimension of flavor and from a culinary perspective should be used in small to moderate amounts in many recipes. But people often forget that it also has fantastic medicinal value too, and is rich in nutrients. Chili spice decreases inflammation levels, as well.

Curry spices are also great at reducing inflammation. They too help prevent cholesterol from being oxidized into arterial plaque. And having cinnamon every day can help lower your blood sugar and reduce inflammation.

The anti-inflammatory ingredients in spices play an important role in the 30-Day Heart Tune-Up in many ways. Keep in mind that inflammation not only grows arterial plaque, but joint pain from inflammation will interfere with your desire to exercise too!

## Fresh Herbs (Even If They're Dried) Are Best

Nothing beats the fragrance and taste of a handful of chopped fresh basil, thyme, rosemary, or parsley. However, sometimes, for the sake of convenience, we have to substitute dried herbs for fresh. Not to worry. Dried herbs still enhance the flavor of your meals and also contain all the excellent nutrients present in fresh herbs. However, be aware that dried herbs have a shelf life of 12 to 24 months. Not only can they lose their aromatic properties, but their health-giving nutrients will also fade in potency over time. So be diligent about clearing your spice cabinet of old, rarely used bottles once a year. Replace and refresh!

3. **Real dark chocolate!** If hot cocoa is good for your cardio-vascular system, it stands to reason that dark chocolate (with at least 70% cocoa mass) is heart-healthy too. Like cocoa, it decreases the oxidation of LDL into arterial plaque, lowers blood pressure, improves artery function, enhances blood sugar control, and is packed with anti-aging and stress-relieving compounds.[16] But read the label. Most products sold as "chocolate" are a combination of sugar, milk, and palm oil, with only a trace of cocoa. Milk chocolate—even the expensive brands—also lacks the benefits of dark chocolate. The first ingredient on the label should be cocoa, followed by cocoa butter, and then sugar. Vanilla and lecithin are acceptable too. But if you see palm oil, milk products, or butter, keep searching.

| A Quick Guide to Better Eating | |
|---|---|
| *If you feel like eating...* | *Have this instead* |
| Cheese | A handful of almonds, pistachios, or walnuts |
| Soda | Iced green or black tea, unsweetened |
| Milk chocolate | Dark chocolate |
| Tuna salad sandwich on white | Salmon salad sandwich on whole-grain bread |
| Hamburger | Sirloin steak |
| French fries | Baked sweet potato fries |
| Chips and ranch dressing | Hummus with whole wheat pita or carrots |
| Caesar salad | Salad with vinaigrette |
| Ice cream | Nonfat plain yogurt with fresh berries |
| White rice | Wild rice, brown rice, or quinoa |
| Rice Krispies, Special K, Wheat Chex | Oatmeal with protein powder, almonds, and berries |
| Bacon and fried eggs | Veggie omelet |
| Coffee with sugar and cream (even worse, creamer) | Coffee with skim milk, almond milk, coconut milk, or soy milk |
| Pretzels | Dry-roasted edamame or soy nuts |

Now that you know the foods that you need to fuel your heart and body for great health, let's show you how to use that fuel to enhance your activity levels and get moving. Yes, food is essential to a healthier heart. Yet consider two facts as we shift to getting fit. The #1 cause of heart disease now is metabolic syndrome—defined as having three of the following: an expanding waistline; elevation of blood sugar, blood pressure, or triglycerides; increased inflammation; or low HDL. While food is important in reversing this epidemic, getting fit is the fastest and most effective way to reverse metabolic syndrome quickly, and to achieve a younger, stronger heart!

*Chapter Five*

# Take Your Heart for a Spin

**W**hat single thing in your life:

- burns away fat
- makes you mentally sharper
- builds muscle to make you look sexy
- improves blood sugar control
- lowers inflammation
- enhances your sleep
- improves multiple aspects of your cholesterol profile
- lowers your risk for cancer
- lowers your risk for death
- reduces stress
- fights constipation
- strengthens your bones
- sweats away internal toxins *and*
- builds stamina and circulation to make you a better lover?

It isn't sleep, dark chocolate, or an expensive supplement. You know the answer in your heart. Yes, exercise is *that* important. So the next time you think about skipping your workout, recite the many benefits listed above and think again. There is no excuse good enough to overcome all these great advantages. So get going! You can thank me later.

# EXERCISE IS KING!

Of all the options for preventing and treating cardiovascular disease, including drugs, food, and supplements, the single most effective tool is exercise. People who exercise regularly have 40% fewer heart attacks, strokes, and cases of sudden death. Remember, the federal government's definition of "inactivity" is *less than* 30 minutes of moderately aerobic movement a day. So a 20-minute stroll to the grocery store won't cut it. As 78% of adults engage in less physical activity than is currently recommended, simply walking briskly (walk until you get a little sweaty and out of breath, to the point that you can talk but not sing) 30 minutes daily would be of some cardiac benefit and would cut the risk of all cardiovascular events in the United States by at least 33%.

Why is this so? Exercise improves your blood pressure, blood sugar, cholesterol levels, weight control, mental speed and performance, sleep, clotting factors, and lowers inflammation.[1] It also enhances the function of the critical cells that line your arteries, ensuring that they dilate even when stressed. In reality, arteries are just muscles in tubular form. Like any muscles, they must be exercised to function optimally. Regular exercise can help to turn a sick, stiff, plaque-coated artery into a healthy one.

*Heart power* is a new term I use to describe the ability of your heart to pump nutrients and oxygen to your cells. Your heart power will depend on the strength of your heartbeat and the ability of your arteries to dilate and allow blood to flow easily to your tissues. In Chapter 3, we reviewed how you can assess the age of your heart. In this chapter, we will delve deeper. I will explain how to perform some of the tests I outlined earlier. I'll highlight how you can tune up your heart by improving your aerobic capacity, heartbeat, and heart rate recovery after exercise. The key is designing a program that combines aerobics with strength training, plus a touch of stretching as well. Each has special benefits, and medical evidence suggests the combination is much more powerful than any single part alone.

## ASSESS YOUR CAPACITY BEFORE GETTING STARTED WITH AEROBICS

In Chapter 3, we looked at some tests that are helpful in measuring your cardiovascular fitness. In this chapter I'm going to give you instructions on how to do them. Knowing your baseline will help you determine where you can begin your workouts. It will also give you a way to measure your progress over 30 days as you follow the program.

One of the other important benefits of clarifying your fitness level before you start working out is that it will help you tailor your activities to your body's capacities. Many people devote hours a week to exercise, but they don't get much of a bang for their buck. Either their workout is too easy, reducing the calorie burn and metabolic burst they deserve for the time spent, or they overexercise and exhaust themselves. They end up feeling worse than before they started. Keep in mind that the heart rate tables at gyms based upon age are merely estimates. That means they get it right for one third of us. But for nearly one third, the targets are too low, and for the final third they are too high. Without determining your own peak workout zone, you may find that you're working against yourself.

That's what happened to Jennifer, who was 45 when she first came to see me. Boy, was she frustrated. She reported to me that she walked for an hour every day with her pulse at 122 to 140 beats per minute—precisely the zone recommended for her age on the heart rate table at the gym. (That number is reached with the following formula: 220 minus one's age multiplied by 70% to 80%.) She had a better-than-average diet, yet despite this and her exercise regimen, she couldn't lose weight. Her blood sugar was moderately elevated. She felt flabby, and in fact she was clearly overweight, since we measured her body fat at 35%. We also determined that she had metabolic syndrome—a situation that made her very unhappy. "What am I doing wrong?" she wanted to know. "I thought I was doing all the right things!"

So we went ahead and measured Jennifer's fitness level. Her METs score of 7.8 put her at the 20th percentile for her age—not very good. That made her mad. "How can I be only at the 20th percentile if I'm putting in so much time walking every day?" Her stress test score was low, her heart rate recovery was only 18; it needed to have dropped by at least 25 beats at one minute to be normal. Her blood pressure response was flat, meaning the diastolic blood pressure didn't drop during exercise, something you would anticipate in somebody who is fit. In fact, none of this made sense for someone who "exercised" for an hour a day.

But during Jennifer's stress test in our office, we discovered something interesting. Although the tables told her to keep her pulse in the 122 to 140 zone, until she got to a heart rate of 140, she didn't even start to get aerobic. Our equipment told us that her calorie burn, oxygen burn, and $CO_2$ production looked great at 150 to 160 beats per minute. Now, this was a level she had never attempted to achieve, because the gym table told her she shouldn't go there! In fact, Jennifer's peak heart rate went clear up to 200! If she had only known that her peak heart rate was 200, even without my help, she could have used the "exercise at 70% to 80% of your true maximum heart rate" rule to show that she needed to work out at least in the 140 to 160 heart rate range.

## I Don't Get It...

Calculating your maximum heart rate and aerobic workout zone can be complicated, I admit, yet it can be so beneficial. In fact, the next ten pages are by far the hardest part of this whole book. But I promise you that it will be worth the effort to understand your fitness and how to get the most out of your workouts. If you find it all too confusing, I recommend spending $40 to $80 to hire a trainer for a one-hour gym appointment to take this test. If you know you'll be seeing your doctor in a month but want to get started right now, you can rely on the gym table calculation tool for your desired heart rate (220 minus your age times 60% to 80%) for five days a week until you see your doctor. It isn't great, but it's still better than sitting at your desk, doing nothing. In the pages to follow, I will show you how to find your maximum workout zone. With that feat accomplished, it should get easier and, over time, working within your zone will become second nature to you.

Once she made the adjustment and really gave her heart a workout in the zone that made sense for her, Jennifer quickly turned her situation around. Within a month, she was losing weight, her heart rate recovery improved, her blood sugar went back to normal, and her HDL2 increased. Perhaps most important, her metabolic syndrome disappeared. Jennifer had been sputtering metabolically. She needed to take her heart for a spin. The only real change for her was revving up!

Jennifer's predicament is very typical of the people I see in my office. And it emphasizes how important it is not just to put in the hours, but to exercise at a rate appropriate for your own body's metabolic requirements. Those charts at the gym can be misleading. They're designed to be safe and to match the "average" person, but few of us are actually average.

So my goal is for you to feel terrific after your workout, and for you to burn as many calories as is realistic for your current aerobic capacity. In this chapter, you'll discover how to assess your aerobic fitness, maximum heart rate achieved, and heart rate recovery scores to customize and optimize a workout plan for yourself.

But before I explain how to measure your aerobic capacity, a word of caution. In my clinic, I teach my patients how to capitalize on their exercise investment, but first I need to clarify the risks and benefits of maximal exercise testing. If you push yourself to your highest effort during exercise, there's a very small risk (1 in 10,000) that you could have a cardiovascular accident (a fainting spell, heart attack, or much more rarely, sudden death).[2] The worse your health and fitness level, the higher your risk becomes.

That tiny risk of having a significant cardiovascular event exists in my clinic too. But in truth, if you were to encounter a problem during testing, what better place to have it than at your doctor's office with medical equipment and trained staff immediately available? This is why I recommend you do this type of testing either with your doctor, or with your doctor's permission, or that you schedule this test in a gym with an *exercise physiologist* (which is a fancy name for a well-educated trainer).

## HOW TO GET THE MOST OUT OF YOUR WORKOUT

In Chapter 3, I explained that physicians worldwide rely on the MET (metabolic equivalency level) score taken during a standardized treadmill test to gauge cardiovascular function. They commonly use what's known as the Bruce Protocol, increasing the speed and incline of the running surface every 3 minutes, until the point you feel you are at maximum exertion. This means you will be pushing yourself on a stationary bicycle or treadmill (one that shows you a MET level on the screen) to the point where you are breathing hard, puffing, and just barely able to talk in short sentences, but are clearly unable to sing. Your stride is still steady (you aren't stumbling), your color is good, and you could keep on going a few more seconds. Once you get to this point, you will know your MET level.

## HOW TO DO THE BRUCE PROTOCOL

Start the treadmill at 1.7 miles per hour with a 10% elevation. (This should be an easy walking warm-up speed.) After exactly three minutes, increase the speed to 2.5 miles per hour and the elevation to 12%. Continue to increase the settings every 3 minutes, as shown on the "Bruce Protocol Fitness Calculation Tool" table, page 127. When you reach your maximal comfortable exertion level (breathing hard and just barely able to talk in short sentences), check your pulse. This is your maximum heart rate, which is extremely beneficial for you to know.

Some treadmills and exercise machines do have heart-rate measuring devices in the handgrips, but these may not be accurate enough, as they usually record only a three-beat sequence and yield varying heart rates. So for this test, the most efficient way to measure your pulse is to use a heart rate measuring tool or monitor, such as a chest band and a wristwatch that shows your heart rate precisely. This is easily purchased at a sporting goods store. A basic model costs about $45 to $50.

If you're really adept at taking your pulse while you're working out on the treadmill and want to go low-tech, you can gently place your fingers over the radial artery on your inner wrist. Looking at your watch, count the number of heartbeats for 15 seconds. Let's just say it was 42 beats. Multiplying that number by 4 gives you your pulse rate for a minute. (42 beats × 4 = 168 beats per minute.) This is your maximal achieved heart rate. Most exercise machines at the gym can calculate your MET score for you. If you do this test with a trainer, he or she will ensure that your MET is calculated properly.

While you're in the midst of the METs test, you may also want to assess your perceived exertion level: How hard are you actually pushing it on the treadmill? This will help you notice the intensity of your aerobic workouts. You should get to the point where you are sweating, puffing, and nearly spent, but still capable of running well without stumbling, and are able to talk in short sentences. This is your maximum heart rate zone, so record it and then stop. If you were unable to speak in one- to two-word sentences, you'd be near collapse, so don't go this far!

If feasible, identify your heart rate when you feel you are exerting yourself somewhat. This would be at a level where you are able to speak in short sentences but unable to sing. Regardless of what the gym tables tell you, this is a great range for sustained exercise. It's the level you should be trying to reach during your daily aerobic workouts.

## Bruce Protocol Fitness Calculation Tool

Physicians typically use this treadmill exercise protocol to look for signs of heart disease, yet it can also be used to measure aerobic fitness. To calculate your score, you need to determine your MET level based upon when you stop the treadmill test. The longer you last, the higher your score will be. But before you begin, ask your doctor if it is safe for you to do this test with a physician, an exercise physiologist, or on your own.

| Minutes Completed | Speed (mph) | Elevation (% grade) | MET Level for Men | MET Level for Women |
|---|---|---|---|---|
| 1 | 1.7 | 10% | 3.2 | 3.1 |
| 2 | " | " | 4.0 | 3.9 |
| 3 | " | " | 4.9 | 4.7 |
| 4 | 2.5 | 12% | 5.7 | 5.4 |
| 5 | " | " | 6.6 | 6.2 |
| 6 | " | " | 7.4 | 7.0 |
| 7 | 3.4 | 14% | 8.3 | 8.0 |
| 8 | " | " | 9.1 | 8.6 |
| 9 | " | " | 10.0 | 9.4 |
| 10 | 4.2 | 16%* | 10.7 | 10.1 |
| 11 | " | " | 11.6 | 10.9 |
| 12 | " | " | 12.5 | 11.7 |
| 13 | 5.0 | 18%* | 13.3 | 12.5 |
| 14 | " | " | 14.1 | 13.2 |
| 15 | " | " | 15.0 | 14.1 |

*If your treadmill doesn't go beyond 15% elevation, at 10 minutes adjust the incline to 15% percent and increase your speed to 4.4 miles per hour, and at 13 minutes maintain the 15% incline and increase the speed to 5.4 miles per hour.

Tyler has been my patient for three years. At the age of 58, he could sing for the first 9 minutes on the treadmill using the Bruce Protocol elevation and speed guide I outlined above. That meant he wasn't exercising at an aerobic level. From the 9th through the

12th minutes, he was moderately winded, sweating, and could talk in only two-word sentences. He felt he was working pretty hard, but he could still keep going. This is his best workout zone. He noted his heart rate. By 13 minutes he was spent. He couldn't talk without taking a breath. He calculated his maximum heart rate and stopped. He scored 13.3 METs.

If a woman lasts 13 minutes and stops, her score would be 12.5 METs. On average, women achieve a slightly lower score with this table, partly because they are usually smaller than men, so they have less weight to carry uphill and less muscle mass. A slim man might choose the optimal score from the women's table and a heavy, muscular woman could choose a score from the men's table. Keep in mind that these are only estimates, and you'd have to do a real oxygen-burning treadmill test with a physician like me to calculate your score with 100% accuracy. See the aerobic capacity testing tables for men and women as samples to help you calculate where you stand in METs, compared to other people of your gender and age.

| Aerobic Capacity Testing Table for Women | | | | | |
|---|---|---|---|---|---|
| Maximum Aerobic Capacity Achieved (in METs), by Age | | | | | |
| Percentile | 20–29 | 30–39 | 40–49 | 50–59 | 60+ |
| 90 | 12.5 | 11.7 | 11.3 | 10.1 | 10.0 |
| 80 | 11.7 | 11.0 | 10.4 | 9.2 | 8.9 |
| 70 | 10.9 | 10.5 | 9.7 | 8.8 | 8.4 |
| 50 | 10.0 | 9.7 | 8.8 | 8.1 | 7.4 |
| 30 | 9.2 | 8.7 | 8.1 | 7.3 | 6.8 |
| 10 | 8.1 | 7.6 | 7.2 | 6.4 | 6.0 |

Adapted from the American College of Sports Medicine's Guidelines for *Exercise Testing and Preparation*, 6th Edition, 2000. Data provided by Institute for Aerobics Research, Dallas, TX.

| Aerobic Capacity Testing Table for Men | | | | | |
|---|---|---|---|---|---|
| **Maximum Aerobic Capacity Achieved (in METs), by Age** | | | | | |
| Percentile | 20–29 | 30–39 | 40–49 | 50–59 | 60+ |
| 90 | 14.7 | 14.4 | 13.8 | 12.9 | 12.1 |
| 80 | 13.8 | 13.4 | 12.6 | 11.7 | 10.9 |
| 70 | 13.4 | 12.7 | 11.9 | 11.0 | 10.1 |
| 50 | 12.1 | 11.7 | 10.9 | 10.1 | 9.1 |
| 30 | 11.3 | 10.7 | 10.0 | 9.2 | 8.2 |
| 10 | 9.9 | 9.3 | 8.8 | 8.0 | 6.6 |

Adapted from the American College of Sports Medicine's *Guidelines for Exercise Testing and Prescription*, 6th Edition, 2000. Data provided by Institute for Aerobics Research, Dallas, TX.

After performing your aerobic fitness test with a machine that can calculate your maximum MET score, compare your actual achieved score with your age and gender in the aerobic capacity testing charts. For example, if 45-year-old Michelle runs on the treadmill for 11 minutes and 15 seconds, she reaches 10.9 METs, just above the 80th percentile for her age group; this means she is in good but not excellent physical condition. In contrast, 58-year-old Tyler ran for 13 minutes, scoring 13.3 METs, in the 90th percentile for someone 5 to 10 years younger than he is, so he is in very good but not excellent athletic shape.

You'll note the test stops at 15 minutes. If you reach this level, you are in excellent condition. From a safety perspective, you shouldn't go beyond 15 minutes without your doctor or an exercise physiologist. Equally important, after 15 minutes, the estimated MET scores vary greatly, so if you are this fit and want to know your true MET level, you'll need to do a $VO_2$ max test (which measures maximum oxygen burn rate at peak exercise) at a facility like mine. Most physicians and hospitals don't offer this testing; high-end fitness and age management facilities do.

If you're at this level of fitness, it's pretty certain that you have excellent cardiovascular health. To reassure you further, only 3 of my 600 patients have had an elevated carotid IMT score (more than 0.8 mm) if they reached 15 minutes on the stress test. Importantly, I have never met a patient who consistently ate more than 30 grams of fiber daily *and* exceeded 15 minutes on the Bruce Protocol who had an elevated IMT score, nor have I met one who had any signs of cardiovascular disease.

Hopefully, you finished in the 70th to 90th percentiles for someone your age. If not, take heart; this program is designed to help you improve your score over time. Your long-term goal would be to achieve scores in the top third for someone ten years younger, although that might take several months and sometimes up to a year to reach.

## HEART RATE RECOVERY TEST

In the Bruce Protocol I described above, I asked you to take your pulse at your level of maximum exertion. After you achieve maximum exertion, immediately decrease the speed to 1 mile per hour with no elevation. You'll do this because another good predictor of your heart's ability to accommodate varying levels of physical effort is to track how quickly your heart rate drops after peak exercise. Your heart can race as high as 160 to 200 beats per minute. When you stop exercising, the quicker your heart rate drops, the better. Here's what to do to find out:

After reaching your maximum exertion rate, walk at 1 mile per hour without incline for one minute and take your pulse again. A minimum 25-beat drop at 60 seconds is normal, but I'd prefer more than a 30-beat drop. That would show good heart rate recovery. However, if you have had heart surgery or are taking medication that alters your heart rate, then your recovery may not meet these guidelines and you should clarify your targets with your own physician. Athletes will often observe that their heart rate drops by 40 to 60 beats at one minute. On the other hand, if it drops less than 20 beats at one minute, this would be concerning, and if it drops less than 12 beats, I'd call that alarming. At two minutes, your heart rate should drop by at least 45 beats. This too indicates a good cardiac recovery level.

## STEP TEST

If a gym or treadmill is inaccessible to you, you can still measure your estimated MET score at home with a 3-minute step test. Again, be sure to get your doctor's permission before doing this on your own, especially if you have health issues or are in poor physical condition. You'll need a step—a 16.25-inch sturdy box that won't move or be crushed by your weight, a stopwatch, a metronome (optional), and a heart rate monitor (optional, but recommended). The step test I have chosen is called the Queens College Step Test. You can take the YMCA 3-Minute Step Test at your local Y.

To take the Queens College Step Test, follow the instructions below or, better, hire a trainer who can calculate this for you:

- Warm up for 10 minutes with mild to moderate, not strenuous activity
- Set the metronome, if you are using it, to the required pace, 22 beats per minute for women and 24 beats per minute for men.
- Step up and down on the box at a rate of 22 steps per minute for women and 24 steps per minute for men. Use a four-step rhythm: "up-up-down-down" for 3 minutes. Stop immediately after 3 minutes, and count your heartbeats for 15 seconds, using the stopwatch. Multiplying your 15-second reading by 4 will give the beats per minute

(bpm) that you'll use in the calculation below. Or use the heart rate monitor to get an accurate reading of your pulse. Heart rate is the same as beats per minute.

- Men: Multiply your heart rate by 0.42. Then subtract that number from 111.33. Divide your answer by 3.5 to get your estimated MET score.
- Women: Multiply your heart rate by 0.185. Subtract that from 65.8. Divide your answer by 3.5 and that gives you your estimated MET score.

As an example, after 3 minutes on the step test, Mary had 38 heart beats in the first 15 seconds. Here is the calculation:

38 times 4 = 152 beats per minute

152 beats per minute times 0.185 = 28.1

65.8 minus 28.1 = 37.7

37.7 divided by 3.5 = 10.8.

Thus, her estimated MET score is 10.8. At age 45, this put Mary at the 80th percentile for fitness for her age group.

Once you have your MET score, look to the men's and women's aerobic capacity testing tables on pages 128 and 129 to see how you did.

## AEROBIC EXERCISE BY PHASES

Aerobic exercise focuses on speeding up your heart rate and maintaining it for a minimum of 20 minutes, and preferably for 30 to 40 minutes. It strengthens your heart, helps you burn calories, and revs up your metabolic rate. Studies in my clinic show that it makes you mentally sharper too. In addition to helping your heart, aerobic exercise can reduce mental stress and decrease cancer risk. Weight-bearing activities such as fast walking build strong bones—the benefits are endless!

You can perform aerobic exercise by walking briskly, jogging, cycling, swimming, or exercising on an elliptical machine. Anything that raises your heart rate into your target aerobic heart rate zone will do. The first workout question is usually, "Where do I start?" You can think about developing an exercise routine in manageable phases. But please don't pick a phase based upon your activity from 5 or 10 years ago. Be sure to check with your doctor and choose your routine from what has been typical activity for you over the last month or two and base it on the information you've discovered in the fitness tests you've just taken.

- **Phase One** is for people who don't exercise at an aerobic level. For instance, they never reach 70% of their maximum heart rate. If you are a "couch" or "office credenza" potato, or if you stroll when you walk, this means you! People with a heart rate recovery that is less than 25 beats per minute should also start in Phase One, as this low heart rate recovery is below normal and often means they are unfit and have low exercise tolerance.
- **Phase Two** is for people who:
  o can only sustain their heart rate in the low end of their aerobic workout zone
  o can push it for 30 minutes to 80% to 85% of their heart rate zone, but only work out for 20 to 30 minutes two to three times per week
  o have a heart rate recovery of at least 25 beats after one minute, which is normal exercise tolerance.
- **Phase Three** is for people who are able to work out for at least 30 minutes at a time, typically at the top of their aerobic zone, meaning above 80% of their maximum heart rate. Most people ready to start in Phase Three have a heart rate recovery that is more than 30 beats per minute, which shows good exercise tolerance.

As you've seen, these calculations are detailed and a bit complicated, although very doable. But if you pay for a one-hour assessment with an exercise physiologist, he or she can help you calculate your MET score and safely determine which of the three phases best matches your current condition.

## YOUR AEROBIC WORKOUT PLAN

- Pick an activity you enjoy, such as fast walking, jogging, treadmill or elliptical machine exercise, or playing a fast game like racquetball.
- If you are walking or jogging, be sure you have good quality shoes and, for women, a good exercise bra.
- You'll likely have better success sticking to it if you have an exercise partner.
- Plan to use a heart rate monitor on occasion. It will give you a reading of your average and maximum heart rate during your workout and also of the calories you've burned. It will even keep a record of your exercise activity level. It's a good investment. You don't need it every day, yet it helps as your fitness improves to ensure you optimize the time you spend exercising.

**If You Are in Phase One:** start exercising at 60% to 70% of your maximum heart rate. (See page 126, if needed, to review the heart rate calculation tool.) Twenty minutes, five days a week may be plenty for the first week, with 30 minutes daily five days a week thereafter. If you repeat your fitness test and your 1-minute heart rate recovery is still less than 25 beats, stay in Phase One another two weeks to be safe.

**After the first two weeks, move to Phase Two.** Work out 5 to 6 days a week for 30 to 45 minutes at 70% to 85% of your maximum heart rate. After one or two weeks, you'll find you have to exercise harder and faster to keep your heart rate in the same zone. This is good, because it means you are rapidly growing fitter!

**After two weeks, you can move into Phase Three.** In addition to continuing the Phase Two plan, now you can add *interval training.* This consists of short bursts of intense exercise, typically for 1 to 2 minutes, followed by a slow easy zone for 1 to 2 minutes. At the middle of your aerobic workout, determine your heart rate. Then push yourself to 85% to 90% of your maximum rate, and keep your heart pumping like that for 1 minute. Then slow back down to your normal aerobic zone. Repeat this burst five times, and you have completed an interval workout session! Interval training is great for many reasons. It burns calories and fat rapidly, while it revs up your metabolism. If you are always short of time, interval training also allows you to shorten your workout—from 30 to 20 minutes, and you will still get similar benefits. After a while, interval training will begin to feel easy. That's when you'll have to retest your maximum achievable heart rate, because your heart will be responding as if you were years younger.

Here is how the aerobic workout plan worked for Stephanie. She had only been exercising one day a week and had never reached her aerobic zone, so she needed to start at Phase One. Stephanie had a treadmill at home that sat idle in the garage, gathering cobwebs. As part of her 30-Day Heart Tune-Up, she agreed to get on it for 30 minutes, five days a week. Her walking shoes were several years old, so she bought a new pair. She already had a heart rate monitor (an old, but unused birthday present), a good exercise bra, and some comfortable clothes, so she was ready to start. She had done the fitness tests I've outlined above with the exercise physiologist at our clinic.

During her test, Stephanie's maximum heart rate reached 160 beats per minute, and her 1-minute heart rate recovery was 26 (normal), so for the first two weeks, her goal was to get her heart rate up to 96 to 112 (60% to 70% of her maximum) and keep it there for at least 20 minutes. Day One, she woke up 40 minutes earlier than usual, having gone to bed 40 minutes earlier the night before, made and drank a quick protein, almond milk, and berry smoothie, and turned on her treadmill. She set it for 2.5 miles per hour without any elevation and started walking for 2 minutes. Her heart rate was 90 beats per minute, just right for a warm-up. At 2 minutes, she increased her speed to 3.5 miles per hour, but after 2 minutes her heart rate rose to only 95 beats. This was not enough, so she increased the elevation to 5 degrees. Two minutes later, her heart rate was 110 beats per minute, and she maintained that speed, elevation, and heart rate for 20 minutes. She slowed back to 2.5 miles per hour for 3 minutes with no elevation, in order to calm her heart. She stretched her calves and hamstrings (as I'll share later) for 2 minutes, jumped in the shower, dressed, and headed to the office. Driving to work she realized, "Wow! I feel alive, sharp. This is great!"

She kept up the routine 5 days that week, but by the second week, she noted she needed to go faster, to 4 miles per hour, to keep her heart rate in the right zone. She continued that pace during Week Two.

Week Three, she gradually pushed up her speed and elevation to keep her heart rate at 112 to 136 beats per minute, and by 30 days, she had to jog at 6% elevation and 4.5 miles per hour to keep her pulse in the right zone. Stephanie was not just getting fitter; her heart was getting stronger, her weight was dropping by about a pound or two a week, and her energy level was dramatically higher. Even her husband noted a difference, as her libido strengthened nicely.

We repeated Stephanie's weight, blood pressure, and laboratory measurements after 30 days. She smiled broadly when we reviewed her results. I was so proud to see her improvement. It was obvious to everyone in the office, because her clothes didn't fit—they were at least one size too big—and instead of the person we'd met 30 days ago, she now glowed.

At just one month, Stephanie was ready to start interval training. Her transformation had begun.

# THE POWER OF STRENGTH TRAINING

Strength training stresses your muscles and stimulates them to build mass. Most of us lose far too much muscle mass as we age, and as a result, we have frequent muscle and joint pain, our growth hormone and testosterone levels drop, our bone mass decreases, and our resting calorie burning rate plummets—promoting weight gain.

Building muscle mass is essential to preventing and reversing metabolic syndrome, which you now know is the #1 cause of cardiovascular events. That's why it is also essential to your heart. Extra muscle decreases inflammation, lowers blood pressure, and helps you control your blood sugar and insulin.[3] Muscle power is absolutely essential for stopping heart attacks and strokes.

Women, in particular, benefit from the effects of weight and strength training, mostly because they usually have much less muscle mass than men. (And no, you won't end up looking like Arnold Schwarzenegger!) The 30-Day Heart Tune-Up won't make you big and bulky, but will help you add tone, definition, and shape—all essential for a fit, sexy, and healthy look. The key is pushing your muscles to exhaustion. This encourages muscle mass to rebuild and make itself stronger.

Muscle mass is like money in the bank—something to retire on. Otherwise, you'll experience a poverty of health. It prevents fractures later in life by building bone that is denser and stronger. It provides the amino acid building blocks you require to fight infections and accelerate healing of injured tissues. A bigger muscle mass burns more calories, even at rest; in fact, add 1 pound of extra muscle and you'll burn an extra 40 calories every day, enough to burn off 4 pounds of fat over one year. In volume, that means losing one football of fat. Muscle also produces anti-aging compounds such as interleukin-10, a protein that blocks inflammation.

# ELEMENTS OF STRENGTH TRAINING

Most people think of their arms and legs doing all the work when it comes to strength training. But in the 30-Day Heart Tune-Up program, you will be focusing on your trunk or torso too. Trunk strength (also referred to these days as "core strength") is essential to preventing back pain, maintaining good posture, and gaining balance.

Fixed-weight machines such as Nautilus or Hammer Strength systems at a gym flex and extend your muscles. But that's not enough. In real life, you need to keep your joints from twisting and falling from side to side. That means you have to stabilize them, not just flex and extend. In my functional training program, you'll be building the stabilizing muscles in your core as well as those big power muscles in your arms and legs. That is why I prefer for you to work with free weights rather than machines. In many of the exercises I recommend, you will be standing on the floor or you'll use an exercise ball. These strategies will help you to strengthen the little muscles that provide balance and joint stability. You'll also find twisting exercises to strengthen your trunk. Taken together, these activities will help you function optimally every day.

If strength training is a new activity for you, check with your doctor. An advantage of gym membership is that the facility will have all the equipment you need. That will make it easier for you to start. And once you get into the habit—a four-week membership might be enough for you to get the hang of it—you will be able to continue at home with your own equipment. You'll have to buy some tools, though. Different parts of your body require different weights, so you'll need various sizes of dumbbells. These will help you work 8 to 12 body parts. I also recommend buying an exercise ball, especially if you're not using a gym. Get one that's the right size for your height. Your knees should be bent at a 90-degree angle with your feet flat on the floor in front of you when you sit on the ball. An exercise bench might be useful, but don't worry if you don't have one. In the program below, you'll find moves that don't involve one.

One of the first steps is to identify how heavy a dumbbell you need for each movement. This varies from one individual to another and will change as you grow stronger. One person might need to start with 3 pounds, while another might be comfortable with 30 pounds. I've noted an average starting weight for many of the exercises below, but the sensible thing to do is experiment to find the ideal weight for you.

To begin, choose a weight that you can arm curl at least 8 to 10 times. The last couple lifts should make your biceps feel very fatigued—you'll feel a little shakiness at the end, and that's good. If you can't lift the weight at least 8 times, it is probably too heavy. This would increase your risk of injury. If you can lift the weight 15 or 16 times, it is too light. You won't stress your muscles enough to strengthen them.

You'll find that I've provided several options for some muscle groups such as your abs (abdominal muscles) or your chest; the exercises become progressively harder as you advance in your program. So you should begin working your abdominal muscles with simple crunches but then move on to crunches on the ball, which are more challenging and much more fun!

Here are your 30-Day Heart Tune-Up strength-training guidelines at a glance. Aim to work out two or three days a week. You can do strength training on your own, but many find it more fun to do with an exercise partner. In addition, you are less likely to skip your session if you know your partner is waiting for you.

## YOUR STRENGTH-TRAINING WORKOUT

- Start with a 5- to 10-minute warm-up. If you haven't done aerobic exercise on a treadmill or elliptical machine, run up and down the stairs or do some jumping jacks—get a bit sweaty 5 to 10 minutes before you start lifting weights.

- Exercise at least 8 to 12 body parts during each session and balance your workout. That means if you strengthen your biceps (elbow flexors) with arm curls, you'll also need to strengthen your triceps (elbow extenders). If you do lots of crunches for your abs, balance them with back extension exercises.
- Lift your weight 10 to 15 times. If you can't do at least 10 reps, the dumbbell is too heavy. But if you can lift it more than 15 times, it's too light. When you are first starting, you can count out the up-and-down motions to slow yourself and also keep a good rhythm. You can say, "one one thousand" for "up" and "two one thousand" for "down."
- Lift the weight smoothly and lower it slowly. Jerky movements can cause injuries, so avoid them. If you can't lift the weight without jerking, then it's too heavy for you. Go back to a lighter weight. Aim to feel a gentle burn as you lower the weight.
- With leg exercises, keep your knees bent. When exercising your arms, bend them at your elbows. This will help you avoid injuries.

## HOW TO AVOID INJURIES

Simply put, injuries wreck all of your good intentions to exercise. As soon as you're hurt, you stop the activity...you get out of the habit of exercising, lose momentum, and end up back where you started. This is definitely unproductive! So it's wise to avoid injuries in the first place. The following tips will help you avoid injuries:

- Always begin with a warm-up.
- Unless you are a semicompetitive athlete, don't exceed 85% of your maximum heart rate. Exceeding it increases the

release of inflammatory agents and will limit the benefits of exercising.

- Cross-training (working on different aerobic exercise machines, or alternating swimming, bicycling, walking, and running) during the week can prevent injuries associated with overuse.
- Wear good-quality exercise shoes. If you are flatfooted (have fallen arches or pronate to excess), get arch supports for your shoes. You can obtain custom-made orthotics from an orthopedist or standard ones from medical supply or sports shops.
- Many strength-training injuries occur when people are using weight machines. Make sure they are set up appropriately for your size. (A trainer can help you with this.) And don't overload the weights. Lifting free weights, though it requires more skill, is more functional and safer.
- Avoid squats and knee contortions. Don't bend your knees more than 90 degrees.
- If you're new to strength training or if you have a history of injuries, consider working with a trainer, at least in the beginning. You don't need to hire this person for every workout, because that can become quite expensive. Meeting once a week, even if only for the first month, will help you learn safe and effective moves. It is also a good way to be sure that you are pushing yourself hard enough to keep improving, but not so hard that you hurt yourself. Just ask your trainer for homework assignments so you keep on working your muscles safely between sessions.

## THE POWER-YOUR-HEART MOVES

*Pick twelve of the following activities and repeat them two to three times a week.*

## ABDOMINAL CRUNCHES

Most people should be able to do 75 crunches every day. If you're not up to that yet, this exercise provides a great opportunity for you to strengthen your core muscles. But don't go back to the old-fashioned sit-ups you might have done in high school, where you sit up and touch your elbows to your knees. These are now out of favor, as they can strain your back. Stick to crunches instead.

*Benefits:* Crunches build abdominal muscles and provide critical support for your spine.

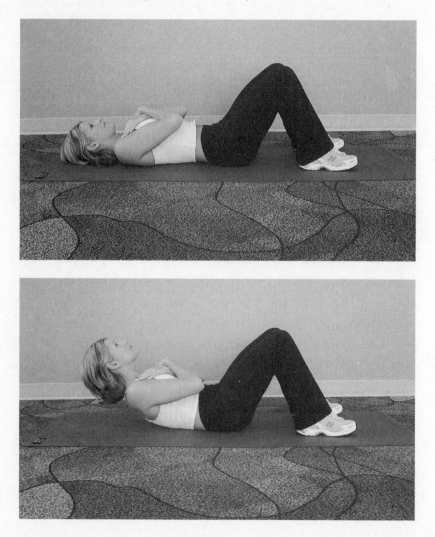

*What you'll need:* A floor mat or other comfortable surface.

- Lie on your back with your feet flat on the floor and your knees bent at an angle of 30 to 45 degrees. Your arms are folded across your chest, one hand on each shoulder.
- Flex your pelvis, pushing your lower back into the floor and tilting your pelvis up; this protects your back during crunches.
- Now raise your upper back and head off the floor, lifting your shoulder blades about 1 to 2 inches from the ground. Be sure you're looking up at the ceiling. Hold for 1 second, and then lower down slowly. Repeat until you feel your abdominal muscles strain. Then take a break for 5 to 10 seconds and perform at least 10 more crunches.
- Exhale through your mouth on the upward motion (the most strenuous part of an exercise) and inhale through your nose on your down motion. And don't forget to breathe on each movement!

*Tip:* Once you can easily reach 75 crunches, try this exercise with your feet lifted gently off the ground, keeping your pelvis flexed. This works your lower abs. Also, be sure your pelvis remains flexed with your back firmly pressed against the floor throughout your routine.

## ABDOMINAL CRUNCHES ON THE BALL

Once you've mastered abdominal crunches on the floor, advance to the ball. It forces you to use your whole trunk, subtly working your oblique stomach muscles as you balance yourself. This makes the exercise more difficult, but also much more effective. You are building the balance and strength you need every day to lift and carry objects.

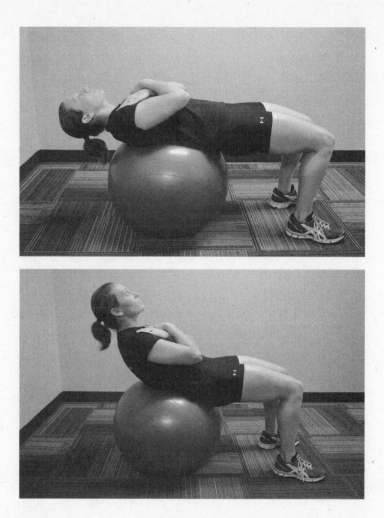

*Benefits:* These are wonderful for people with back problems, and they give you a firm tummy. As with the regular crunches, these will help to give you that sexy six-pack look, when combined with proper weight control.

*What you'll need:* An exercise ball.

- Sit on the ball with your feet on the ground and your arms folded across your chest. Now walk your feet forward and lean backward until your lower and mid-back are against the ball and your feet are a foot or two apart in front of you on the floor.

- With your pelvis flexed, curl up and lift your chest and head toward the ceiling until only your lower back pushes against the ball and you feel a strain in your abdominal muscles. Hold the up position for 3 to 5 seconds; then slowly lean back. Repeat until your abdominal muscles tremble.

*Tip:* As these get easier, bring your feet closer together, until they are side by side, forcing you to recruit more trunk-twisting muscles for balance.

## BACK EXTENSIONS

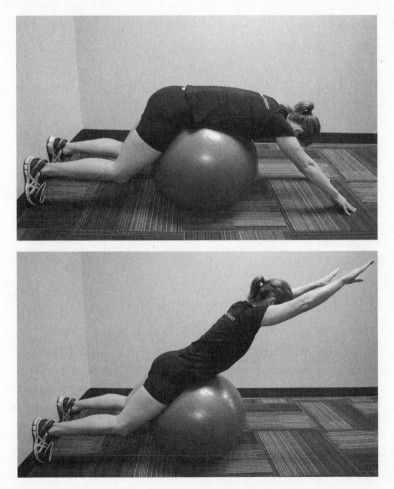

This exercise balances the muscle groups used when performing crunches.

*Benefits:* Back extensions stabilize your spine and prevent back pain by building your lower and upper back muscles. Doing back extensions on an exercise ball also helps to build your trunk's twisting muscles because you are forced to balance. Back exercises should also help with your posture and give your back a sculpted look.

*What you'll need:* An exercise ball. If you are more advanced, you'll also need some small free weights.

- Lying facedown over the ball, brace your toes against the wall or another object. Your feet should be at least hip-width apart, if not a bit wider. (The wider apart your feet, the easier it is to perform this exercise. With time, you can bring your feet closer together.) Place your hands gently on the floor and bend your abdomen over the ball at about a 30-degree angle.
- Now lift your arms so they are extended out in front of you, as if you were Superman flying. Your trunk and arms should be in a straight line, with only your mid-tummy touching the ball. Be careful not to overextend or arch your back into a V. Hold for 1 to 2 seconds.
- Slowly and smoothly, lower your arms and allow your stomach to bend so that your hands touch the floor again. Your feet should remain against the wall during the whole exercise.
- Repeat 12 to 16 times.

*Tips:* If you can't achieve 10 to 12 smooth extension lifts, make the exercise easier by holding your arms behind your back, over your buttocks, or along your sides. Lean forward until you are bent over the ball, then extend so that your trunk is straight, again keeping your toes against the wall. Once you've easily reached

16 back extensions, add a 2- or 3-pound weight to each hand. Continue to add weight as needed over time.

Note: If you have back problems, avoid extending your back beyond the straightened neutral position.

## CHEST PRESS

You can choose this exercise or, as you advance, do the chest press on the ball or do push-ups. They all work the same muscle groups—your triceps, deltoids, and pectoral muscles.

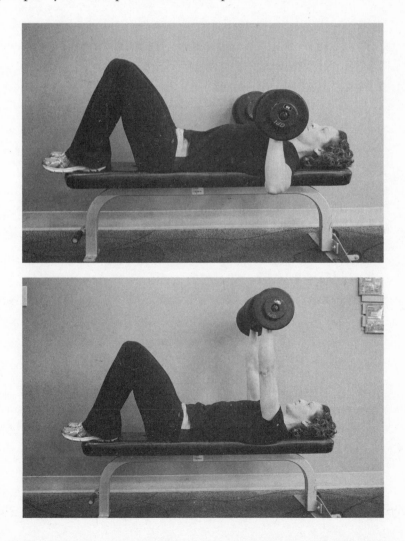

*Benefits:* This builds your chest muscles and is also good for your triceps and shoulders. For women, the chest press helps to tone up the muscles under the breast, adding firmness, lift, and shape to the breast area. For men, it builds pec muscles that help you look great with or without a shirt on.

*What you'll need:* A bench (or you can also perform this on the ball or on the floor) and two free weights that you can lift 10 to 15 times with smooth, even movements. Average starting weight, 10 to 30 pounds.

- Lie on your back on the bench with your knees bent and your feet resting on the end of the bench. Your legs should be bent at an angle of 30 to 45 degrees.
- Press your lower back into the bench, flexing your pelvis.
- Hold the weights next to your chest at breast level with your palms facing toward your knees. Your elbows are pointing down toward the floor.
- Now straighten your arms up into the air so they are perpendicular to your body. Don't let the weights touch at the top of the motion; this keeps your muscles working. Don't lock your elbows. Keep your body and wrists steady and pelvis flexed.
- Raise and lower the weights with smooth motions, counting "one one thousand" for up and "two one thousand" for down. You should just barely be able to lift the correct weight 10 to 15 times smoothly without jerking your arms or trunk.

*Tips:* As these get easier, advance to chest presses on the ball for an even tougher workout.

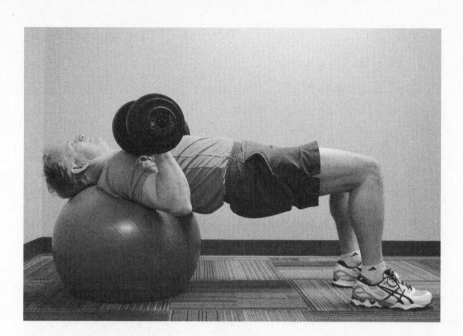

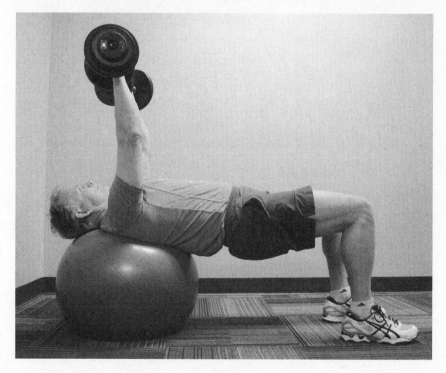

## PUSH-UPS

You can perform either this exercise or the chest press.

*Benefits:* Push-ups build triceps and pectorals (chest) muscles. They help create firm and shapely chest, shoulder, and upper arm muscles, similar to the chest press.

*What you'll need:* A smooth, clean floor surface.

- Lie facedown with your palms on the ground, directly below your shoulders. Beginners can start by doing the

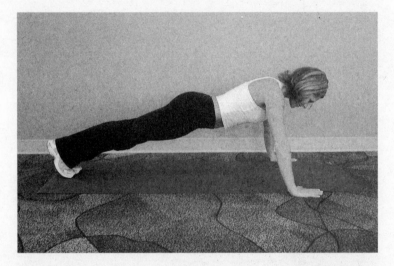

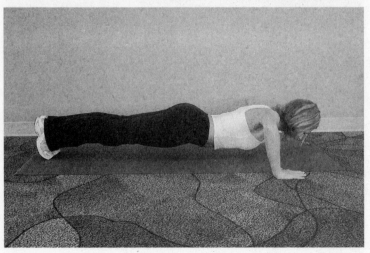

push-ups with weight on your knees. As you build strength, you can perform the push-ups with your weight on your toes, as shown in the photos.

- Inhale and straighten your arms, keeping your back straight and pushing your trunk up and away from the floor.
- Now slowly exhale and lower yourself back down until your chin just touches the floor. Your back remains straight at all times. (If your tummy or chest touches the floor before your chin, despite keeping your back straight, be sure you drop low enough that your elbows are bent to at least 90 degrees in the down position.)
- Continue raising and lowering yourself until you break form. Rest a few seconds, and then perform at least a few more.

## ONE-ARM ROW

This exercise balances the muscles used in the push-up and chest press exercises.

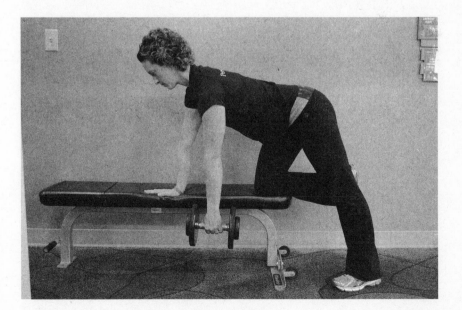

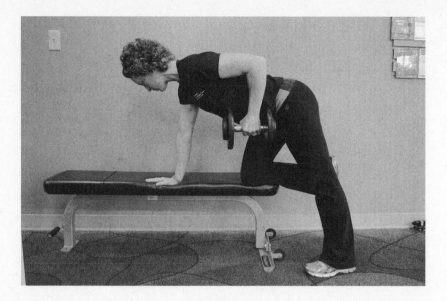

*Benefits:* Builds upper back and rhomboid muscles. This exercise provides you with a shapely upper back and helps your posture by pulling your shoulders back.

*What you'll need:* One free weight (average starting weight, 10 to 25 pounds) and a bench or chair.

- Place your right knee on the bench or a chair and rest your right hand on the bench in front of your knee.
- Hold the weight in your left hand.
- Lean forward so that your trunk is parallel to the floor and your left arm dangles toward the floor, your palm facing your standing leg.
- Inhale and pull your left elbow as high as you can, pointing toward the ceiling without shifting or rotating your trunk. Keep your arm close to your body.
- Exhale and slowly lower your left arm to the starting position.
- Repeat 10 to 15 times.
- Change sides and repeat, holding the weight in your right hand and your left knee and hand on the bench or chair.

# Biceps Curls (with Free Weights)

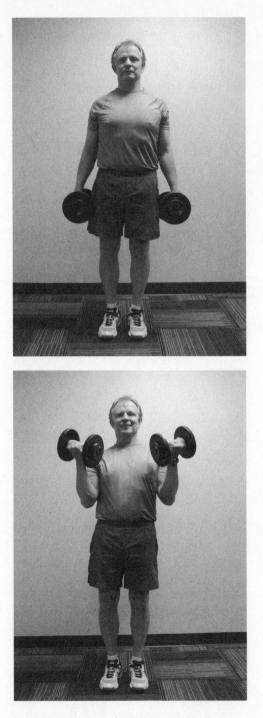

*Benefits:* Builds the biceps and the brachioradialis (upper forearm), giving you nice, shapely arms.

*What you'll need:* Two free weights (average starting weight, 8 to 25 pounds).

- Stand with your knees slightly flexed and arms extended, holding a free weight in each hand, with your palms facing your legs.
- Keeping your upper arms stable and your elbows at your side, raise your forearms upward, until your hands nearly reach your shoulders. Your palm rotates as you lift your arm so that it is facing your chest at the end of this motion.
- Next, lower your hands smoothly to the starting position. Repeat 10 to 15 times.
- Keep your trunk stable during your movements, your pelvis and knees flexed, and your abs tight to protect your lower back.

## TRICEPS EXTENSIONS

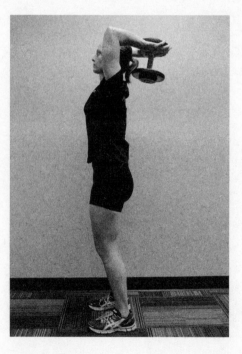

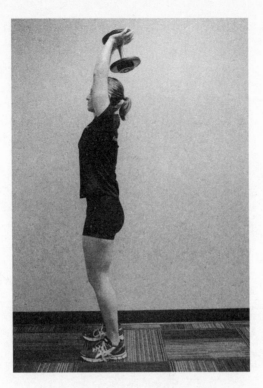

This exercise balances the muscles used in the biceps curl.

*Benefits:* Good for building triceps muscles, helping to create shapely but not bulky arms.

*What you'll need:* One free weight (average starting weight, 10 to 20 pounds).

- Hold a dumbbell vertically by one of its knobs with both hands behind your head, making sure your elbows are pointed forward and up (see photo).
- Extend your hands above your head, straightening your elbows and keeping them close to your ears, but do not lock your elbows.
- Count "one one thousand" on the up motion; then, slowly lower your hands behind your head and count "two one thousand" as you drop the weight to the down position. Repeat 10 to 15 times.

- Watch to make sure your head is clear of the dumbbell. Keep your neck aligned with your spine.

## OVERHEAD PRESS

This exercise balances the muscles in your shoulders.

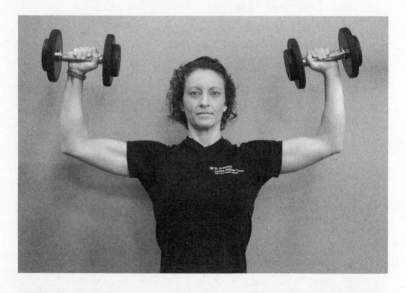

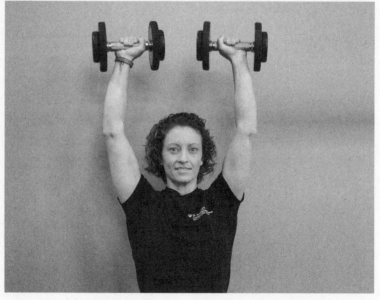

*Benefits:* This builds your deltoids and trapezius (shoulder and neck) muscles and triceps to give you a shapely neck and shoulders.

*What you'll need:* Two dumbbells (average starting weight: 5 pounds for women, 20 pounds for men).

- Stand erect with your pelvis flexed. If you find you are arching your back, perform this lift sitting instead to avoid back strain. Hold a weight in each hand at shoulder height with your palms facing forward and your elbows out to your sides. To prevent shoulder strain, make sure your elbows don't bend more than 90 degrees.
- Now slowly press the weights up until your arms are nearly straight, directly above your shoulders, without locking your elbows. Do not allow the weights to touch.
- Keeping your trunk still, lower the weights slowly.
- Perform 10 to 15 reps.
- If you note pain or popping in your shoulder, stop immediately.

## BALL SQUATS

These are not difficult. When you get stronger, you'll move on to the lunges. They work the same muscle groups, but require more strength and balance.

*Benefits:* These are a great exercise for shaping and firming your buttocks (gluteals) and thighs (quads).

*What you'll need:* An exercise ball and an unobstructed wall.

- Stand with your back to the wall, your feet about shoulder-width apart.
- Place the exercise ball between the wall and your lower back and upper gluteal muscles.
- Flex your pelvis forward to protect your back throughout the movement.

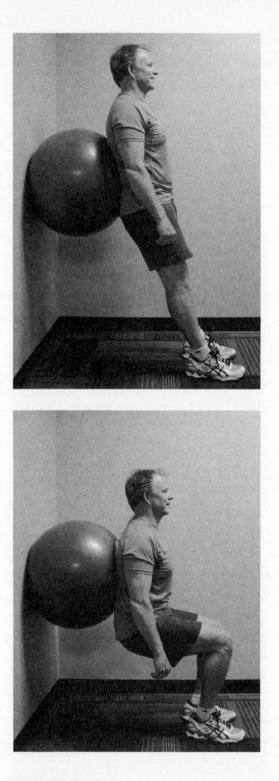

- Lean back against the ball and walk your feet forward several steps. Walk far enough away so that your knees don't go over your toes when you squat.
- Bend your knees until they're at 90 degrees, and lower your body so the ball rolls down the wall. If you feel you want an extra push and you don't have a history of knee problems, bend your knees to 120 degrees, but no further.
- Make sure your weight is in your heels as you squat.
- Straighten back up to standing, tightening your glutes as you stand.

## LUNGES

This exercise works your quads and glutes (buttocks) and also adds some work for your hamstrings.

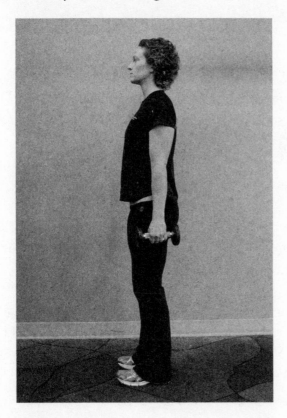

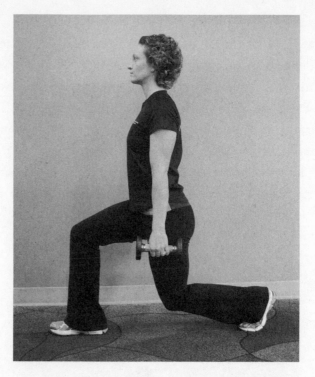

*Benefits:* Lunges help build your quads (thighs) and gluteal (buttock) muscles. They also enhance your balance. This is an excellent exercise for building shape, tone, and firmness in your thighs and buttocks.

*What you'll need:* Two free weights (average starting weight, 1 to 15 pounds).

- Be sure to perform lunges with your pelvis flexed forward. If you extend your back and pelvis, you can irritate your lower back and spine.
- Stand with your feet shoulder-width apart.
- Holding one weight in each hand (or not), take a big step forward on your right foot, bending your right knee and lowering your left knee toward the floor. Stop when your left knee is just above the floor, and make sure your right

knee doesn't extend beyond your toes. Your right knee should be bent at about a 90-degree angle when your left knee is close to the floor. Keep your weight in your front (right) heel. You want to feel a smooth dropping motion.

- Next, push back smoothly to your initial standing position.
- Repeat with your left foot lunging forward while slowly dropping your right knee.
- Once you can perform 20 to 25 lunges with each leg comfortably, add an extra 5-pound weight to each hand. Gradually increase the weight, so that reaching 15 to 20 lunges with each foot produces some moderate strain.

## HAMSTRING BRIDGE

This counterbalances the squat and the lunge.

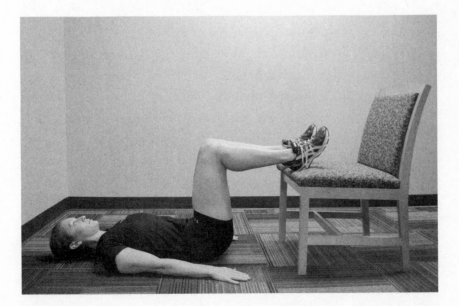

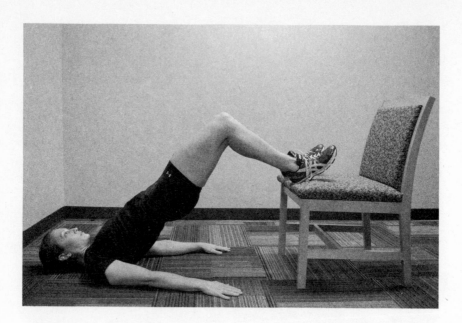

*Benefits:* You're working your buttocks and hamstrings to achieve well-toned and shapely thighs.

*What you'll need:* A chair or an exercise ball and an unobstructed floor surface.

- Lie on the floor with your back flat.
- Place your hands on the floor next to your hips.
- Place your heels either on the ball or on a chair.
- Lift your pelvis and buttocks off the floor as high as you can, pushing with the backs of your heels against the ball or chair. You may need to rely on your hands for balance and strength at first. Feel the pull in your hamstrings as you go up.
- Hold the position for 2 seconds; then lower your buttocks slowly back toward the floor.
- Lift again without resting your buttocks on the floor, keeping your muscles contracted between repetitions.
- Repeat 10 to 15 times.

# Calf Presses (with Free Weights)

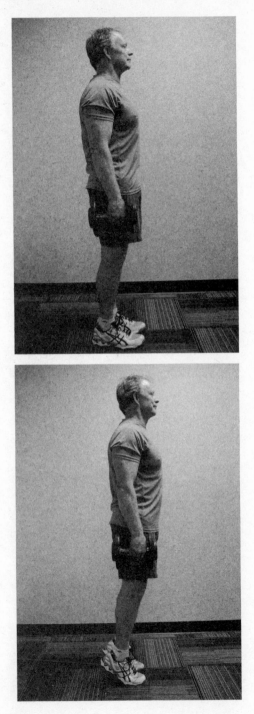

*Benefits:* This builds your calf muscles and develops nice, shapely calves.

*What you'll need:* Two free weights (average starting weight, 10 to 30 pounds).

- Stand erect, holding free weights in each hand, with your feet pointing forward, shoulder-width apart.
- Slowly rise up on your toes, holding for one half second, and then slowly lower back down. Repeat with a weight you can lift 10 to 15 times.

## SHOULDER ROTATOR CUFF LIFTS

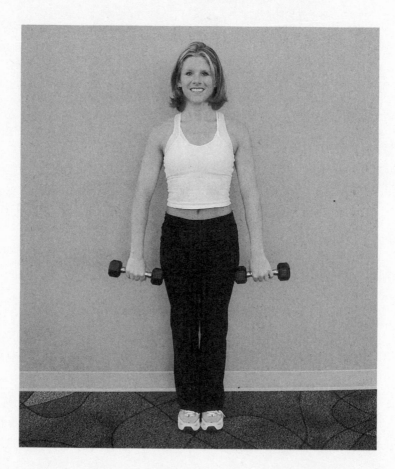

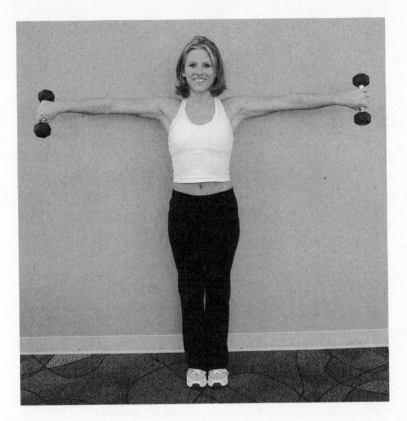

*Benefits:* This strengthens the small muscles beneath the larger deltoid muscles of the shoulder, which are critical for maintaining healthy shoulder function. This exercise won't make your shoulders look shapelier, but it will protect them so you can use them into your golden years.

*What you'll need:* Two small free weights (average starting weight, 2 to 4 pounds).

- While standing with your pelvis flexed, hold a small weight in each hand with your thumbs pointed directly down toward the floor and your hands resting beside your thighs.
- Slowly lift your arms upward with your hands more than shoulder-width apart, and with your thumbs pointing to the floor, until they're shoulder height and parallel to the

floor. Don't raise your arms above shoulder height; doing so can pinch tendons inside the shoulder.

- Now slowly lower your arms and repeat 12 to 15 times.

## STRETCH FOR FLEXIBILITY

Even if stretching doesn't offer the benefits of aerobic activity or strength training, it is very important, because it will help you improve your athletic performance and reduce injuries. The key is to stretch after a workout, not before. A 2- to 5-minute stretch is enough for most people, and optimally you would add one or two yoga sessions a week as well. Some stretching can be harmful, such as bouncing or vigorous stretching prior to warming up. You can do the following four stretches in just a few minutes.

### HAMSTRING STRETCH

- Sit on the floor with your legs shoulder-width apart in front of you. Slowly lean forward and reach toward one foot at a time, feeling the stretch in your hamstring muscle, which runs from just below the back of your knee to your buttock.
- If you can, hold your toes, one foot at a time, then feel the pull as you take deep breaths in and out. If you can't reach this far yet, then just hold your ankle. With each exhalation, slide gently deeper into the stretch, and with each inhale, you'll note an added pull.
- Don't bounce. Maintain a steady stretch for at least 10 seconds, and preferably 20 seconds.

### CALF STRETCH

- Stand facing a wall with your arms extended out in front of you so that you touch the wall. Your palms will lie flat against its surface.

- Now step backward about 1 to 2 feet with one foot, keeping the other foot in place.
- Keeping the extended leg behind you straight, feel a pull in your calf muscles as you press the heel against the floor. Hold it steady for 10 to 20 seconds.
- Bring the extended leg back to center and switch, stretching the other leg.
- After completing the calf stretch on both legs, step back with one foot at a time into the same position, but this time keep the leg extended back slightly bent. This will help you feel a different stretch, lower on your calf. Repeat for each leg for 10 to 20 seconds.

## LOWER BACK STRETCH

This stretch can be useful when you feel tightness in your lower back.

- Lie on your back.
- With your knees bent, pull your legs toward your chest with your hands behind your knees. Feel a gentle pull in your lower back as you hold this stretch for 20 seconds.

## HIP AND ILIOTIBIAL (IT) BAND STRETCH

The IT band is a strip of connective tissue extending from the hip to the outside of your knee, along the outside of your thigh

- Lie on your back with your arms out to your sides, perpendicular to your body.
- Pull your knees up, and let them fall to the right side. You should be able to touch your knees to the floor on your right without lifting your left shoulder off the floor, feeling a stretch along your lateral left hip and down to the knee. Feel the stretch for 10 seconds.

- Now roll your knees over to the left, keeping your right shoulder on the floor, feeling the stretch over your lateral right hip and down to the knee. Hold it for 10 seconds. Repeat both sides.

---

When used in conjunction with the 30-Day Heart Tune-Up eating plan, these exercises will help you look better, feel stronger, and walk sexier. But perhaps more important, they'll help your heart and cardiovascular system over the long haul. And that is your ultimate goal, after all.

Now that I've stressed you with this exercise chapter, let me help you find some peace and calm with the next chapter—about managing your stress.

*Chapter Six*

# De-stress Your Heart

Modern living can be packed with stressors: nonstop work deadlines, incessant e-mails and texts, marital woes, financial worries, competing for a promotion, juggling work with child care, insomnia, needy family members, moving, bad traffic, rebellious teenagers...you name it! Unfortunately, a stressed soul leads to poor eating, inactivity, and angst. Who looks forward to steamed broccoli and a grilled chicken breast when overstressed? Just about nobody. More likely, you'll seek out comfort foods like ice cream, chips, alcohol, candy, cookies, or a big hunk of cheese. Often, this leads to a downward spiral: The worse you feel, the less you exercise, the more poorly you eat, the worse you feel, and on it goes.

High levels of uncontrolled stress are not just psychologically uncomfortable. They also cause many major health problems throughout your body, because of increased levels of cortisol. These problems can include brain cell death, decreased memory and learning, bone density loss, muscle mass loss, reduced skin healing and growth, impaired immune function (which can lead to more frequent infections and even cancer), elevated blood sugar levels, increased visceral fat, a drop in levels of DHEA (dehydro-epiandrosterone, an important adrenal hormone), and shortened telomeres, which speed destruction of our own cellular DNA. In fact, studies suggest that high levels of unmanaged stress accelerate DNA aging by at least ten years.

In particular, stress can damage your cardiovascular system. Because it leads to a jump in adrenaline levels, it increases your blood pressure and heart rate. These factors irritate your arteries and can trigger the accumulation of more plaque, thereby boosting your chances of having a heart attack or stroke.

---

### Some Stress in Your Life Is Good

I am not proposing that you walk around in a Zen state 24/7. I actually believe we all need some stress in our lives, because it gives us purpose, challenge, and a sense of achievement. For instance, you may experience stage fright before a big presentation, but then feel a sense of triumph after you've knocked it out of the park. You may feel the burn while running a marathon, but then celebrate your accomplishment when you cross the finish line. You may fret over a huge project with a looming deadline, but then gain recognition and big promotion with its successful completion. There's even a term, "eustress," which describes the positive, exciting physiological reaction that occurs when you're beside yourself with joy.

---

Charles Darwin would say it isn't the strongest species that survive, but those that adapt best to change. It is essential to point out that stress is not all about the situation we are in, but rather, how we respond to it. Often we can't change our environment, but we can change our reaction to it. In this chapter, I want you to discover how to manage your stress, but even more, how to proactively transform stress toward healing your heart.

## STRESS ISN'T JUST EMOTIONAL, IT'S HORMONAL

Excessive unmanaged stress increases cortisol and adrenaline hormone production, which can lead to heart attacks and strokes.

This is not just theoretical! The Los Angeles County Coroner reported a 500% increase in cardiovascular deaths on January 17, 1994—the day of the major earthquake in Northridge, California. Clearly, a sudden increase in stress is highly associated with your risk for death.

Making matters worse, people who are too stressed often fail to follow an optimal nutrition and exercise regimen. As a result, they gain weight, feel worse, and experience even more stress.

How does your angst affect your hormonal system? When you're initially stressed, the adrenal gland makes extra cortisol to cope. But over time it can't keep up this overproduction. That causes cortisol to drop and eventually crash. Without it, we can't handle the extra stress. Chronic stress engenders similar problems with DHEA, a hormone produced in the adrenal gland. This hormone gives us drive, energy, and libido. If DHEA levels decrease, our ability to handle stress plummets even further. Unbalanced hormonal control feeds itself, contributing to the downward, self-reinforcing spiral that in the end creates even greater hormonal imbalance.

Your goal here will be to reverse the spiral biochemically. One of the hormones that helps reduce stress is oxytocin. You can think of it as the "cuddling" hormone, as it enhances that warm, delicious feeling mothers experience when they are nursing their infants, and that lovers feel when they are caressing one another. Another group of brain chemicals that modulate stress are endorphins, which are released when you exercise. Both of these neurochemicals will help control cortisol production and ease your transition toward a greater sense of serenity.

As you reduce your stress, you'll eat more wisely, you'll work out more, and you'll feel better all the way around. With time, your cortisol, DHEA, and adrenaline levels will stabilize, and you'll feel calmer. As your stress management improves, it will become easier for you to maintain a healthy diet and to work out regularly.

For you to achieve balanced stress hormones, you will be guided by the pillars of the 30-Day Heart Tune-Up—adding revitalizing foods, getting fit, meeting key nutrient needs (see Chapter 7), and managing stress in your life. In this chapter, I'll focus on specific aspects of how these pillars help restore hormone balance so that you can better handle whatever life throws at you.

This is an excellent opportunity to share a patient story from my clinic on how stress can make the difference between life and death.

## JACKIE CAN'T TAKE IT ANYMORE!

Jackie had been my patient for many years, yet she had managed to avoid a comprehensive assessment. She never had the time to schedule a full-day evaluation, even though her employer paid for her annual testing. But at 55, Jackie started having chest pain when she felt stressed, two or three times a week for up to 10 minutes per episode. She did not have any of the classic risk factors for heart disease: she never smoked, she had no family history of cardiovascular disease, and her regular cholesterol profile was normal, as was her blood sugar. Her blood pressure was only modestly elevated. All reassuring.

In the past, Jackie had always been a little reserved in my office, but the day she came in to see me about her chest pains, she was crying and scared, even though she wasn't having any symptoms at the moment. I had to take Jackie's complaints seriously, because she described the pain as heavy, like someone was sitting on her chest. It didn't radiate, but when she experienced this particular discomfort she also became nauseated, short of breath, and sweaty. This sounded enough like angina for us to schedule a stress test and carotid IMT testing. As a precaution, I also had her take a baby aspirin daily (see Chapter 3) and reviewed with her detailed instructions on what to do if the pain persisted or worsened.

Jackie's stress test was normal—somewhat encouraging. Yet her carotid IMT score showed advanced arterial plaque—closer to that of a woman of 70 rather than one of 55. After several days, her advanced lipid profile and inflammation markers came back normal as well. The good news in Jackie's case was that she ate very well. We had discussed her dietary habits several times over the years, and she had been following my recommendations closely. But in a way, this confused me even further. I was puzzled as to why she had so much plaque and a history suggestive of angina if she followed such a healthful regimen.

Women, more than men, can have artery spasms, causing angina without a major blockage. Jackie's history of chest pain that accompanied stress appeared to be the most important clue, as stress can cause arterial spasms. To find out whether stress was the culprit, I checked objective physiological measures: Jackie's fasting cortisol and DHEA levels. Not surprisingly, her cortisol level was very high, showing ongoing stress, but also showing that her adrenal function hadn't crashed yet (in that case, the cortisol level would have been low). Her DHEA level was quite low, indicating that her adrenal function had dropped and that these stressors had been gnawing at her for a long time. Combined with the angina history, it seemed clear that stress was killing Jackie, and it was accelerating the growth of plaque in her arteries too!

As we talked about what was going on in her life, Jackie shared that her job as the vice president of research for a large company had created a great deal of pressure for her. But the problem wasn't the stress—it was that she wasn't handling it well. To make matters worse, she was also upset at home. She burst into tears when she explained that her husband expected her to do most of the housework (cleaning, cooking, and taking charge of home repairs), especially now that their children were grown and on their own. The fact that she also spent occasional weekends watching the grandchildren added to her burden, although the children brought her joy.

Jackie wasn't coping well with all of this. She had tried various antacid treatments for the chest pressure, but they had offered no relief. No surprise there! This wasn't a case of acid reflux. She admitted that her job performance had slipped over recent months, as she often felt tired and dull at work. She slept poorly, averaging only six hours a night, which she was sure was inadequate. She felt she didn't have the time to exercise, as her work, family, and home responsibilities always came first. Clearly, Jackie had little peace and calm in her day. She drank 4 to 5 cups of coffee daily, mostly so she could function at work. She didn't imbibe alcohol at all during the week, but overdid it on weekends, consuming a whole bottle of wine by herself on Friday, Saturday, and Sunday nights to blow off steam. When I asked about her romantic life, she rolled her eyes and replied, "Who has the time or energy for sex?"

Unfortunately, sex was the least of Jackie's problems. The stress-induced spasms in her arteries were clearly life-threatening. With time, her symptoms would worsen or she would simply die from a heart attack, stroke, or sudden death (arrhythmia). I thought long and hard about several approaches to our next course of action. There was probably some value in starting her on cholesterol-lowering and blood pressure–lowering medications, yet that was not going to fix the underlying cause of her heart disease. (I review the indications for cholesterol-lowering statin medications in Chapter 7.) Besides, because her advanced cholesterol profile looked good, I believed that stress management would bring her blood pressure back to normal without any medication. With Jackie's permission, I called her husband, Mark, and asked him to come in that afternoon to join us in a discussion of her diagnosis of stress-induced angina. I wanted him to participate in the creation of a treatment plan for his wife. I sighed with relief when Mark agreed to leave work and come in immediately. He really did care about Jackie; he just didn't know how to show it.

# THE SIX STEPS TO OPTIMAL STRESS MANAGEMENT

In discussing Jackie's situation with her, I asked her the six questions you'll see in the "How Stressed Are You?" box. I use these in my practice to assess how stressed my patients are feeling, and I ask you now to think about how you would answer for yourself.

---

## How Stressed Are You?

1. Do you feel loved and supported?
2. Are you getting enough good quality sleep?
3. Do you get a workout most days to burn off the stress?
4. Do you schedule some time for peace and calm every day?
5. Do you overuse stimulants and alcohol?
6. Are you having fun and experiencing joy?

---

Sadly, Jackie answered, no, to most of the stress management questions and yes to overdoing it with alcohol, so we had our work cut out for us. But what about you? Let's review the six steps to optimal stress management. I hope that taking the right kind of action will help you avoid the situation Jackie found herself in. Life is hard enough. There's no point in being stressed to death—especially if you can do something about it!

## Step 1. Feeling Loved and Supported

Of all the executives I've met in my medical practice, those who have been highly successful feel loved and supported at home, allowing them to thrive in a pressure-cooker work environment. Those whose stressful jobs are coupled with marital problems often don't fare well in the workplace for long. By contrast, in the Harvard Study of Adult Aging, a stable marriage was one of the six most important predictors of aging well. People need to feel needed and loved.

To be loved, first we need to love. Loving another requires us to share openly of ourselves, to care, and to nurture—without seeking anything in return. This is the act of loving. A loved one could be a spouse, a partner, a parent or other relative, or a friend. We all flourish when we have loving and supportive relationships. Studies have shown that even interacting with a pet improves life spans and enhances the quality of our lives.

Interestingly, some of the benefits of intimacy are biochemical. As you know, stress raises cortisol, but oxytocin (the bonding hormone) reduces it. Any activity that increases oxytocin (including intimacy and sex) is great for stress reduction. I'll talk more about this in Chapter 8. Just bear in mind that you don't have to be sexual to enjoy the benefits of this hormone. Caressing touch, a 20-second hug, cuddling the new grandchild in your family, and playful interactions with your children or pets will help release it.

Beyond loving relationships, we also benefit from being connected to our community. When we share our positive energy with others, we feel bonded and supported in achieving our goals. That is why being involved with a religious group (church, synagogue, temple, or mosque) or being actively engaged in a charity we believe in can be so powerful. Besides, we reap rewards that we never expected when we give of our time and energy. We forge meaningful relationships, assist those in need, and create opportunities that never existed before, all of which can help us feel good about ourselves. Indeed, research has shown that an individual who lives a generous, altruistic life can discover deeper relationships, happiness, health, and even longevity.[1]

> ## When You Have High Levels of Stress in Your Life
>
> Spend time with loved ones and community projects you believe in. For the greatest benefit, generously share random acts of love and kindness with others without seeking anything in return.

Some of the most common barriers to developing loving and satisfying relationships are traumas from our past. Sometimes we are unaware of how a disturbing event that occurred during childhood or young adulthood can affect us decades later. A mental health therapist, psychologist, or psychiatrist can be incredibly insightful in showing us how these past events can create stress-filled personal relationships today, and how to heal from them. Many of us have forgotten the triggers that make us feel anxious or afraid, but working through these can enhance intimacy and soothe relationships.

## Step 2. The Benefits of Good Quality Sleep

I find it hard to imagine how any of us can function without a good night's sleep. People need a fresh start each day, but for many, a good night's sleep is fleeting. They may suffer from a combination of insufficient sleep and poor quality sleep.

Sleep deprivation results in poor brain performance, increased appetite, decreased calorie burning capacity (low basal metabolic rate), and weight gain. On the other hand, research with college students has shown that those who sleep 7 to 8 hours nightly have better memory retention than those sleeping less than 7 hours, even if the extra waking time is spent studying. Sleep helps store memory in the brain and renders those memories more functional. It also increases growth hormone production, helping the body to repair itself. With inadequate sleep, your brain will be sluggish. Shut down your mental computer, restart it the next morning, and it will run more efficiently.

## SUGGESTIONS TO OPTIMIZE SLEEP QUALITY

Below is a list of suggestions that can optimize the quality of your sleep, helping you sleep better.

- Our natural sleep patterns don't synch without regular sleep cycles. Having an irregular bedtime is like being jetlagged all the time. So aim to go to bed and rise on a schedule that deviates by no more than 1 hour daily (2 hours maximum), even on weekends.
- Use your bed for sleep, rest, and/or romance, but not for office work, video games, iPads, or watching TV. Reading or working a crossword puzzle for 15 to 30 minutes before sleep while lying in bed is okay.
- Since the dawn of modern human life, we evolved while living in dark caves. We don't sleep well with light! So when you turn out the lights to sleep, be sure to keep the bedroom dark and quiet. The darker the better. Wear earplugs and a sleep mask if necessary.
- Avoid sleeping in a warm room. Ideally, you want your body and extremities warm but the air cool. Some people do best with the thermostat set between 68°F and 72°F. If you use a fan, ensure that it's ultra-quiet. If you feel cold at this lower temperature, then wear socks to bed; warm extremities help you to fall asleep.
- Be sure you have a high-quality pillow, which you may want to replace annually. If you have neck problems, consider an orthopedic, shaped pillow. If you use a down pillow, check the label for a fill power of 650 to 775 $cm^3$/gram.

## Tips to Reduce Insomnia or Poor Sleep

If you have problems with insomnia and/or poor quality sleep, keep these tips in mind:

- Avoid bringing pets or children into your bed at night, as they can awaken you.
- Have no more than 1 to 2 servings of caffeine in the morning, and no caffeine after noon.
- Don't drink more than 2 servings of alcohol at night, and preferably none within 2 hours of going to bed, as a drop in alcohol levels when you are sleeping (often around 2 a.m.) causes a startle response, which will awaken you. Most people find it difficult to fall back into dreamland thereafter.
- Exercise for 30 to 60 minutes daily, but not within two hours of going to bed.
- Warm skim milk or herbal teas before bed raise body temperature and help you to fall asleep.
- Tryptophan-rich foods such as bananas, turkey, peanut butter, or nonfat milk will help you to fall asleep if eaten 30 minutes before bedtime. If you suffer from heartburn, keep the servings size to a minimum and avoid eating within 2 hours of bedtime.
- Don't nap after 4 p.m. If you take a nap daily, limit it to no more than 30 minutes.
- White and blue light tells your brain to wake up. Orange and red light tells your brain to make melatonin and to get ready to sleep. This all goes back to our former cave-dwelling habits. For 85,000 years, orange-red sunsets before dark told us it was bedtime and bright light told us it was dawn. The light from TVs, computers, and tablet screens stimulate the primitive parts of the brain, blocking hormone release that helps us fall asleep. So avoid white or blue light 2 hours before sleep. Change the computer, iPad,

or tablet screen to a red background, or wear orange-red tinted glasses for 2 hours before bedtime.

- Don't engage in work or stressful activities within 2 hours of bedtime.
- Try meditation before going to sleep. (See Step 4, page 181.) Consider buying a 20- to 30-minute CD to help get you started.
- Dim the lighting 30 minutes before going to sleep, to help ease you into a sleep pattern.

If you have trouble waking up in the morning, realize that you need some form of bright, full-spectrum light (such as sunlight or a full-spectrum bedroom light that activates with your alarm) first thing in the morning for 5 to 30 minutes to stimulate your morning wake cycle.

If you have tried falling asleep to no avail, don't watch the clock and fret. Get up, get out of bed, go to the living room, and look for something calming to do for 10 to 20 minutes. You can have cup of herbal tea, meditate, write in your journal, or pray. If you decide to read, be sure to select material that's soothing (even boring), not stimulating. Then return to bed. You could also consider a tryptophan-rich snack and warm beverage, as noted above.

If menopause issues disrupt your sleep, talk to your doctor about both natural as well as bioidentical hormonal options for better sleep. Extracts of Siberian rhubarb root can be very helpful for night sweats or hormonal sleep issues.

If none of these suggestions makes a difference, sleeping supplements/medications can help, but are best used on occasion rather than every night. Talk to your doctor about treatment options that might be appropriate for you. Keep in mind that over the long term, sleeping meds disrupt sleep cycles and are often habit-forming. It becomes more difficult to sleep without them.

### Step 3. Regular Exercise

I have covered the importance of exercise extensively in Chapter 5. In addition to helping your heart in every other way, daily exercise is also the most powerful therapy for burning away stress. Tension tends to pour out of us just like sweat during a vigorous workout. No drug is as effective as exercise in reducing stress in our lives. A good workout gives you a surge of compounds called endorphins, which promote pain relief and relaxation. Many people don't sleep well unless they are physically tired, not just mentally fatigued. A daily workout is absolutely required for optimal stress management.

### Step 4. Enjoy Peace and Calm

Many of my patients eat well and exercise, yet they don't schedule any time in their day for peace and calm.

If you don't have a daily relaxation routine—15 to 30 minutes of soul-calming activity—in place to manage the stress in your life, it probably won't happen on its own, as the demands of work and family life will encroach. The key is to be organized. Make sure to schedule some relaxation every day. Give yourself enough time to recharge your batteries. Gentle sounds, soft lighting, sweet fragrances, and massage bring sensory relief to different parts of the brain. If you don't create a relaxation routine for yourself, the grinding away of continuous stress will age you and hurt your heart. Below are some tips that will help you carve out some time for peace and calm.

#### BE FORMAL ABOUT IT! SCHEDULE SOME TIME

- Make an appointment for a massage once or twice a month, or better yet—how about once a week? Massages help release oxytocin.

- Sign up for a yoga class. If hot yoga or athletic yoga programs are too strenuous for you, opt for an "easy" or relaxation yoga class. Some are even given by candlelight in the evening.
- If these organized activities don't appeal to you, then at least tell the family you are going to take a hot bath by candlelight every night. That will give you 10 to 20 minutes for peace and calm each day. Of course, make sure to plan your relaxing bath after your kids have gone to bed.

## RECHARGE YOUR BATTERIES

Enjoying peace and calm also means recharging your batteries. Consider how your cellular phone goes dead once you've used up all of the stored energy. Well, you're not all that different. In today's world, with the constant stimulation of 24/7 phone calls, e-mails, texting, Tweets, Facebook, and more, we have the potential to deplete all of our energy reserves, if we don't take the time to recharge our batteries. Otherwise we stress ourselves mentally and physiologically with the consequential jump in cortisol and adrenaline levels and drop in DHEA (the adrenal hormone that gives us drive and energy)—leading to hormonal imbalance.

Vacations are a great opportunity to recharge your batteries. I believe everyone should aim for at least two to four weeks of fun and vacation time yearly to enhance productivity as well as quality of life. Leave your work phone and projects at home and have a blast!

But don't forget your weekends! The end of the week was designed for fun, plus some quiet. Plan to go for a bike ride, socialize with friends, plant flowers, have a picnic, watch the latest movie, enjoy a concert or ballgame—do whatever will bring you pleasure. Have some fun in the kitchen too! Weekends are a wonderful time to cook with friends and loved ones. Invite your friends over and prepare some of the delicious, heart-healthy recipes you'll find in Part III of this book, and have a great time. But don't forget to leave some time for peace and calm. Every major religion calls for a day of prayer, reflection, family time, and rest from work. Your challenge is to schedule the time for yourself. If you don't consciously make a point to create space for some fun, pleasure, peace, and calm, it is likely your to-do list will consume you.

## MEDITATION

Dr. Dean Ornish has made a tremendous contribution to the field of cardiology by emphasizing how proper stress management reduces cardiac risk. One of his recommendations is the practice of meditation, which provides an effective means to reduce stress. Meditation lowers blood pressure, decreases heart rate, relaxes muscles, lowers cortisol levels, and enhances sleep. It can be hard work, requiring mental focus and direction. In fact, you will find that it is different from "trying to relax." Learning how to meditate can be difficult once you are stressed out, so it's best to gain the needed skills before that happens. In some ways, it is like riding a bike, as it initially seems impossible, but once you get the hang of it, it's easy to resume at any time.

There are many forms of meditation, some easier and less time-consuming than others. Below are two options that can help you de-stress your heart.

1. *Simple breathing exercise:* The 1-minute meditation. Breathe in 5 seconds, breathe out 5 seconds. Repeat 6 times, and you create a peaceful mind, slowing your heart rate. You could perform this while in a hot bath, watching the sunset daily, or when your head first hits the pillow.

During *each* breath, recall a highly positive memory (holding a baby; a warm, safe, sandy beach), something specific that brings joy and love to your senses.

**2.** *Prolonged breathing-meditation exercise:* This 10- to 20-minute version drops your blood pressure by 10 points, lowers anxiety, reduces chronic pain, and leads to transformation. My suggestions are based, in part, on Herbert Benson's well-known concept of the relaxation response. Here's what to do:

- Shut off your phones. Close your door if you have to. Create a peaceful space where there will be no intrusions.
- Close your eyes.
- Find a comfortable sitting position. Let your shoulders drop, sit up straight, and become aware of your breathing as you inhale and exhale rhythmically.
- Beginning with your toes and working your way up your body, slowly relax each muscle group: toes, calves, thighs, buttocks, abdomen, back, chest, shoulders, neck, jaw, scalp. Try to keep your muscles in this relaxed state as you continue.
- The goal while meditating is to focus on your breathing and avoid thinking about your to-do list or other mental priorities. Usually you'll have fleeting thoughts—don't fight them or dwell on them. Rather, let them pass through you, and go back to focusing upon your breathing.
- As you take in a deep breath, use a *mantra*, similar to a repetitive prayer. The word mantra in its most literal sense means to free the mind. A mantra is a sacred word, chant, or sound that is repeated to promote relaxation and cultivate inner peace. It could be the repetition of a word like *Jesus, Sh'ma, Rama, Om, One, Let go—feel love,* or many others. Develop a mantra to use prior to potentially stressful situations. Repeat it several times when anxious, going to a meeting, when falling asleep, when angry (especially with insomnia).
- Continue for 10 to 20 minutes. You can open your eyes to check the clock.
- After the allotted time, don't rush to stand up. Just let yourself sit quietly. After a few minutes, you can open your eyes. And then gradually move about.

Repeating a mantra has many positive effects on your health. It:

- improves heart rate variability
- decreases sympathetic tone, which is associated with rapid heart rate and can sometimes be dangerous. Sympathetic tone is a measure of your sympathetic nervous system activity, the fight-or-flight response. If it is high all the time, it is hard on your health.
- synchronizes respiratory and heart rate cycles
- frees your mind from daily thoughts and worries

Learning to meditate is like acquiring any new skill. It takes time and patience. Most people spend a couple of weeks practicing daily before they get efficient at it. Many classes, DVDs, and videos are available to help you on your way.

If you can't face meditation, maybe a computer "game" will help you relax. HeartMath is a new kind of biofeedback program you install on your own computer or as an app on your smart phone and practice anywhere (see www.heartmath.org). The program promises to teach you to control your physiological stress response by breathing along with your heart rhythms as you concentrate on positive emotions. Hardware measures your pulse and translates it into computer graphics. As you practice the protocol, the graphics will change to reflect how your heart rate, mind, and emotions have become balanced and synchronized, leaving you in a much more peaceful and creative place. I have found this very useful for patients who feel like they are under the gun, yet can't bring themselves to meditate.

## Step 5. Don't Overuse Stimulants or Alcohol

### CAFFEINE

To manage your stress, you will have to put limits on stimulant use. When we're tired or burned out, many of us turn to a steaming cup of coffee for relief. While a wake-up cup may be helpful first thing in the morning, too much is sure to make you feel agitated. Not only that, excessive caffeine can lead to a racing heart, stiffening arteries, and higher blood pressure. In fact, rather than helping you, too much coffee will stress you all the more. How much is too much? It's best to limit yourself to no more than 2 cups a day, and clearly no more than 3.

What to do instead? As I mentioned in Chapter 4, to enhance your heart health, you'd benefit by drinking 3 or 4 cups of green tea daily. Iced or hot, it will calm you, and it also has many benefits for your heart. Indeed, green tea consumption is associated with a drop in heart attack and stroke rates. Even a cup of hot cocoa is a better choice than coffee, because of its heart-healthy effects: It decreases the risk of clotting and the oxidation of LDL into plaque, helps dilate your arteries, and lowers your blood pressure. Cocoa is rich in magnesium and fiber and is packed with anti-aging and stress-relieving compounds. Though green tea and cocoa have some caffeine, it occurs in much lower amounts than in coffee—especially the strong filtered coffee available at Starbucks and other gourmet coffee shops.

## TELEVISION AND OTHER MEDIA

If you're overly stressed, remember that the media can act as a stimulant too—especially at bedtime. Limiting media stimulation (including the 24/7 news and electronic communication) is critical. Probably one of the worst things you can do for yourself is watch the late news before going to bed. All of the world's problems are better handled in the morning, when you've had enough rest and your mind is ready to process the daily crises we confront. Besides, the media sells news that is controversial and frightening—remember their motto, "If it bleeds, it leads." It's not meant to provide peace and calm.

On the other hand, if you enjoy the late night talk shows

because the hosts and guests make you laugh, why not enjoy the humor and relax?

## ALCOHOL IS A DEPRESSANT

Excessive alcohol can be a worse stressor than excessive use of stimulants. Alcohol depresses your brain; in excess it can lead to a major depression. Drinking right before you go to bed typically causes you to wake up with a startle 2 to 3 hours later, making it hard to fall back to sleep. While a single serving of wine with dinner is of benefit to your heart, there is nothing healthy about having more than two drinks a day. Excessive alcohol intake disrupts loving communication with family, friends, and worsens job performance too.

Typically, when people are stressed, they reach for a drink to calm themselves. This has been programmed into us through decades of movies, TV viewing, and advertising. Yet alcohol does not help us deal with our stressors or their causes. It is more like a bandage covering a wound, dulling our awareness of problems that should be dealt with more actively. So when you are highly stressed, the last thing you want to do is pour yourself an extra drink.

## Step 6. Have Fun and Experience Joy

Having fun and experiencing joy sets off biochemical reactions in the brain akin to lighting sparklers on a dark night. Joy stimulates the brain to release powerful endorphins that promote relaxation, calm, pain relief, and happiness. Norman Cousins famously stated that laughter is the best medicine. There's nothing like watching a few episodes of a favorite sitcom to get your endorphins going. Playing with your children, nephews and nieces, grandchildren, or pets can also bring a smile to your face and a lift to your spirits. Sharing love creates joy and contributes to your physical well-being.

Having a sense of purpose in your community also creates joy. Those who participate in community-related activities, people who practice altruism, enjoy better health than people who are isolated. We all need some volunteer involvement to keep us in touch, to be of service, and to benefit ourselves internally in the process. To increase joy and love in our lives, practice random acts of love and kindness.

When it comes to experiencing joy, don't forget the importance of attitude. Whether or not we seize the opportunity, the truth is that even if we can't control the situation we're in, we do have control over how we deal with it. We can be optimistic or pessimistic. We can beam or scowl. We also have choices about our companions. When we are depressed and/or stressed, it's helpful to look for happy people who bring cheer, and to limit time with those who are irritable or glum. When we're overstressed, violence in the news or in our entertainment choices will only exacerbate tension and distress. Rather, turn to lighter, comfort fare: comedies, classic movies that soothe and amuse us—even though we already know the outcome. There's nothing wrong with enjoying animated films and the newspaper comics.

## JACKIE'S PLAN

At this point, you should be able to guess my 30-Day Heart Tune-Up treatment plan for Jackie, the woman I discussed earlier. First of all, she needed to feel loved and supported. Her husband, Mark, agreed to take over the shopping, cooking, and cleaning for one month, with the proviso that they would split those activities in the future. When he made this offer Jackie breathed an enormous sigh and started crying again—not quite tears of joy, but obviously tears of relief.

Holding Mark's hand, she agreed to get at least 7 to 8 hours of sleep every night, with an extra hour on weekends. Instead of going to bed at 11:00 p.m. every night, she changed that to 10:00, so she would arise earlier and have 40 minutes for working out moderately at home in the mornings. Since her adrenal function indicated that she was physically stressed, I cautioned her to keep her exercise moderate, stay in her low aerobic workout zone, and avoid interval training for at least the first three months.

She balked when we discussed scheduling 20 minutes of peace and calm every day. "I don't have that kind of time to waste," she told me. I had to emphasize that this was not wasted time. Instead, I reiterated that peace and calm were medical treatments and critical for her heart, her adrenal function, and her mental state. After reviewing some options, Mark volunteered to buy a meditation DVD they could follow together for 20 to 25 minutes daily. They agreed to practice this when they both came home from work, before he started making dinner.

With the extra sleep, Jackie thought she could limit her coffee to 2 cups every morning. I encouraged her to have 1 to 2 cups of green tea each afternoon. We also drew the line at one bottle of wine split between the two of them on the weekends. Mark was at least 70 pounds heavier than Jackie, so a better split was 2 glasses for her and 3 for him, and not more.

They didn't go out much, so we talked about planning something fun each weekend. They agreed to schedule a weekly Saturday night dinner date with a movie or other activity they both enjoyed. I also wrote out a prescription for a massage each week and passed it to Mark. We then talked about their romantic life, or lack thereof. They were both interested, but they had drifted apart physically. I did prescribe an adrenal hormone (DHEA) supplement for Jackie, as low DHEA levels reduce sex drive and libido, especially in women. Jackie also shared that she had experienced vaginal dryness since she'd hit menopause (definitely a disincentive), so I recommended a vaginal delivery form of DHEA that would be well absorbed. It has been well-studied in the scientific literature and would restore normal vaginal function and lubrication. I encouraged Jackie and Mark to enjoy sex 2 to 3 times a week, noting that sex has many health benefits. Jackie's normal stress test reassured me that sex was safe for her to enjoy.

To finish, we discussed starting a series of medications if the symptoms were to persist or worsen. But guess what! Jackie never needed them. She and Mark took my stress management recommendations to heart. She never had another episode of angina. Their relationship blossomed, and so did their lives.

*Chapter Seven*

# Tune Up Your Heart with Revitalizing Foods and Supplements

Everyone needs a personalized plan to meet their key nutrient needs, because no one eats well all the time. Just bear in mind that the vitamins, minerals, herbals, and other valuable treatments that I'll discuss in this chapter can only enhance a healthy eating plan and an optimal lifestyle. They can't replace it. They will never make up for snacking on junk food or being stressed or inactive. Nevertheless, supplements can benefit your heart health substantially even if you eat well, exercise regularly, and manage stress. They can also provide some nutrients that you may otherwise be lacking. At least 80% of Americans are nutrient deficient. Yes, we get plenty of calories, but we don't consume enough vitamins and minerals. Nutrient content has been dropping in our highly processed food supply. That's why nutritional supplements are an integral part of your 30-Day Heart Tune-Up. And, as you'll see, they may boost your heart health in ways that food alone cannot. In this chapter, I aim to answer many of the questions you may have about this vital issue.

## MULTIVITAMINS

Taking a multivitamin is a familiar and convenient way to meet many nutrient needs. If these supplements are properly formulated, they can provide your vitamin D, B, and K and trace minerals nicely. In fact, a recent study showed that even taking a poor-quality multivitamin daily decreases cancer risk.[1] However, while taking a multivitamin is important, I believe people should take one that is *customized* to their unique medical needs. As always, review your supplement program with your doctor.

Keep in mind that a multivitamin won't supply fiber, fish oil, magnesium, and potassium in a significant way. These are critical heart nutrients. You can get each of these from following the 30-Day Heart Tune-Up eating plan, or by taking supplements if needed. Moreover, most multivitamins purchased at the grocery store or pharmacy contain vitamin D, vitamin B12, and vitamin K, but *not* in adequate amounts, and these too are essential heart nutrients.

What should a high-quality multivitamin contain? To begin with, 1,500 to 2,000 IU (international units) of vitamin D. (You can also get your vitamin D separately. It is often combined with calcium and fish oil supplements, so it's important to read labels to determine exactly how much you're taking. You don't want to overdo the vitamin D.) If the pill has vitamin E, it should contain 40 to 100 mg of mixed tocopherols—not just alpha tocopherol— and should contain more delta and gamma than alpha. I'll explain why below. You'll also want a pill that has mixed carotenoids, not just beta carotene, as well as mixed forms of folate, especially 5-MTHF (5-methyltetrahydrofolate), not just folic acid. If you're over 50, you'll need adequate vitamin B12—at least 100 mcg (micrograms) daily, but if you take an acid blocker, a minimum of 500 mcg is recommended. Vitamin K should come as a mixture of vitamin K1 and K2, as I'll discuss; you should be taking 250 to 500 mcg altogether. And finally, you should take 75 to 150 mcg of iodine.

Be sure the minerals in your pill are protein-bound. These are very well absorbed and don't cause gastrointestinal distress. Ideally most minerals, such as zinc, selenium, manganese, and magnesium, would come in protein-bound form. Examples of protein-bound magnesium include magnesium malate, glycinate, or Albion brand chelated magnesium. Iron should be included for menstruating women and growing children, but not for women after menopause or for men.

Companies producing supplements have asked me to design a multivitamin for my patients. The table below reflects my recommendations. This ingredient list assumes that people follow at least 75% of my eating plan. *Premenopausal women are asked to take an iron pill (ferrous bisglycinate-chelate, such as Ferrochel) on the days they menstruate.*

| Recommended Multivitamin Ingredients | | |
|---|---|---|
| Compound | Form | Daily Dosage |
| Vitamin A | Palmitate | 2,000 IU |
| Mixed carotenoids | | 3,000 IU |
| Vitamin D3 | | 2,000 IU |
| Mixed tocopherols | | 50 mg |
| | More as gamma and delta tocopherol | 30 mg |
| | Less as d-alpha tocopherol | 20 mg |
| Vitamin K | Total vitamin K | 500 mcg |
| | Vitamin K1 | 300 mcg |
| | Vitamin K2 | 200 mcg |
| Vitamin C | Ascorbic acid | 250 mg |
| Thiamin (B1) | Thiamin HCl | 50 mg |
| Riboflavin (B2) | Riboflavin 5-phosphate | 12 mg |
| Niacin | Niacinamide | 80 mg |
| Pyridoxine (B6) | Pyridoxal -5-phosphate | 20 mg |
| Folate | More than 50% as 5-MTHF | 400 mcg |

*continues*

| Recommended Multivitamin Ingredients (continued) | | |
|---|---|---|
| Compound | Form | Daily Dosage |
| Vitamin B12 | Methylcobalamin | 500 mcg |
| Biotin (B7) | | 500 mcg |
| Vitamin B5 | Calcium pantothenate | 45 mg |
| Boron | Bororganic glycine | 2 mg |
| Copper | Copper glycinate chelate | 500 mcg |
| Chromium | Nicotinate glycinate chelate | 400 mcg |
| Iodine | Potassium iodide | 100 mcg |
| Magnesium | Magnesium glycinate chelate | 20 mg |
| Manganese | Manganese glycinate chelate | 3 mg |
| Molybdenum | Molybdenum glycinate chelate | 100 mcg |
| Selenium | Selenomethionine | 150 mcg |
| Zinc | Zinc glycinate chelate | 15 mg |

Multivitamins seem to cover a lot of nutritional ground. So why take additional supplements? The fact remains that even the best products don't supply everything your body needs in the dosages that are essential to your health. In particular, molecules like magnesium and calcium are very bulky (especially when combined with salt or protein), and the dosages required for daily health won't fit even in a 2-a-day multivitamin. Besides, medications; your diet; activities; and health conditions such as diabetes, high blood pressure, bone density loss, and memory loss all impact which nutrients you should include. That's why you'll want to personalize the supplements you take.

Also bear in mind that an excess of certain nutrients can create potential heart health problems. For instance, despite the fact that iron deficiency is widespread, too much is even worse for you from a cardiac perspective, as it inflames your tissues and ages your heart and arteries. Therefore, it's important to know what to take in what amounts. In this case, the bottom line is: Men and menopausal women should not take an iron supplement (unless they have anemia from iron deficiency).

Calcium is another mineral that can be bad for your heart when taken in excess. Most people should get 800 to 1,000 mg of calcium daily. If you have lost excessive bone mass and have osteopenia or osteoporosis, 1,200 to 1,500 mg are recommended daily. Yet this should come from a combination of diet and supplements. Far too often a doctor might say you need 1,200 mg of calcium and ask you to take 600 mg twice daily. But if your diet also includes 900 mg of calcium, your total intake will now be 2,100 mg—far too much. Excessive calcium is associated with a greater risk of both cancer and heart problems, so clearly the goal is to take the correct amount. For details on how to calculate your calcium needs, dietary intake, and supplement recommendations, please see Appendix III, "Calcium Requirements," page 356.

You can't depend on supplements chosen from advertising, press releases, or personal recommendations from your friends to be right for you. All too often, you read in the paper that supplement "A" is terrific, so you are convinced to take it; then a friend mentions that supplement "B" is wonderful, so you take that too. Soon you're swallowing 15 to 20 pills a day, but without any real guidance. In fact, some supplements can be dangerous when combined inappropriately with others or with certain medications; therefore your first step is to get the right information.

## Safety First! Choose High-Quality Products

Compared to the regulations governing prescription and over-the-counter drugs (such as Advil and Tylenol), those controlling the production of supplements are much more lax. This can lead to tremendous variations in quality.

In general, even though you might assume the mass market, national brand vitamins and supplements you buy in the pharmacy, grocery, discount, or health food store are safe, they may not be, unless they meet the quality rating standards I explain below. Some can be produced in outdoor "labs" in China or India. These pills might contain fillers and contaminants but few active or safe ingredients. Even if the product is manufactured in the United States, there is no guarantee of purity. Although the bottle may say that each tablet contains 500 mg of active ingredients, the true content can vary from 100 mg to 1,000 mg. No government agency is monitoring exactly what is in each pill. I know of vitamin distributors that sold supplements that swelled and leaked from their capsules into something resembling pink marshmallows. Disgusting! They were willing to continue unloading potentially harmful pills on an unsuspecting public, because they wanted to make more money and collect on every last item in their inventory. The bottom line: Quality varies immensely.

Fortunately, some companies produce excellent products in pristine, pharmaceutical-grade laboratories. They manufacture pills that contain the exact dosages stated with no contaminants. Still, it can be hard to tell the difference between these superior products and those that are below standard, because the bottles may look similar. So how are you to know which pills to buy with confidence?

To find the very best products, seek those that have been audited and approved to produce drugs in the United States, in FDA-approved facilities listed as following "drug good manufacturing practices, (drug-GMPs)," or those that are approved by Australia's pharmaceutical regulatory agency, the Therapeutic Goods Administration (TGA), considered the toughest regulatory agency in the world. TGA inspection and certification is similar to the criteria the U.S. Food and Drug Administration (FDA) requires for drug production.

As of this writing, brands such as Thorne and Metagenics meet TGA standards. Integrative Therapeutics has been audited as a drug-GMP facility. Other good-quality supplement producers on the market include: Designs for Health, Pure Encapsulations, Douglas Labs, ProThera, and Xymogen. However, they will only remain the best brands to buy if they continue to earn their high ratings. If you can't find out which companies meet these standards, one way to check their general production quality is to compare their contents with the "Recommended Multivitamin Ingredients" list on pages 193 and 194. If the ingredients and dosages are close, then the product is promising.

When shopping for supplements, realize you're unlikely to purchase these brands at your usual retailers. Look for them from licensed medical providers or on the Internet. Medical providers such as chiropractors, nutritionists, and some physicians offer them for sale. When you buy these supplements, make sure the rating is on the label. Try to confirm that your pills meet or exceed the FDA's requirements for drug production. If not, perhaps you should be seeking out a different product. Also, good brand supplements may be sold online at a discount but they have exceeded their expiration date, so if you see what looks like a deal that is "too good to be true," be cautious.

If you're buying supplements, be sure they're safe. They must meet your specific needs, and they should be state-of-the-art in their formulation. Of course, the cheapest, mass-produced supplements often are not the best, but the most expensive ones may not be the best either. What you want is a supplement that provides superior ingredients, reliability, and value. Ideally, you should have a physician or medical expert guide you through these decisions.

## KEY NUTRIENTS FOR HEART HEALTH AND THEIR SOURCES

The discussion above refers to all supplements in a general way. So now let's turn to those key nutrients that you may need for the sake of your heart and cardiovascular system. My aim will be to meet your personalized requirements with food whenever feasible, and give you a good supplement alternative if the food options are not realistic for you. The clinically important deficiencies that have an impact on your heart are fiber, fish oil, magnesium, vitamin D, vitamin K, and potassium. Let's look at these individually.

## Fiber

### FOOD SOURCES OF FIBER

As I explained in Chapter 4, most people in the United States don't meet their requirements for fiber. Yet this is perhaps the single most important deficiency, and it can be easily corrected. I recommend 30 to 50 grams of fiber daily (with at least 15 grams from fruit and vegetables and 10 to 15 grams from beans). As examples, a medium apple has 3.3 grams of fiber, a cup of broccoli has 2.3 grams, a cup of cooked black beans has 15 grams, and a cup of cooked brown rice has 3.5 grams. You don't get any fiber from eating animal protein. Unfortunately, most Americans only manage to get 10 to 15 grams altogether.

Fiber is important for your intestinal function, but it also lowers bad cholesterol, cuts blood sugar levels, decreases inflammation, and provides nutrients that allow your arteries to dilate and function beautifully. And the more colorful your fiber choice, the better, because those plant pigments are fantastic for both heart and brain health.

In Chapter 4 and in Appendix IV, "Fiber Content of Common Foods," page 360, I've listed excellent fiber sources, and on page 199 you'll find a quick table that will help you boost your fiber to 40 grams daily with supplements.

### FIBER SUPPLEMENTS

If you don't consume all of your recommended fiber from food, you'll be glad to know that several good supplements exist. You need both soluble and insoluble fiber. The latter is good for your intestinal function, while the former drops blood sugar, decreases bad cholesterol, and lowers inflammation. I recommend supplements that are

60% to 75% soluble fiber. In the "Fiber Supplements" table, you'll find several easy-to-use products and suggested daily amounts. Just keep in mind that, when mixed with water, the supplement will absorb the liquid and swell. This same action is very healthy when it occurs in your intestinal tract, since it makes you feel full and satisfied. But swelling fiber has a slimy (Jell-O-like) texture, which offers an unpleasant sensation in the mouth. So if you mix fiber powder with fluid, drink it immediately; don't put it aside for later.

| Fiber Supplements | | |
|---|---|---|
| *Fiber Source and Daily Amount* | *Fiber Content (Grams)* | *Special Benefits, Comments* |
| Ground flaxseed (1 Tbsp) | 2 | Contains cancer-fighting compounds too. |
| Chia seeds (1 Tbsp) | 2.6 | |
| Metamucil (1 Tbsp) | 3 | |
| Psyllium (1 Tbsp) | 3 | |
| PGX (2 softgels), many brands carry PolyGlycopleX in supplement form | 1.5 | Excellent to control sugar and cholesterol levels |
| Medibulk (1 scoop, 11 grams) | 8 | |
| UltraMeal Plus 360 shake (2 scoops, 50 grams) | 4 | Improves cholesterol, blood pressure, and blood sugar levels as well |
| FiberMend (1 scoop) | 9 | 8 grams soluble fiber, 1 gram insoluble |
| Sunsweet Supra Fiber (2 Tbsp, 10 grams) | 5 | 3 grams soluble fiber |

## Long-Chain Omega-3 Oils (Fish Oils)

### FOOD SOURCES OF OMEGA-3 OILS

Long-chain omega-3 fatty acids are good for your health, and especially for your heart. The easiest way to get these special healthy fats is by eating cold-water seafood. Eating these sources of omega-3 fats decreases your risk for heart attacks, strokes, blood clots, sudden death, arterial plaque formation, and inflammation.[2] In addition, omega-3 fats improve brain function and are involved in hundreds of anti-aging reactions. The best sources are wild salmon, sardines, herring, sole, trout, mussels, and oysters.

However, beware of products sold as "good sources of omega-3s" that come from plants such as flax, soy, and canola. These are healthy plant foods, but they have medium-chain omega-3 fats that do not have the same beneficial properties as the long-chain omegas that come from seafood. See the "Best Seafood Choices for Omega-3 Fats" and "Good Seafood Choices" tables, below and on page 201, for detailed listings.

## Best Seafood Choices for Omega-3 Fats

The following seafoods are high in omega-3s, fairly low in saturated fat, and low in mercury. Enjoy 3 to 5 servings a week. All are based on a 3.5-ounce serving, unless noted.

|  | Omega-3s (grams) |
| --- | --- |
| Herring, Atlantic | 2.1 |
| Mussels | 0.7 |
| Oysters | 0.6 |
| Salmon, Atlantic, wild | 2.2 |
| Salmon, coho, Pacific, wild | 2.4 |
| Sardines (water-packed) | 1.9 |
| Sole/Flounder | 0.5 |
| Trout, rainbow, wild | 1.2 |
| Trout, rainbow, farmed | 1.2 |
| Whitefish | 1.8 |

## Good Seafood Choices

The following seafoods are low in mercury, but also low in omega-3 fats. They aren't as healthy as salmon or sole, but better protein sources than chicken or turkey breast choices. Enjoy 2 to 3 servings a week. All are based on a 3.5-ounce serving, unless noted.

|  | Omega-3s (grams) |
| --- | --- |
| Calamari (squid) | 0.3 |
| Catfish, channel, farmed | 0.2 |
| Clams | 0.3 |
| Cod, Atlantic | 0.3 |
| Crabs, Dungeness | 0.4 |
| Halibut | 0.5 |
| Lobster, spiny (or shrimp) | 0.5 |
| Mahi mahi (dolphinfish) | 0.1 |
| Pollock | 0.5 |
| Scallops (6 ounces, raw) | 0.3 |
| Tilapia | 0.1 |

If you try to get your omega-3s from seafood, don't forget that big-mouth fish (tuna, grouper, snapper, bass, and swordfish) are high in mercury. Excess mercury is clearly bad for your brain, so unless you have checked your whole blood mercury level to confirm that you don't suffer from mercury toxicity, I recommend you eat big-mouth fish no more than 2 or 3 times a month. Avoid fish with high levels of mercury if you are pregnant. Nearly one third of my patients do have high mercury levels. The irony is that they ate more fish to be "healthier," but they chose the wrong types and inadvertently decreased their brain speed and performance as a result.

Also a cautionary word about farm-raised salmon. Although

I have emphasized the importance of eating salmon, farm-raised fish can contain high levels of mercury, as well as other harmful compounds, including PCBs. It depends upon what the fish farmers use for feed. If the fishery is located in pristine water, and the salmon are fed herring and shrimp, this farm-raised product will be excellent. But if the salmon are fed ground-up by-catch from shrimping, their flesh could have high levels of mercury and other chemicals. Yes, this is maddening to think about. So the best solution is to buy only "wild caught" fish, unless you know how the farm-raised fish were produced. See the table "Limit Your Intake of These High-Mercury-Content Seafoods," below, for details.

## Limit Your Intake of These High-Mercury-Content Seafoods

The following are moderately high in mercury (more than 0.2 parts per million), so limit your intake to no more than 2 to 3 servings monthly. Avoid altogether if you are pregnant. In general, large-mouth fish are higher in mercury levels than small-mouth fish. All are based on a 3.5-ounce serving, unless noted.

|  | Mercury (parts per million) |
|---|---|
| Chilean sea bass | 0.35 |
| Bluefish | 0.37 |
| Grouper | 0.45 |
| Lobster, Maine | 0.15 |
| Tuna, albacore* | 0.35 |
| Tuna, bluefin (ahi)* | 0.7 |
| Tuna, yellowfin* | 0.3 |

*In contrast to albacore and yellowfin tuna, skipjack or light tuna is lower in mercury than the other kinds of tuna (0.1 to 0.15 parts per million). Bluefin tuna is the highest in mercury.

Adapted from the FDA's U.S. Food and Drug data base, 1990–2010.

| Stay Away from These Very-High-Mercury Fish |
| --- |
| The following are very high in mercury (greater than 0.5 parts per million). You should avoid these fish as much as possible. |
| King mackerel<br>Marlin<br>Shark<br>Swordfish<br>Tilefish |

## DOES FISH OIL CAUSE PROSTATE CANCER?

Many of my patients have asked about the relationship between prostate cancer and fish oil, so let me make sense of the headlines for you. A scientific paper was published July 2013 in the *Journal of the National Cancer Institute* that induced widespread concern for people taking fish oil supplements, despite the fact that this study wasn't even about supplements.

There are serious problems with this type of study if you hope to draw any conclusions:

- First, the researchers could not distinguish between eating fish and taking a fish oil supplement.
- Second, the study could not tell the difference between eating wild fish and fish raised in polluted waters that might be packed with carcinogens.
- Further, cheap fish oil that is commonly sold in the United States is loaded with rancid fats (lipid peroxides) and these bad fats are believed to cause cancer.

For years, I have believed that taking a cheap fish oil supplement puts people at risk for cancer. This study certainly could not distinguish between good fish oil intake and bad fish oil intake. Consider that close to 90% of fish oil produced in the United States is illegal in Europe because the quality is so bad. Three or four other studies have shown similar findings between EPA and DHA blood levels and prostate cancer. Yet, importantly, one of these studies was able to distinguish between fish oil intake and fish intake. One study[3] compared fish intake and fish oil intake separately with prostate cancer risk in 2,268 men in Iceland. In this study, high-quality fish oil was shown to decrease the risk for prostate cancer (this was a European study that had quality standards for fish oil). Eating salted and smoked fish was shown to increase prostate cancer risk.

In light of these studies, even though the benefits likely outweigh the risks, there is the chance that fish oil intake may increase prostate cancer risk slightly. To minimize this potential risk, follow these steps:

- Avoid eating farm-raised fish unless you know its source and feed.
- If you take fish oil, pay a little extra for high-quality fish oil, or skip it. Don't risk taking cheap, rancid fish oil.

Bad fish oil by the spoonful tastes rancid and gives you a yucky belch, so people won't buy it from a bottle more than once. It is much harder to determine the quality of fish oil that comes in a capsule. But it can be done! Just poke a needle into one capsule and gently squeeze out a drop of the oil. Smell it, and if it smells acceptable, then taste one drop of the oil that surfaces. If it tastes rancid, then the oil is bad, and you should return it. Of all the supplements available, fish oil is perhaps the most important when it comes to high quality. That's because quality varies greatly, and rancid fish oil is likely harmful. Some brands will add lemon or orange flavoring, which is fine—you can't hide the foul taste with a little lemon flavor.

Once you have found a fresh product, make sure it also has the right ingredients. For general and heart health, you should aim for 1,000 to 1,200 mg per day of the omega-3 fats that come specifically from a combination of EPA and DHA. Some supplements can achieve this dosage of EPA and DHA with 1 or 2 capsules, while for others 4 to 6 are required. In natural, high-quality fish oil, expect to see about 500 mg of EPA and 400 mg of DHA listed on the label, with 1,200 mg of total omega-3 content. Avoid brands that don't list EPA or DHA content. Since they may be inferior products, buy something else.

Also keep in mind that most excellent fish oils with appropriate EPA and DHA may cost $15 to $25 a month. If this is beyond your price range, then the least expensive way to get your recommended fish oil is to eat a 3-ounce can of wild salmon or sardines, 4 to 5 days a week. Not only do you get your EPA and DHA, but you get protein and a meal out of it too!

If you are trying to lower high triglyceride levels or are battling excessive inflammation, then large dosages of long-chain omega-3s are recommended: 2,000 to 4,000 mg of EPA and DHA daily. EPA has more power than DHA to lower inflammation and triglyceride levels; DHA may provide more benefit for your brain and eyes. So if you need a higher anti-inflammatory or triglyceride-lowering supplement, you will get more benefit from oil that has extra EPA.

You'll also find krill oil on the supplement shelf, but even though it's sold as a "fish oil," it usually doesn't have much EPA or DHA. An advantage of this supplement is that it contains astaxanthin, a red pigment found in algae that provides the same kinds of benefits as blueberries and other brightly colored plant foods. This pigment gives salmon and shrimp their pink or red color. But to get 1,000 mg of EPA and DHA daily, you'd need to swallow 6 to 8 capsules. The price becomes exorbitant. That might make this a poor choice if you're looking to quickly increase your long-chain omega-3s with only 1 to 2 pills per day.

## Omega-3 Supplements

Most Americans do not meet the minimal requirements for long-chain omega-3s for optimal health, largely because they dislike oily, cold-water fish. If you fall into this category, then a fish oil supplement makes excellent sense. In my publication "Emerging Lifestyle Factors That Predict Carotid IMT Scores,"[4] we found that the "best" and "good" seafood options (noted on pages 200 and 201) were much better for your heart than fish with high mercury content. Sadly, buying a good-quality supplement with an adequate dosage of the essential long-chain fats is far more complicated than it should be because:

- Most fish oil sold in the United States is of poor quality.
- Most fish oil doesn't have adequate EPA and DHA, the most important ingredients.

In Europe, fish oil supplements must meet specific quality standards or they cannot be sold. We don't have these regulations in the United States. Here marketers are free to sell junk if people will buy it. In the old days, fish oil could be contaminated with mercury or other heavy metals, but fortunately this is seldom the case now.

---

### Caution! What to Look for When Buying Fish Oil

- **Is it rancid?** If so, it will be harmful, because it will be filled with free radicals. These damaging molecules can cause cancer and accelerate aging. See text for details.
- **Does it have the right amounts of the active agent?** Be careful, as many companies sell omega-3 fats that don't have adequate EPA and DHA.

---

The biggest issue is simple these days: Is the fish oil fresh or is it rancid? Fish oil is delicate and needs to be fresh and processed carefully. Stale oil tastes bad (sometimes horrible) and is loaded with free radicals that accelerate aging. The sad truth is that some people likely do themselves harm by taking rotten fish oil. Clearly this creates controversy, as clinical studies that don't control for these damaged fats will not detect differences in products. This, in turn, skews outcomes. Only the best brands sell the same fish oil in capsules as in liquids swallowed by the spoonful. As of this writing, I recommend Thorne, Nordic Naturals, Metagenics, and Designs for Health.

## Magnesium

Magnesium is an essential mineral for health; it is required for hundreds of anti-aging reactions. Unfortunately, at least half of the people in the United States do not meet their minimal recommended magnesium intake and consequently suffer from the following symptoms:

* constipation
* elevated blood pressure
* elevated blood sugar levels
* muscle cramps
* wheezing (asthma)
* heart arrhythmias (which occasionally include sudden cardiac death)[5]

Adequate magnesium intake has also been shown to lower your risk for a stroke.[6] Most doctors don't measure magnesium levels unless their patients are in the hospital, as it requires a special test (red blood cell magnesium level or RBC Mg). Each year, I see several patients in my office with symptoms related to a magnesium deficiency. Cindy was one such patient. She came for her first visit, complaining of daily palpitations. She was a full-time homemaker with a husband and three teenage children—twin 15-year-old boys and a 13-year-old girl. At age 43, she was very pretty, slender, but not fit. She felt like a full-time chauffeur, driving her children to and from school and sporting events seven days a week. They had only one weekly family meal, on Sundays. The other evenings, the family relied mostly on fast food.

Cindy drank a pot of coffee in the morning to get going, and munched on a white flour bagel with cream cheese for breakfast while driving the kids to school. Lunch was something simple, like canned chicken noodle soup. She ran errands, cleaned the house, shopped, paid bills, and did other chores until she picked up the kids from school. Her husband had a great new job, but he was working 50 to 60 hours a week and he didn't help much at home.

Cindy didn't seem worried by her palpitations, even though sometimes they would continue in fast runs for 10 to 15 minutes. They didn't give her chest pain, nausea, or shortness of breath. After looking up the symptoms of a heart attack online, she didn't think it was an issue, and figured it was probably due to the coffee—which she didn't want to give up.

During her assessment, Cindy's history was noteworthy for bad constipation and frequent muscle cramps. Her physical exam was normal, but her food diary revealed that she was grossly deficient for nearly every nutrient. She certainly frightened me during the stress treadmill test I use to check for an abnormal heart rhythm. Her heart rate took off at 180 beats per minute, accompanied with a worrisome electrocardiogram pattern, even though she was only walking briskly. When we halted the stress test, it took 20 minutes for her heart to come back to normal.

Fortunately, Cindy's laboratory studies clarified why she had this dangerous heart rhythm problem; they were not just mere palpitations. Cindy's magnesium levels were excessively low. This can lead to a rare but fatal heart condition—basically sudden death. The combination of poor nutrition and large quantities of coffee had depleted her of magnesium, and her heart couldn't function properly without it. When magnesium supplements and other foods were prescribed to restore most of her key deficiencies, Cindy's palpitation problems were solved.

## Food Sources of Magnesium

Foods rich in magnesium include nuts and seeds, beans, whole grains, and leafy green vegetables—many of which are an integral part of the 30-Day Heart Tune-Up eating plan. Most people should consume at least 400 mg of magnesium daily. From the "Magnesium in Foods" chart below, determine how much you are getting daily. The foods selected have more than 50 mg of magnesium per serving.

| Magnesium in Foods | |
|---|---|
| Food and Portion Size | Magnesium (mg) |
| Pumpkin and squash seed kernels, roasted, 1 oz | 151 |
| Brazil nuts, 1 oz (1 handful) | 107 |
| Oat or wheat bran ready-to-eat cereal (100%), 1 oz | 103 |
| Halibut, cooked, 3 oz | 91 |
| Quinoa, dry, ¼ cup | 89 |
| Spinach, frozen, ½ cup | 81 |
| Almonds, 1 oz | 78 |
| Spinach, cooked from fresh, ½ cup | 78 |
| Swiss chard, 1 cup | 76 |
| Buckwheat flour, ¼ cup | 75 |
| Cashews, dry roasted, 1 oz | 74 |
| Soybeans, mature, cooked, ½ cup | 74 |
| Pine nuts, dried, 1 oz | 71 |
| Mixed nuts, oil roasted, with peanuts, 1 oz | 67 |
| White beans, canned, ½ cup | 67 |
| Pollock, walleye, cooked, 3 oz | 62 |
| Black beans, cooked, ½ cup | 60 |

*continues*

| Magnesium in Foods *(continued)* | |
|---|---|
| *Food and Portion Size* | *Magnesium (mg)* |
| Bulgur, dry, ¼ cup | 57 |
| Oat bran, raw, ¼ cup | 55 |
| Artichoke hearts, cooked, ½ cup | 50 |
| Peanuts, dry roasted, 1 oz | 50 |
| Lima beans, baby, cooked from frozen, ½ cup | 50 |

## MAGNESIUM SUPPLEMENTS

If you don't obtain enough magnesium from food, then you need to take a supplement. The combined dosage from food and your supplement should reach at least 400 mg daily. I recommend the same brands for magnesium that I do for multivitamins.

## Avoid Gastrointestinal Distress

Let's face it, magnesium is the primary ingredient in Milk of Magnesia—so it has the potential to act as a strong laxative if taken in the wrong form. The best absorption is achieved with magnesium bound to protein. Look for:

- Albion's magnesium chelates
- Magnesium malate
- Magnesium glycinate

More common than protein-bound magnesium are magnesium salts (magnesium oxide, magnesium citrate). Avoid magnesium oxide. It is cheap but it acts as an intestinal irritant. I have met hundreds of people who have had gastrointestinal cramping related to it. In the past, it was used as a bowel prep before surgical procedures!

Magnesium citrate does not cause intestinal irritation, and some people use it to relieve constipation. However, it isn't as well absorbed as protein-bound magnesium, so you would need to consume about 600 mg (2 to 3 pills) to achieve the same blood level.

## Caution! Calcium Blocks Magnesium Absorption

Consider a typical heart disease patient who is low in magnesium. She adds a calcium supplement at her doctor's request to combat osteoporosis. The extra calcium will lower her magnesium levels further, worsen blood sugar levels and blood pressure control, and cause constipation to boot. It might even induce dangerous cardiac arrhythmias that can cause sudden death—so clearly she should take calcium and magnesium together. No study has absolutely confirmed the optimal dosage of magnesium when taken with calcium, but most experts recommend using a 2:1 or 3:1 calcium to magnesium ratio. In other words, if I recommend 800 mg of calcium supplement daily, I will also recommend 300 to 400 mg of magnesium to go with it.

## Vitamin D

Vitamin D is called a fat-soluble vitamin, but once converted to its active form, it functions like a hormone. Every cell in the body appears to have vitamin D receptors, so having adequate amounts in your bloodstream is absolutely critical to your health. Studies now show that people with higher blood levels of vitamin D have lower rates of heart attacks and strokes and better blood pressure and weight control. Clearly vitamin D is essential for optimal heart and general health. As a hormone, vitamin D communicates directly with your genes, influencing how they function, and tells the cells which proteins to produce.

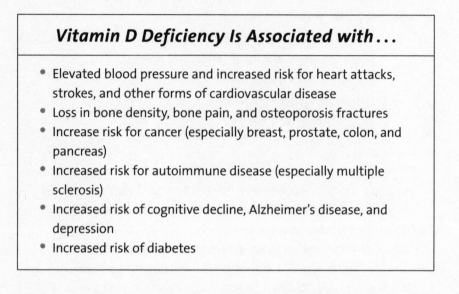

## *Vitamin D Deficiency Is Associated with...*

- Elevated blood pressure and increased risk for heart attacks, strokes, and other forms of cardiovascular disease
- Loss in bone density, bone pain, and osteoporosis fractures
- Increase risk for cancer (especially breast, prostate, colon, and pancreas)
- Increased risk for autoimmune disease (especially multiple sclerosis)
- Increased risk of cognitive decline, Alzheimer's disease, and depression
- Increased risk of diabetes

Most Americans today are in danger of developing these major conditions, because of their low vitamin D levels.

How much vitamin D do you need? That would depend on your current blood levels, as I'll discuss below. However, for most people, optimal dosages vary from 1,500 to 3,000 IU daily, with the goal to achieve a blood level of 40 to 70 ng/mL (nanograms/milliliter). Our bodies absorb vitamin D from the sun and also from the foods we eat, but as you'll see, these sources don't provide enough to satisfy our needs.

## THE SUN

When the sunlight hits your skin, the ultraviolet rays penetrate and convert cholesterol into vitamin D. For the last 85,000 years, vitamin D was produced in just this way, as our ancestors hunted and gathered all day, often wearing no more than a skimpy deerskin for cover. But today, only a rare person receives enough sunlight on the skin to produce vitamin D adequate to his or her needs. I live in Florida, the Sunshine State, but when my patients first come into my office, nearly all are vitamin D deficient.

Can you get 1,000 to 2,000 IU of vitamin D daily from the sun? Yes, but you should not! That would require excessive sun exposure, at least one hour a day without sunscreen in a region such as Southern California. That much sun, as we all know, may cause sunburn, skin cancer, and aging. We're advised to slather on the sunscreen, and most of us do, but anything more than 8 SPF blocks nearly all vitamin D formation. If it is cloudy, vitamin D production is reduced to 50% when compared to full sunshine, and our bodies generate almost no vitamin D when the sun's rays pass through glass. So don't count on sunshine for your vitamin D.

## FOOD SOURCES OF VITAMIN D

We find many products on the grocery store shelves—dairy, orange juice, packaged breakfast cereals—that advertise that they're fortified with vitamin D. But read the labels. You'll only get 100 IUs in a cup of milk, so you'd need to drink 15 to 20 cups of milk a day to get the recommended daily dosage. Egg yolks also have vitamin D, but you'd need to eat a bucketful—75 to 100 yolks—definitely not recommended.

---

### *Foods Containing Vitamin D*

- Cold-water fish, 3.5 oz: 100 to 350 IU per serving (fattier fish such as salmon have the higher range of vitamin D)
- Milk, calcium-fortified orange juice, calcium-fortified soy or almond milk: 100 to 125 IU per 8 ounces (1 cup)
- Egg yolk (1): 25 IU
- Cheese, 1 oz: 5 to 10 IU

---

## Vitamin D Supplements

You may meet some of your vitamin D needs with sunshine or food, but it's clear that for most people neither source will provide adequate amounts (at least 1,500 to 2,000 IUs a day), so you must use a supplement. Just be aware that two forms of vitamin D are available for purchase: vitamin D2 and D3. Vitamin D2 is a vegetarian form of vitamin D and has only 20% to 50% of the activity of D3, so I'll be referring to vitamin D3, which is clearly more effective. Since people who choose a vitamin D2 supplement have more variability in the blood levels they achieve, it is more important for them to have their vitamin D blood levels checked after several months of use.

How much vitamin D3 should you take? That depends. If you're on several supplements, such as multivitamins and calcium with vitamin D3, be sure to calculate your total intake before you add any more. You may only need a single 1,000 IU capsule a day or less, because you're already filling some of your nutritional requirements.

## Should You Check Your Vitamin D Level?

The optimal range of vitamin D in your bloodstream is 40 to 70 ng/mL. Less than 32 ng/mL is deficient. If you don't take at least 1,000 to 2,000 IU of vitamin D3 daily, your levels are probably low. I would suggest trying 1,500 to 3,000 IU for three months. Then ask your doctor if you should check your level. If you've been taking vitamin D3 supplements for at least three months, there is a good chance it will look good. In that case, you simply need to maintain the regimen you're on.

If your level is very low, then taking 5,000 IU daily for 2 to 3 months will probably bring you back to normal. Once stabilized, consider 1,500 to 3,000 IU daily for the long term. Some people with limited vitamin D absorption from their gastrointestinal system may need to take 3,000 to 5,000 IU daily to maintain a normal level. If you require more than this, please check with your medical provider as this could be a sign of the following:

- You don't convert 25-OH vitamin D to 1,25 dihydroxyvitamin D properly, which can cause immune suppression if missed.
- Gastrointestinal absorption problems, which can cause many other health issues that need to be addressed, such as gluten intolerance
- Decreased genetic activity to transport vitamin D. This means you simply need to take more vitamin D to meet your needs.

---

## Caution! You Can Take Too Much Vitamin D

A blood level of vitamin D higher than 100 ng/mL is associated with several medical problems. I don't recommend a level greater than 70 ng/mL unless your doctor specifically recommends it for a particular medical problem. Keep in mind that it's fine if you are started on 10,000 IU for three months to bring your vitamin D back to normal. But once your blood level normalizes, vitamin D levels will keep going up if you maintain this high dosage. So recheck to ensure you are in the appropriate range.

---

### Vitamin K

Vitamin K is essential for cardiovascular health, because it prevents calcium from shifting from your bones to your arteries. Not surprisingly, then, vitamin K is essential to keeping your bones strong. It was originally named for its relation to clotting, as in the German word for coagulation, which begins with a *K*.

With vitamin K deficiency, artery walls calcify, blood pressure increases, and the lining of your arteries grows more plaque.

The minimum dietary intake of vitamin K for proper clotting is around 100 mcg per day (90 mcg for women and 120 mcg for men). Yet bones and arteries function much better with at least 250 mcg and preferably 1,000 mcg of vitamin K daily.

There are two primary forms of vitamin K, K1 and K2. K1 comes from leafy green vegetables and provides most of the dietary intake in the United States. K2 comes from fermented cheeses and in particular from fermented soy products; most Americans won't consume enough K2 to provide any real benefit. Both forms aid bone and artery health, and both are available as supplements.

## FOOD SOURCES FOR VITAMIN K1

Foods—especially dark green leafy vegetables—are an excellent source of vitamin K. See the "Good Sources of K1" chart, below, for foods rich in Vitamin K.

| Good Sources of K1 | | |
| --- | --- | --- |
| Food | Measure | K1 (mcg) |
| Kale, cooked, drained | 1 cup | 1,062 |
| Collards, cooked, drained | 1 cup | 1,059 |
| Spinach, cooked (or about 7 cups raw) | 1 cup | 889 |
| Beets, cooked | 1 cup | 697 |
| Broccoli, cooked | 1 cup | 220 |
| Brussels sprouts, cooked | 1 cup | 219 |
| Onions, raw | 1 cup | 207 |
| Parsley | 10 sprigs | 164 |
| Cabbage, cooked (or about 3 cups raw) | 1 cup | 163 |
| Asparagus, cooked | 1 cup | 144 |
| Lettuce, iceberg | ¼ head | 33 |

## Vitamin K Supplements

If you are following the 30-Day Heart Tune-Up eating plan, you will be enjoying many foods that are packed with vitamin K. Most nutritional experts suggest that for optimal functioning you need 500 to 1,000 mcg daily.[7] Keep in mind that calcium supplements may already provide some of the vitamin K your body needs, as some calcium sources also provide magnesium, vitamin D, and vitamin K with the calcium. Calculate how much vitamin K you're getting from your diet and other vitamins, and then supplement accordingly.

---

### What If I'm Taking Warfarin (Coumadin)?

Physicians typically prescribe warfarin (brand name Coumadin, and other names) or other blood thinners for people at risk of clotting. (The patients may have atrial fibrillation or deep venous thrombosis in the legs. A blood clot would cause major health problems or even death.) Warfarin blocks our ability to recycle vitamin K, so as a result, patients taking warfarin may suffer from vitamin K deficiency. People taking warfarin often have arterial calcification and loss in bone density. The most practical solution would be for them to eat at least 1 cup of leafy green vegetables every day. They would get some consistent vitamin K for their arteries and bones, and the warfarin would still limit and control their clotting process. However, many doctors tell patients on warfarin *not* to eat leafy green vegetables. Here's why: If you are inconsistent with how much you eat, your anticoagulation levels will rise and fall. This exposes you to the risk of excessive or inadequate clotting, which can cause a stroke or bleeding. So if you're eating greens to add vitamin K, be sure to do so every day. Ask your doctor if this approach would be appropriate for you, but be aware that 100% consistency is required. Don't forget that if you modify your leafy green intake while taking warfarin, your physician initially may need to monitor your blood levels more frequently and change your warfarin dosage as well. So you absolutely need to involve your doctor with this type of change.

---

## Potassium

Every cell in your body requires potassium to function. In particular, your arteries need potassium to dilate and keep blood pressure levels normal. Very low and very high potassium can cause your heart to stop beating or can lead to irregular heart rhythms that may result in death. Low potassium most commonly occurs as a side effect of medication, but it can also occur with low intake of potassium-rich foods. High potassium levels typically occur with kidney failure or as a side effect of a variety of medications. I have never seen a problem if a healthy person ate too much potassium-rich food.

### FOOD SOURCES OF POTASSIUM

We require at least 3,500 to 4,000 mg of potassium daily, yet typically most people in the United States only get half that much. As a consequence, our heart and arteries don't function properly, which can lead to hypertension and muscle cramps too. Beans, fruits and vegetables, and seafood are good sources of potassium, as are some other lean protein sources. See the "Food Sources of Potassium" chart, below, for details.

| Food Sources of Potassium | |
|---|---|
| Food | Potassium (mg) |
| Beans (1 cup cooked) | 1,000 |
| Fish, salmon (6 ounce) | 1,000 |
| Dark green leaf veggies, spinach or kale (1 cup cooked) | 840 |
| Dark green leaf veggies, spinach (1 cup raw) | 170 |
| Baked potato, with skin (1 medium potato) | 930 |
| Sweet potato, baked with skin (1 medium potato) | 550 |

*continues*

| Food Sources of Potassium | Potassium (mg) |
|---|---|
| Dried apricots (½ cup) | 750 |
| Baked squash, acorn or butternut (1 cup cooked) | 900 |
| Yogurt, plain, nonfat (1 cup) | 625 |
| Avocado (½ cup) | 550 |
| Banana (1 medium) | 420 |
| Mushrooms (1 cup sliced) | 420 |

## POTASSIUM SUPPLEMENTS

If your potassium levels are low despite eating the healthy foods listed in the "Food Sources of Potassium" chart, then this requires a visit to your doctor for evaluation. Since potassium must be given in the correct dosage, a prescription is necessary. Your potassium levels should be monitored. Too much or too little can create dangerous irregular heart rhythms. So I do not recommend that you take potassium supplements on your own.

## The Vitamin E Question

Often I'm asked about vitamin E. This was all the rage some years ago—everyone seemed to be taking this supplement. Vitamin E is made up of several molecules: four tocopherols (alpha, beta, gamma, delta) and four tocotrienols (alpha, beta, gamma, delta). But the sad truth is, studies have shown that the most commonly sold type of vitamin E, alpha tocopherol, lowers healthy HDL cholesterol levels, decreases its beneficial activity, and therefore may actually contribute to arterial plaque growth.[8] In contrast, gamma and delta tocopherols and tocotrienols improve the advanced lipid profile, so if you are taking multivitamins that contain vitamin E or a vitamin E supplement, make sure it has "mixed forms of vitamin E"—in particular, more delta and gamma than alpha, and ideally it would contain both tocopherols and tocotrienols as well. Eating foods that contain vitamin E, such as almonds, avocado, and extra virgin olive oil, is your safest bet. They have a mixture of all forms of tocopherols and tocotrienols.

## IF YOU TAKE CHOLESTEROL-LOWERING STATIN MEDICATION

Cholesterol-lowering (statin) medications (marketed as Lipitor, Crestor, Pravachol, Zocor, Atorvastatin, Pravastatin, and Simvastatin) decrease not only cholesterol but also compounds in the body that are derived from cholesterol, such as testosterone, coenzyme Q10 (CoQ10), and other substances that repair muscle. Yes, cholesterol-lowering medications help reduce heart attacks and strokes in people with known heart disease and for those at high risk for the same, but they can also produce a variety of symptoms. Most people assume the benefit from taking a statin medication is related to its cholesterol-lowering effects, but other important benefits are due to the fact that statins also decrease artery inflammation and they make your blood less sticky, so it's less likely to clot.[9]

Statin medications cause multiple side effects, so let's discuss the most common ones: a reduction in CoQ10 levels, a rise in blood sugar, memory loss, muscle aches, and a decrease in testosterone. All of these have health and nutritional implications. Statin medications can also impact liver function and cause liver inflammation, but as this is rare and your doctor should be following your liver function while taking these medications, I'll leave that to you and your doctor.

### Reduction in Coenzyme Q10

Coenzyme Q10 (CoQ10, also called ubiquinone and ubiquinol) is a substance produced by our tissues that is essential for energy production, especially for heart cells. Every cell in the body has tiny energy-generating organelles (think of them as microscopic factories) called mitochondria. The body's mitochondria require CoQ10 to produce energy. Studies have shown that the ability to produce CoQ10 drops by 20% in people who take a statin. No studies to date show that lowering CoQ10 with statin medication kills you or causes cancer, yet the big concern is that it might decrease your energy and mental sharpness and interfere with your quality of life. Despite a lack of clinical studies that prove the benefits of combining a statin with CoQ10, most holistic and integrative physicians, including one of my former professors, Dr. Andrew Weil, recommend that patients on a statin should take CoQ10 with it. This is largely to bring the body back to its normal, prestatin state.

For most people, I find that 50 to 100 mg of a high-quality and well-absorbed product will bring the CoQ10 level back to pre-statin levels. Many companies spend a great deal of energy marketing the advantages of one form of CoQ10 over another, such as ubiquinol versus ubiquinone, although from a clinical perspective, it doesn't make much difference. Yet absorption is a very important consideration, as inexpensive crystalline CoQ10 (sold in a tablet) has only a 1% absorption rate. CoQ10 soluble in oil has 4% absorption, and nanolipid spheres have a reported 8% absorption. To date, even better absorption rates have been published using a fully dissolved, crystal-free, lipid-based form—a product we offer through our medical office. To date, the brands I've found with the best proven absorption are Thorne's Q-Best and Designs for Health's Q-Avail. So although cheap CoQ10 tablets may be one third the cost of more expensive versions, the very poor absorption makes it much more expensive, in reality. Buyers should beware when choosing CoQ10! Fortunately, since absorption is an issue and you may be unsure of your product, blood levels for CoQ10 can be measured. This will help your doctor confirm if your dosage brings your levels back to normal. Measuring CoQ10 in the blood is fairly simple, although it may not be covered by your medical insurance.

### Rise in Blood Sugar with Statins

In addition to experiencing a potential drop in energy when taking a statin medication, many people will also experience a modest increase in blood sugar levels. I tell my patients that if they are on a statin regimen, they need to eat fewer refined carbs and less sugar, and to exercise more to make up for the drug's effect. If you are in this situation, be sure to ask your doctor to check your fasting blood sugar levels.

### Memory Loss with Statins

Memory loss, often described as brain fog, has also been noted by the FDA recently with statin medication use. Adding CoQ10 may help some people with these symptoms, but clearly it does not help all. There are no studies linking an increased dementia risk with statins, yet I recommend that if you notice memory loss while on a statin medication, you should discuss with your doctor whether stopping it is appropriate. You might consider other cholesterol-lowering options, such as healthier eating, as a start.

### Muscle Aches with Statins

Perhaps the most common complaint when taking a statin medication is muscle aches. Very rarely, this can progress to major muscle tissue breakdown, leading to kidney failure and/or death. Much more common are diffuse muscle aches that are associated with decreased muscle repair and muscle atrophy. If you notice these symptoms, which occur in nearly 10% of people taking these drugs, talk to your doctor about potentially stopping the medication.

### Reduction in Testosterone Levels with Statins

Finally, drug companies fail to mention that statin medications lower testosterone levels. After all, your body uses cholesterol to make testosterone. With less cholesterol available, testosterone levels decrease as well. This drop has been reported in several medical studies.[10] On many occasions, I have seen a man start a statin medication for a cardiac problem and note his testosterone level dropping 50 or more points. For someone with a completely normal testosterone level, say 700 mg/dL, this is unlikely to be a problem. But a man with a borderline testosterone level (say 340 mg/dL) who begins a statin could lose erectile function. This person may need to have his physician prescribe testosterone in order to tolerate the statin. Consider talking to your doctor about checking your testosterone level if you take a statin drug—in particular, if you have noticed a drop in energy, libido, drive, and sharpness. This applies to women as well, as both men and women require an adequate amount of testosterone for a normal sex drive.

### When Should You Take a Cholesterol-Lowering (Statin) Medication?

Obviously I can't address this adequately here without knowing your medical history. But below are a few guidelines I use in my practice to help my patients decide when it might be warranted.

* If you have established cardiovascular disease (meaning you have already had a heart attack or stroke, or an abnormal test, such as treadmill stress test), I believe the benefits of using a statin medication are greater than the risks. If you have an elevated carotid IMT (intimal medial thickness) plaque score, a high LDL cholesterol level, and your plaque score keeps growing despite your best efforts, I typically recommend starting a treatment with a statin medication.

- People with multiple abnormal risk factors for developing cardiovascular disease should talk to their doctor about whether a statin is appropriate for them.
- In clinical studies, women have been shown to benefit less from taking a statin medication than men, so women should have a stronger reason (such as multiple risk factors for heart disease) to begin this type of therapy.

### What Is the Difference Between a Statin Medication and Red Yeast Rice Extract?

This is a common question, and it is important for anyone considering cholesterol-lowering medication to know the answer. A red-pigmented yeast, called *Monascus purpureus*, can be grown on rice. An extract from this yeast has been shown in numerous studies in China and the United States to help maintain healthy blood cholesterol levels. The red yeast rice extract produces chemical compounds, called monacolins, that decrease cholesterol production in the liver. The first statin cholesterol medication, lovastatin, was isolated from red yeast rice extract.

In contrast to a drug that contains a high dosage of one type of statin, red yeast rice extract may contain ten or more cholesterol-lowering ingredients. Small dosages of multiple compounds seem better tolerated than a single large dosage of one. In fact, some patients who cannot take a statin medication due to muscle aches or liver inflammation are able to tolerate red yeast rice extract and lower their cholesterol levels.[11]

In my opinion, red yeast rice extract is a cholesterol-lowering drug and should be treated with the same safety concerns as any other medication. The biggest difference between it and a statin medication is that it is available over the counter, while drugs are prescribed by physicians and sold through pharmacies. Please remember that red yeast rice extract has the potential to have all the same benefits, side effects, and complications as any of the other statin medications, if it is given at the same dosage. The biggest challenge is finding a high-quality product that is contaminant free and contains the same "drug" dosage with every package. Due to quality concerns with production, my approach is to prescribe a medication first, and if there are side effects, to use the best quality red yeast rice I can find as a second option. Since we are using this like a drug treatment, I choose a product that meets or exceeds production standards required for medications, such as Choleast-900 from Thorne.

## FOR THOSE WITH CONGESTIVE HEART FAILURE (CHF) AND ADVANCED HEART DISEASE

The purpose of this book and this chapter is to keep your heart healthy and, for those who need it, to reverse heart disease. Anyone who has progressed to the point of heart failure should be under the regular care of a physician.

With heart failure, the heart is starved for energy. Without it, your heart can't pump efficiently, and the fluid from your blood backs up into your lungs. One of the many keys to restoring function, then, is restoring heart cell energy.

Mitochondria produce most of the energy your cells use. Your heart cells have more mitochondria than any others in the body. Stephen Sinatra, MD, a nationally renowned integrative cardiologist, was one of the pioneers in advocating therapy to enhance heart cell mitochondrial function—something Dr. Sinatra called "metabolic cardiology." He focused on three key supplements: CoQ10, ribose, and carnitine. Randomized clinical trials have shown some controversy in quantifying the benefits of this combination, but clinical experience using these agents has shown that they are excellent in improving the quality of life for some people who have heart failure.

If you're in this situation, only your doctor should recommend the supplement treatment options listed below, depending upon your unique situation. Dosages are just for your consideration and to help with your discussion.

- CoQ10: 50 to 200 mg twice daily. I suggest you ask your doctor to confirm that you have a blood level of at least 2 to 2.5 mcg/mL of CoQ10. To reach this level efficiently, ensure you take a high-quality form that is well absorbed.
- Ribose: 5 grams twice daily (powder mixed into liquid is convenient)
- Carnitine: 2 to 3 grams twice daily (powder mixed into liquid is convenient)
- Although not as well studied in clinical trials, two other agents have great promise to enhance mitochondrial function and energy production. These are curcumin and resveratrol. Compounds such as curcumin (an extract found in the bright yellow spice turmeric) and resveratrol (an extract from red grapes and red wine) are essential to controlling artery inflammation and oxidative stress, but are required in such large amounts that it is unrealistic to get an adequate dosage from food (or in the case of resveratrol, from red wine). Curcumin is such an outstanding anti-inflammatory therapy that I even prescribe it for my patients with arthritis, those who want to limit cognitive decline, and for cancer prevention. However, curcumin absorption is highly variable, so it is critical to take a high-quality form with proven absorption rates. Depending upon your situation, taking these supplements makes good sense.

With heart failure, not only does the heart pump poorly, but there is often substantial artery dysfunction as well. If a weakened heart must pump against stiff, calcified arteries, it creates even more stress on the heart. Several agents may improve artery function and help reduce plaque and calcification.

- As noted above, vitamin K prevents artery calcification. If you have advanced heart disease and/or heart failure, ask your doctor about adding extra vitamin K1 (aim for 1,000 mcg from your diet and supplement regimen daily) and vitamin K2. Increase magnesium to 300 to 500 mg twice daily. It will help relax blood vessels and enhance blood pressure control, making pumping easier for the heart. At some point on this dosage, ask your doctor to measure your red blood cell magnesium level to confirm you are in the normal range.
- Arginine is also an excellent nutrient to enhance artery function and improve blood pressure control. It is the building block that the body uses to make nitric oxide, which is essential to arterial health and wellness. Nitric oxide induces the arteries to dilate, and for men it results in erections too. See Chapter 8 for dietary sources of arginine, or take a supplement with 1,000 mg twice daily.
- As people with heart failure are at greater risk for clotting, ask your doctor about increasing your fish oil dosage to 2 to 3 grams of EPA and DHA daily (but don't exceed 2 grams daily if taking Coumadin).

My patient Peter suffered from heart failure, but he benefited greatly by following this regimen. Peter's son, Scott, had been in my practice for years. Following my program, Scott had made terrific improvements in his health. But one day he came into my office, and he talked about his dad with tears in his eyes.

Peter was a retired plumber and widower. At the age of 70, he had taken up surfing and loved it. In fact, the sport became his passion. Unfortunately, one day he had exhausted himself and had a heart attack while out in the waves. By the time he was brought to shore and an ambulance finally got him to the hospital, his heart had sustained massive damage. After being discharged, he was so weak and out of breath, he could barely get dressed and keep himself clean.

Since he had no help at home, Scott had Peter move in with his family. Scott asked me if I could help his dad restore some of his energy and regain his dignity. I agreed to do my best.

Peter was following the advice of a doctor from the community (the head of a local primary care group), and he was getting the best of standard care. He was on at least ten medications to treat his heart failure, angina, high cholesterol, and wheezing. Yet, although these medications improved his laboratory results, they seemed to make him feel worse. His heart didn't have the energy to pump properly, and Peter was clearly suffering and depressed as a result.

Peter was eating fairly well at his son's house, but he didn't take any supplements and couldn't muster enough energy to participate in any activities. He was on a high dosage of a statin medication, without any CoQ10, so it wasn't surprising that his CoQ10 level was very low. On my examination, his legs were swollen, his lungs were partly filled with fluid, and he was short of breath—all the result of advanced heart failure. I hoped that if I gave him supplements to help with mitochondrial energy production, lowered his salt intake to decrease fluid retention, and encouraged him to be more active, his heart might pump better. "What do you hope to achieve if you make the changes I'm suggesting?" I asked. I recall being startled when he replied, "I want to be able to surf again."

As a first step, I started him on 100 mg of CoQ10 daily, along with the supplements ribose, carnitine, magnesium, and fish oil at 2,000 mg daily. I was fairly impressed that at his follow-up visit two weeks later he walked with more energy, had started cooking the recipes I had recommended, and seemed to feel better all the way around. But Peter was still far from being back to normal. His new lab results indicated that his CoQ10 level was still low, so I doubled the dosage, added curcumin, resveratrol, and vitamin K2, and sent him to cardiac rehab to work out with medical supervision three days a week.

Peter's response to this was nothing short of miraculous. By the third month he was discharged from cardiac rehab, and he moved back to his own home. Somehow, the combination of eating better, adding daily exercise, and using supplements to restore energy to his heart had transformed him. Peter was ready to give surfing another try.

---

The combination of eating heart-friendly foods, building your fitness level, managing your stress, and meeting your heart's nutritional needs will not only help you to dramatically reduce your risk for heart disease and strokes, but it will also turn back the clock on aging—allowing you to regain energy and vitality you haven't known in years.

The greatest thanks I've received from my patients have been their frequent observation after the first 30 days: "I forgot how much better I could feel." They were more energized, they slept better, and often commented, "Wow, this has done wonders for my sex life!" Yes, not only is this program good for your libido, in the next chapter you are about to discover that sex is good for your heart too.

## Chapter Eight

# Sexier You

Sex and romance are great for your heart health. So, in this chapter, I'll show you how the 30-Day Heart Tune-Up will also revitalize your sex life.

Most of us recognize that a satisfying sexual experience feels fantastic. But encroaching cardiovascular disease; the use of medications to lower cholesterol and blood pressure; and hormonal decline related to illness or aging can cause even the most active libido to wither. Perhaps you have found your passion waning and have simply come to accept this as "normal" at your stage of life. You may resign yourself to the "inevitable" and ask, "What can I expect after all these years?"

The truth is, lots! There are many things you can do to improve your sexual response—you don't have to consider great sex a distant memory. In fact, if you follow my suggestions, the 30-Day Heart Tune-Up can also be your 30-Day Sex Tune-Up.

In this chapter, I'd like to focus on three key discussions:

* Sexual dysfunction: how poor circulation and other factors lead to a disappointing sexual performance for men and women.
* Why it's so vitally important to maintain your sexuality, both for your general health and also for your heart.

- How the 30-Day Heart Tune-Up can rev up your sex life and your overall sense of vitality and well-being.

Let's look at these issues one at a time.

## YOUR HEART IS AT THE HEART OF SEXUAL FUNCTION AND DYSFUNCTION

In poetry and myth, the heart has always been the seat of emotion, and especially of love. Hearts are plastered all over stores around Valentine's Day. And words like heartstrings, heartthrob, heartbreak, heartless, and heartwarming all refer in one way or another to love or the lack thereof. In Hindu beliefs, the heart chakra is associated with love and compassion, charity, and healing. This is more than a coincidence! To a great degree, sexual function—an expression of love—is dependent upon how well your heart is pumping and on the general health of your circulatory system. In fact, circulatory problems such as decreased blood flow, high blood pressure, and high blood sugar affect sexual function in both men and women.

It may surprise you to know that erectile dysfunction (ED), while perhaps disappointing or embarrassing, signifies more than just the inability to perform in bed. In fact, it has the potential to indicate a life-and-death medical issue. That's because the most common cause for men's ED is cardiovascular disease. As arterial plaque grows throughout the body, smaller arteries become blocked before the larger ones do. So, not surprisingly, the arteries to the penis are often the first to be clogged, thereby causing ED symptoms. This occurs well before a man develops angina. In fact, until proven otherwise, we should assume that most men complaining of ED, especially men under age 60, are showing early signs of cardiovascular disease, since narrowed arteries are the most common cause for erectile dysfunction. A Mayo Clinic study found that men with ED are 80% more likely to develop heart disease compared to men who do not have it. Men ages 40 to 49 with ED are twice as likely to get heart disease as those without ED.[1]

To be safe, I recommend that most men with ED have a cardiovascular workup. Because let's face it, for men, there's no erection without good circulation.

This is no small problem. Twenty million men suffer from ED, which becomes much more common with age. For instance, only 5% of men under 40 have ED, 52% of men between the ages of 40 and 70 have it, and only 30% of men over 70 are able to consistently maintain an erection. These numbers are not confined to the males of our species. About 40% of women also have some degree of sexual dysfunction, some of which can be linked to cardiovascular disease. Healthy circulation improves blood flow to the clitoris, promotes vaginal and labial engorgement, and decreases vaginal dryness.

When diagnosed with ED, most men want to jump to an immediate treatment plan. Although this response is understandable, it is unwise. The best long-term solution requires that you first identify the cause, and once it is identified, then proceed to a correct treatment. Unfortunately, in the interest of saving time, too many otherwise well-meaning physicians will write a prescription for Viagra, Cialis, or Levitra without giving cardiovascular disease much thought. *This can be dangerous!* This class of medications temporarily reverses the symptoms of erectile dysfunction by causing the arteries of the penis, as well as those in the arms and legs, to dilate. Blood shifts from the brain and heart toward these extremities. This is why TV commercials for these drugs appropriately warn that if you have hearing or vision loss, stop taking the medication until you talk to your doctor. Hearing loss or vision loss symptoms, arising from reduced blood supply to the brain, indicate that you may be on the verge of a stroke. Furthermore, the dilation of the arteries in the penis may overcome the early blockage and restore erectile function, but these drugs do nothing to correct the underlying cardiovascular problem— the arterial plaque just keeps growing. As the plaque buildup and blockage worsens, at some point the ED drugs stop working. By missing the critical ED early warning sign, a person with cardiovascular disease could easily progress to a heart attack, stroke, or death without ever recognizing that he has this problem.

At the Masley Optimal Health Center, if a patient complains of ED, we do a cardiovascular workup first. We start our evaluation with a carotid IMT study to clarify arterial plaque growth, followed by a $VO_2$ max treadmill stress test to determine a man's fitness. We look at multiple other cardiovascular risk factors and also confirm that he is safe for a vigorous activity like sex. Comprehensive hormone testing is an important part of that evaluation.

One of my patients, Gregory, had developed problems with ED at age 50. A bowling buddy gave him a few Viagra tablets, which helped greatly. Besides this, his wife was bugging him to get a physical, since he had reached this milestone age. So Greg came to see me at the suggestion of a close friend, planning to get his own ED prescription and to allay his wife's concerns.

Greg's hormonal levels were normal, but, not surprisingly, his carotid IMT score was clearly advanced. A normal score for a 50-year-old man would be 0.66 mm, but Greg's was 0.9 mm. Not only that, but he had a 2-mm plaque pustule growing inside the carotid artery. It wasn't large enough to justify a cardiovascular procedure, yet this was clearly enough blockage to account for his ED. Knowing Greg's plaque score and anticipating an abnormal study, I was a bit anxious when we performed his stress treadmill test. At peak exertion, Greg didn't have any symptoms, but his cardiogram was abnormal, suggesting blockages to his heart.

If I had checked only Greg's cardiac risk factors (smoking, a family history of cardiovascular disease, etc.) and given him a Viagra-like prescription, most likely his heart disease would have worsened over time. Fortunately, we now knew what was causing his problem. And with the 30-Day Heart Tune-Up, we also knew how to fix it. I gave Greg the encouraging news. Once we shrunk his carotid artery plaque to less than 0.8 mm, he'd probably regain his erectile function without medications. Plus we had just saved him from some horrible cardiovascular event that was lurking around the corner. I hoped that if we could reduce Greg's plaque at the rate of 6% a year, within one year his stress test would be normal, and within two he'd have regained erectile function. And, after following my program for two years (which initially included a prescription for his ED), he no longer needed the ED medication.

## ADDITIONAL CAUSES OF ERECTILE DYSFUNCTION

There are other reasons a man can experience ED. These are not mutually exclusive—that is you can have blocked arteries as well as low testosterone and poor fitness. Careful evaluation is required.

### Low Hormone Levels

Men's sexual response depends on testosterone and DHEA, although testosterone seems to be more important for male libido. In fact, the lower the level of testosterone, the lower the sexual frequency men have. Nearly 20% of men between age 50 and 60 have low testosterone levels. This is less common before age 50 and more frequent after age 60. Low testosterone not only causes ED, but typically leads to reduced energy, drive, sexual desire, and even interest in exercising. It can also contribute to night sweats, poor quality sleep, and difficulty controlling weight. The latter is usually characterized by a loss in muscle mass and a gain in fat, especially around the waist. In addition to these symptoms, there are medical concerns that low testosterone can lead to a drop in bone density, which creates an increased risk of bone fractures.

Some epidemiological evidence also suggests that low testosterone may even increase risk for cardiovascular disease and prostate cancer, although these last points remain controversial.

Two kinds of low testosterone can cause ED. The first comes from one's total production—the body simply isn't making enough. The second is a bit more complicated. Hormone production is normal, but the testosterone has stuck to blood proteins and is unavailable to stimulate tissues. Because the treatments for these two causes are different, it is critical that your doctor measure both total and free testosterone levels when evaluating symptoms.

DHEA is an adrenal hormone that can enhance sexual desire and function. However, it is commonly low in men who have endured prolonged, unmanaged stress. Initially Viagra and similar drugs work if DHEA levels are low. But eventually, if not treated properly, a man will have insufficient libido for success— even if the drugs produce an erection.

## Low Fitness

Without fitness, you don't have stamina and energy. You have to be in good shape to have a decent sex life! Unfortunately, some men are just not robust enough to perform. If you scored below the 40th percentile for your age on the MET fitness test in Chapter 5, you may need to get fitter before expecting normal erectile function. Keep in mind that average fitness for a person in the United States (when two thirds of us are either obese or overweight) is not terrific. Your health may be unraveling without you even noticing, because we're surrounded by others who look just like us. But this is not good enough. In truth, if you want great romantic performance you should aim for aerobic fitness in the 80th percentile or better for your age group. The only disappointment for some is that you don't get to count having sex as your workout for the day. You still need focused exercise, but don't hesitate to enjoy some romance too!

## Medications

In Chapter 7, I went into detail about the effects of statin medications on testosterone levels. Beta-blockers and drugs used to control blood pressure can also have many adverse sexual side effects. Many antidepressant medications, especially the popular SSRI (selective serotonin reuptake inhibitor) drugs such as Lexapro, Zoloft, Prozac, Paxil, etc., decrease libido. So clearly, when feasible, it's better for you to control your blood pressure, your mood, and your health issues by following the 30-Day Heart Tune-Up. It may remedy depression without your resorting to libido-dampening drugs. Talk to your doctor.

## Tobacco Use

Every time you smoke a cigarette, it constricts the blood flow to your genitals for at least 4 to 6 hours, limiting your ability to have an erection. Tobacco use also accelerates arterial plaque growth, so *most* smokers will eventually suffer from ED. If you smoke, I strongly encourage you to stop. Please talk to your medical provider about the quitting options that are appropriate for you.

## Excessive Alcohol

James Bond notwithstanding, drinking more than one serving of alcohol a night decreases romantic performance. If you suffer from early signs of low fitness, testosterone deficiency, or cardiovascular disease, extra alcohol just compounds your problems. While the average 20-year-old has almost no problems with erectile dysfunction and might gain a little confidence after a drink or two, most men over 35 will experience a drop in sexual function with the same amount of alcohol—whether it's shaken or stirred.

### High Stress

Too much stress can lead to insomnia, lower DHEA levels, and ED. If stress is affecting your romantic performance, please refer back to Chapter 6 regarding better stress management.

## FEMALE SEXUAL DYSFUNCTION

How many cartoons and jokes have we seen about the complexity of women's needs? Most of these, in fact, are based at least in part on reality. Women have many ways of achieving an orgasm, and for them (more than for men), intimacy is often essential for sexual pleasure. I have been fortunate to have had the opportunity to interview Dr. Anna Cabeca—a gynecologist, international expert on women's sexual health, and close professional colleague—on this topic. As she emphasizes, the need for intimacy is based on the hormonal pattern of human development for the last 85,000 years, which has focused on two reactions:

1. Fight or flight to survive
2. Feed and breed during times of safety

Clearly there are exceptions for both genders, but in general, if a woman doesn't feel safe, secure, and intimate, she won't be comfortable feeding or breeding. It may be impossible for her to relax and receive when she's frightened—her sexual organs simply will not respond and over time may shut down and wither. Men have suppressed some of these basic neurohormonal feelings, but many women have not. In addition, when a woman is stressed, sex is not a priority. Stress increases cortisol and depletes DHEA. This can diminish her sex drive and response. And reproductive and libido hormones drop, because they're being shifted to cortisol production to further manage the stress.

Libido is often an issue for couples, in particular because it varies greatly between the sexes. The most common stereotype is that men want sex more often than women do. Of course, we all know that this is only a stereotype, and that many women initiate and enjoy frequent sex as well. However, it seems that several times a month, when I see a husband and wife for an optimal health evaluation, he wants more sex and she wants less—but she also wants more romance and cuddling. To some degree, this is because men have much higher testosterone levels than women, and yes, they do have a greater libido, partly related to this hormonal difference. Yet, as I explained above, many women are also neurohormonally different than men, and need to feel calm for their desire to be activated. Other factors that can inappropriately drop a woman's libido include:

- **Excess body fat.** Fat cells convert testosterone to estrogen (this happens in men and women). This conversion can lower testosterone levels substantially.
- **High stress.** High cortisol levels adversely affect woman's oxytocin levels. Stress can be related to work, child care, or marital conflict. Any type of prolonged stress plays havoc with women's hormones. With diminished oxytocin, women don't enjoy sex as much.
- **High levels of inflammation.** Inflammation can reduce blood flow, and as a result, women have more vaginal dryness and less enjoyment with stimulation.
- **Medications.** Like men, women can have adverse sexual side effects from medications. SSRI antidepressants can cause a profound drop in libido for women as well as men. If a woman must continue on the medication for medical reasons, clinical studies have shown that taking 3 grams of the herbal supplement maca (*Lepidium meyenii*) daily can help reverse some of this dysfunction.[2] Maca is an herb that grows in the Peruvian Andes. It is sometimes called

Peruvian ginseng because of its ability to enhance sexuality. Maca is also being studied to discern whether it relieves other forms of sexual dysfunction unrelated to medication.

Antihistamines, drugs commonly used to treat allergy symptoms, can also block a woman's ability to have an orgasm. Women with long-term allergy problems should take note!

- **Sleep deprivation.** It's not surprising that insomnia affects libido, yet I'm amazed at how often women who are trying to take care of everyone else in their lives don't get enough sleep—and don't connect this to their diminished sex drive.
- **Low fitness.** Without physical stamina, women often find themselves exhausted by the end of the day. One more physical act may just seem out of the question.

Let's face it: For most women, sex and stress are mutually exclusive. If you're tired, worn out, and sleeping poorly, you won't be interested in responding to the man in your life or initiating sex. And if that man is smart and he wants to get "lucky," *he will need to keep in mind which hormonal system is being activated* and help reduce the stress in your life, before approaching you with romantic intentions.

It's also important to recognize that a woman's pelvic organs are intimately connected to her body's health and wellness. You need healthy blood flow to have healthy sexual organs and intimacy. Clitoral engorgement is diminished by circulatory changes, high blood pressure, and high blood sugar. For both men and women, inflammation decreases circulation and will impair sexual function. Yet for women, inflammation also reduces blood flow, creates hormonal imbalance, and causes vaginal dryness and infections. All of these conditions make intercourse unpleasant, if not painful.

Moreover, menopausal symptoms due to the reduction of estrogen and other female hormones can diminish sexual interest and activity. Vaginal dryness is common after menopause, and in some women it may lead to skin thinning which, like inflammation, makes intercourse painful. At the farthest extreme, the lack of estrogen can cause the delicate tissue to thin and atrophy, which may result in bleeding during intercourse. This can create a rift in relationships. Even if a woman doesn't communicate about her discomfort, her partner may sense that she's tense and hurting, and consciously or unconsciously may be reluctant to impose a distressing experience on her. For her part, she may be thinking, "Every time I have sex, I'm doing it for him, but it's hurting me!" This desire to avoid pain can cause couples to drift apart in the bedroom. Some may even sleep on opposite sides of the house, a sad state of affairs indeed, especially since so much can (and should) be done to remedy these problems. That's because...

## SEX AND ROMANCE ARE TERRIFIC FOR YOU AND YOUR HEART

Now that we've delineated what can go wrong and why, let's look at why you should address these issues and not just resign yourself to the "fact" that low libido and sexual dysfunction are a natural part of aging. Beyond the emotional and sensual pleasure, sex within the context of a happy relationship has many physiological benefits. In fact, it can help you live longer. Research at Johns Hopkins University has demonstrated that people who define their relationships as "loving" were much more likely to live into their nineties than those who do not. In fact, couples who enjoy a loving bond *and* increased sexual frequency have greater physical longevity than those who are sexually inactive.[3]

Why should this be so? The answers are emotional as well as chemical and physical. Sexual activities benefit us in many ways. Human touch, a sense of connection, intimacy, love, and bonding are calming and reduce stress. As I explained in Chapter 6, we need these moments of serenity and pleasure to protect ourselves and our hearts from the damage done by ongoing tension and worry.

Besides that, we hit the jackpot in terms of brain chemistry when we experience sexual intimacy and orgasm. It's like plugging our electrical cord into an outlet and recharging. When we are highly stressed, the adrenal glands make cortisol. If we are exposed to high levels of stress over the long term, this constant influence of cortisol ages our brain, our bones, and our cardio-vascular system. On the other hand, touch and cuddling release oxytocin, the bonding hormone, from the pituitary gland in the brain. In many ways, oxytocin acts as an antidote to stress. It has the following benefits:

- It lowers cortisol.
- It increases endorphins.
- It reduces blood pressure.
- It improves the quality of our sleep.
- It improves our intimate relationships as it stimulates emotional bonding.

Since oxytocin has so much value, then yes, you should work to ensure you have an adequate level of this vital hormone.

Not surprisingly then, I am frequently asked, "How often should we have sex?" Clearly this depends upon you—your health, libido, and relationship. But the biological benefits should encourage you to enjoy sex from 2 to 4 times a week, although many factors can come into play in this important decision. *Also keep in mind that from a health perspective, I'm only talking about monogamous relationships, as the health risk of having multiple sexual partners is much higher than the risk of abstaining from sex.*

Finally, as we age, intimacy becomes equally important as having an orgasm, or even more important. Dr. Anna Cabeca explained to me that research with menopausal women shows that fewer than 30% will experience a climax during each sexual act. And if they do, it's pretty short—from 3 to 5 seconds, in contrast to up to 20 seconds for a 20-year-old. If you're in this situation and having an orgasm is your goal, you may be disappointed on occasion, or even repeatedly. However, all is not lost. There are ways to enhance orgasm, as I'll share shortly. Plus the pleasure of intimacy increases oxytocin. Only 20 seconds of hugging or French kissing releases this important hormone, so you can enjoy its health benefits, even without reaching a climax.

---

### What If I Don't Have a Sexual Partner?

Masturbation is a viable choice. As Dr. Cabeca says, "God designed us with erogenous zones. There's no guilt or shame in masturbating." And medically speaking, this activity will provide several of the health benefits noted above. However, for some people this is not an option for a variety of social and/or religious reasons.

If you are in this situation, realize that there are several steps you can take to benefit your heart and raise your oxytocin levels:

* Share a 20-second hug or embrace
* Enjoy deep, belly-shaking laughter
* Play with a child or a pet
* Schedule a 30- to 60-minute massage. It's a great way to increase oxytocin levels

---

## HOW THE 30-DAY HEART TUNE-UP WILL IMPROVE YOUR SEX LIFE

The good news is that there is a great deal we can do with lifestyle and medical therapies to improve your sexual performance. For both men and women, the ability to enjoy sex at least 3 times a week is a good sign that you are healthy and fit. Intimacy also enhances romantic relationships. So how can you apply the 30-Day Heart Tune-Up to improving your sex life? The first step is to optimize your level of fitness and your diet. Second, especially for men, is to build intimacy and tenderness in a relationship. If these steps don't achieve your goals, then additional medical testing and treatments can be very helpful.

There are four important aspects of the program that will help you: overall fitness, food and supplements, romance, and medical intervention, if necessary.

## FITNESS

Active sexual function is like any other athletic activity. The fitter you are, the better you perform. Romantic activity for both genders requires strength, aerobic capacity, and flexibility. If you can't comfortably keep your heart rate in the 130 to 140 beats per minute range for at least 15 to 20 minutes, lovemaking will become a struggle. The following are elements of fitness that will enhance your sexual experience:

- *Circulation:* Because circulation is such an important part of sexual responsiveness, you'll be happy to know that the fitness aspects of the 30-Day Heart Tune-Up will help sexuality greatly. The heart-healing foods listed in Chapter 4 dilate your arteries. The exercise routines are sure to enhance your blood flow as well. Relaxation also increases circulation to all parts of your body. Meditation will improve blood pressure control and enhance circulation. Without a relaxed state of mind, most women don't feel romantic, which obviously affects men too!
- *Endurance:* If their endurance is inadequate, some couples just can't make it long enough to climax. They are too worn out. Or they're so exhausted, they can't enjoy

romance the way they should. The fitness plan will bring your endurance to a new level, so you can both enjoy all types of activities.

- **Strength:** During a long-term loving relationship, you might find yourself in all types of positions. Your partner may not want you to just collapse because you're too fatigued. To be a good lover, you need enough leg, arm, and trunk strength to support yourself for extended periods of time.

- **Flexibility:** Men tend to be less flexible than women, and as they age, they can get stiffer because this aspect of their fitness is often ignored. Sexual activity encourages flexibility, or as my age management medicine colleague and author Dr. Jeff Life has said, "The flexible man is a sexual man." Stretching, Pilates, and yoga are great for your love life. Of course, remaining agile applies to women too.

- **Pelvic Floor Strengthening:** Don't forget Kegel exercises, which strengthen the pelvic floor. In women, these exercises enhance sexual function, increase orgasm frequency and intensity, and help prevent urinary incontinence. In men, Kegel exercises can render erections stronger and harder and help avoid premature ejaculation. To perform a Kegel lift, sit on the toilet to urinate. After the flow starts, squeeze and lift the pelvic floor to stop the urine. This pelvic floor lift is one Kegel contraction. Once you have the feeling down, try 10 Kegel lifts in a row several times a day. With time, build to 30 lifts several times a day. Nobody will know that you are practicing your Kegel exercises each time you stop at a red light, send an e-mail, or chat on the phone.

*Your bottom line is that the 30-Day Heart Tune-Up fitness program will result in a dramatic improvement in your circulation, endurance, strength, flexibility, and mental focus—making you a great lover.*

# NUTRITION AND NATURAL SUPPLEMENTS THAT SUPPORT SEXUALITY

The nutrition arm of the 30-Day Heart Tune-Up will clearly lower inflammation levels and improve circulation. The following nutrients, essential for optimal sexual function, can be augmented by your diet or with supplements:

- arginine for circulation
- zinc for adrenal function
- tyrosine for dopamine production and pleasure

## *Arginine for Better Circulation*

For both genders, sexual arousal and function depend on adequate production of a compound called nitric oxide, which increases blood flow. In men this improves erections. Raising nitric oxide levels is the therapeutic goal of drugs used to treat ED. In women, increased blood flow enhances engorgement, lubrication, and receptivity. Although medications like Viagra, Cialis, and Levitra have become very popular, they also have rare but serious adverse reactions. The good news is that some natural compounds increase nitric oxide levels in your bloodstream and cause your arteries, including those to the genitals, to dilate without any worrisome side effects.

Nitric oxide production depends on the foods we eat. In particular, arginine is an amino acid (protein building block) that converts into nitric oxide. Eat foods high in arginine and expect better arousal. Lean meats, nuts and seeds, dark green leafy veggies, and beans are all high in arginine. Soy protein and shellfish have the greatest concentrations. Happily, all of these foods are an integral part of the 30-Day Heart Tune-Up eating plan.

## Foods with the Highest Arginine Content Per ~200-Calorie Portion[4]

- Soy protein isolate: 3,500 mg per 2 ounces
- Shrimp, clams, oysters, mussels, and crab: 3,000 to 3,500 mg per 5–6 ounces
- Frozen spinach: 3,300 mg (that is a lot of spinach, about 3 cups frozen)
- Turkey breast: 3,000 mg per 4–5 ounces
- Game meat (venison, elk, ostrich): 2,500 to 3,300 mg per 5–6 ounces
- Chicken breast: 3,200 mg per 5–6 ounces
- Fish, white meat: 2,500 mg per 6 ounces

Some of the arginine in food is broken down during digestion. So aim for 3,000 to 5,000 mg of arginine from food daily. Studies have shown that taking 2 to 5 grams of arginine daily in supplement form improves erectile dysfunction symptoms. Very rarely, some men might notice dizziness with this dosage and should contact their physicians. But I've had excellent results treating men with ED by prescribing a 500-mg arginine supplement (Perfusia) twice daily. Don't be surprised if over-the-counter herbal products for ED include arginine in their list of ingredients.

## Caution! If You Have Herpes

People who have herpes may notice more frequent infection outbreaks if taking high dosages of arginine. Many with this condition take lysine daily to prevent outbreaks, because lysine blocks the virus from using arginine to grow and divide. An arginine supplement can potentially reverse this blockage. If you believe arginine helps your sexual function, but you have had more frequent herpes outbreaks when taking arginine, talk to your doctor about using an antiviral medication to prevent infections. This strategy may allow you to continue taking arginine.

Another caveat. You might have heard of other products on the market, about which I urge caution. For instance, clinical studies of ginkgo and ashwagandha (called male ginseng in Asia) show that these supplements don't appear to be more effective than a placebo. What about yohimbine? The bark of the West African yohimbe tree is a source of this compound, which has been found to stimulate blood flow to the penis, increase libido, and decrease the rest period between ejaculations. I do not recommend that you use yohimbine without consulting your medical provider, however, because it has the potential for several adverse reactions, even in small doses. Side effects may include dizziness, anxiety, nausea, a significant drop in blood pressure, abdominal pain, fatigue, hallucinations, and paralysis.

### Don't Forget Zinc for Adrenal Function

As you may recall from Chapter 6, the adrenal glands produce DHEA and cortisol—hormones that help us to deal with stress. If we don't manage our stress, it usually has a negative impact on our sexual function. DHEA is an essential hormone for libido, especially in women. Deficiencies in zinc can lead to poor adrenal performance. A good quality multivitamin will ensure your intake of zinc. But foods on the "Foods Rich in Zinc" list on page 248 provide good sources for this mineral as well.

## Foods Rich in Zinc

- Oysters (The number one source. It's little wonder oysters are called an aphrodisiac!)
- Wheat germ
- Lean beef (zinc isn't in the fat, so select lean cuts from free-range, grass-fed)
- Pumpkin and squash seeds; they are also very rich in magnesium
- Dark chocolate and cocoa (Happily, another reason to enjoy dark chocolate every day!)
- Peanuts
- Crabs

## Don't Miss Tyrosine to Enhance Pleasure

The brain relies on a chemical compound called dopamine to create the sensation of pleasure. This, of course, includes climax. With inadequate dopamine, your ability to experience any kind of physical delight (including that which comes from sexual activity) may be limited. The body requires protein building blocks (amino acids) including tyrosine, L-dopa (levodopa), and/or phenylalanine to make dopamine. But, in fact, tyrosine is by far the most important source. See the "Foods Rich in Tyrosine" list below for food sources.

## Foods Rich in Tyrosine

- Seaweed
- Soy protein
- Egg whites
- Salmon

- Turkey
- Wild game
- Shrimp
- Fish eggs (caviar)

Once you review the heart-healthy recipes in Chapter 10, you will notice that many ingredients rich in arginine, zinc, and tyrosine are featured prominently.

## ROMANCE

Although food and fitness are great for enhancing sexual performance, intimacy is an essential component for wonderful romance. For many men, arousal can start with minimal stimulation. For most women, it is more complicated and depends upon the overall relationship and being relaxed. Most men already know that acts of kindness are essential to building trust and tenderness. A day enriched with a surprise breakfast, hand holding, a bouquet of flowers, a warm cup of tea, and a tidy home go a long way to setting the mood.

It should now be clear to you that having sex is part of stress management because it decreases cortisol while increasing oxytocin. However it is also true that the ability to feel sexual pleasure depends on proper stress management. So remember that the relaxation activities I suggested in Chapter 6 can help in lovemaking. And yoga not only triggers the relaxation response but also contributes to greater flexibility—an asset when you're rolling around in bed.

Your bottom line: Your bedroom should be a playground! Sex should be comfortable, sporting, loving, and fun. Your goal is to create soft, intimate, energetic connections that go a long way toward keeping your heart and the rest of your body healthy.

# MEDICAL THERAPIES TO ENHANCE LOVEMAKING

The lifestyle recommendations I've made will often do wonders for romance. However, if making those fitness, nutrient, and environmental changes doesn't achieve the desired effect, be sure to have your hormone levels checked. Are you ever too old for hormone replacement? No! There are appropriate ways to metabolize them safely. Several medical options can help, although lifestyle treatments should always come first. However, before starting any medical therapy for sexual function, first talk to your doctor. You will need to do the following:

- Ensure that your health screening is up-to-date, as a major illness will appropriately lower your libido. You don't want to delay the diagnosis of a life-threatening problem like cancer or kidney disease because you focused on your sexual function first.
- Learn whether your hormone levels warrant medical intervention.
- Be sure your relationship is nurturing and fulfilling. Consider couples counseling if there are unresolved stressors.
- Be sure that you meet your nutrient and exercise needs. None of these treatments can offset a bad lifestyle, poor diet, and inadequate fitness, yet they can work wonders for people trying to live well.

## For Women

Because women and men have very different sexual equipment and responses, it is not surprising that their treatment options vary too. Women are far more dependent on DHEA for desire and drive than men. This hormone also increases muscle strength and enhances the tissue of the pelvic floor. It is produced by the adrenal glands and drops with chronic, unmanaged stress. It is the "mother hormone" that the body converts to testosterone and estrogen. (Typically, 3 parts of DHEA are converted into testosterone for every 1 part of estrogen formed.) If DHEA levels are low, then taking steps to reduce your stress and/or a supplement is warranted. However, please don't try supplementing with DHEA therapy without seeing your doctor and checking your hormone levels first, as inappropriate hormone manipulations can wreak havoc with many aspects of your hormone balance.

Testosterone levels can also impact drive, energy, and libido in women and are worth testing and treating if they are too low.

Menopause-related and perimenopause-related vaginal skin thinning can be easily treated with either a DHEA or an estriol cream applied just a few times a month. For menopause-related vaginal thinning, there are a few advantages to DHEA compared to estrogen. Both improve lubrication and vaginal dryness. But only DHEA effectively:

- increases vaginal muscle tone
- decreases problems with incontinence (urinary leaking)

These hormones should be prescribed by your physician. DHEA vaginal tablets and cream have been well-studied, and both appear safe and effective. Many of my patients have benefited from using vaginal DHEA tablets, which are less messy than creams. Keep in mind that DHEA will convert to testosterone and estrogen. Even though it's applied on the skin, some will absorb into your bloodstream. So if systemic hormones are dangerous for you (if, for instance you've had estrogen-positive breast cancer) then this may not a viable choice. Again, consult first with your doctor. For people taking a DHEA supplement, I always suggest a blood test at some point to confirm they have reached a safe level, typically aiming for the upper half of the normal range.

If your doctor does recommend vaginal estrogen, estriol is an option to consider. It does not have many of the worrisome side effects of its sister estrogens (estradiol and estrone) that are used to treat hot flashes and insomnia, although it won't reduce hot flashes either. The clinically proven benefits of estriol are mostly related to treating the skin. If your doctor is unfamiliar with estriol, ask him or her to do some research regarding it. Keep in mind that estriol may only be available through a compounding pharmacist.

Like men, women need an increased blood supply to the genital area for stimulation, to enhance receptivity. My colleague Dr. Anna Cabeca has developed a topical sensitivity cream, which I have recently started offering to patients in my clinic. It is an ointment that can be applied 10 to 60 minutes before intercourse. It boosts blood supply and sensation, and helps stimulate lubrication, arousal, and function. The ingredients include a mixture of arginine, naltrexone, pentoxifylline, DMSO (dimethyl sulfoxide), and peppermint oil. It must be prescribed by a physician and is usually sold at a compounding pharmacy that deals with women's health issues.

A prescription for the hormone oxytocin is another possible aid to arousal. It can be taken in several forms, the simplest being 10 units (supplied in a liquid or in a lozenge) administered under the tongue, 10 to 60 minutes before intercourse. As with other medical treatments, it must be prescribed by a physician. Oxytocin enhances bonding, desire, libido, and lubrication. As an extra bonus, it intensifies orgasm. Accordingly, it can be especially helpful for women who have difficulty achieving an orgasm. It also helps with insomnia and anxiety. Remember oxytocin promotes bonding, so make time for cuddling when you take it. And also be sure you're using it with the right man!

### For Men

Men's sexual function also depends on testosterone and on DHEA, although testosterone seems to be a more important hormone for male libido. If these hormonal levels are low, treatment can work wonders.

In 20-year-old men, normal testosterone levels may reach as high as 1,100 mg/dL. But for middle-aged men, the normal range is from 300 to 800 mg/dL. There are two kinds of low testosterone: low *total* testosterone and low *free* testosterone. The first involves one's total testosterone level. The second has to do with how much testosterone is circulating freely. (In this case, the total testosterone level may be normal, but because some of the hormone is bound up with protein, too little is available to do its job.) Because of this factor, some men have low-testosterone symptoms when their testosterone levels are on the low side of normal (below 400 mg/dL), while others don't have symptoms at all even with an abnormally low count of 250 to 300 mg/dL.

If you have symptoms of low testosterone (they include decreases of energy, drive, libido, mental sharpness, sexual function, plus difficulty with weight control) and you have low *total* testosterone, then taking additional testosterone will very often restore normal hormonal function. Keep in mind, though, that this is a long-term treatment plan. Once you begin hormone therapy, your own production may be suppressed over time. This means that therapy is usually lifelong. If you are receiving long-term testosterone therapy, you'll also need more comprehensive medical assessments to monitor how your hormone levels are affected by treatment, and to be sure that related health issues are all well controlled.

For men with normal *total* testosterone levels (preferably levels above 500 mg/dL) but low *free* testosterone, the first step is to optimize their lifestyle, by following the 30-Day Heart Tune-Up. Then reassess levels and function.

In either case, appropriate testosterone therapy will do much more than improve their sexual function, though this may be their primary motive. Men who opt for therapy often notice big improvements in their quality of life as well.

DHEA gives men energy and drive and, as with women, helps with libido and sexual function. The body uses it to produce testosterone. Normally, DHEA levels drop gradually with aging. But if you live with chronic stress for prolonged periods of time, eventually your blood work will show a drop in DHEA levels.

So if you experience low energy and drive, especially if you've been subjected to long-term high stress, I recommend that you have your DHEA measured. Both topical and oral treatments are available, although for your overall well-being, it's also essential to reduce the stressors that caused your hormone levels to drop in the first place.

A warning: In contrast to testosterone, which is only available with a doctor's prescription, you can buy over-the-counter DHEA in tablet form. Yet, because it is a hormone that modifies many others, I recommend taking it only while under a doctor's supervision. You should have your hormones measured before and after treatment. Your physician will know the optimal levels. Without laboratory testing, your DHEA and other hormones may be either too high or too low—resulting in a poor outcome for you.

### What about Viagra, Cialis, Levitra, and Similar Medications?

Once you have talked to your doctor and you've had your medical, cardiovascular, and hormonal evaluation and all the appropriate medical issues have been dealt with, you certainly can use these drugs. (This class of medications are called phosphodieterase-5 inhibitors.) For many men with erectile dysfunction, they provide tremendous benefits. Just make sure you and your doctor discuss all the side effects and options. Keep in mind that if you follow my recommendations for the 30-Day Heart Tune-Up over the years, you may discover you don't need these medications anymore.

All of these treatments can be helpful to restore wonderful sexual function. However, at the risk of repeating myself, I need to emphasize that the primary cause of male erectile dysfunction is cardiovascular disease. So your first step is to assess cardiovascular risk factors and arterial plaque growth.

---

I can summarize this chapter with a simple question: What's better for your health than an apple a day? Well, clearly it's regular sex! And as you now know, it's great for your heart, as well as for your mind, body, and soul.

I hope you've seen how the 30-Day Heart Tune-Up is fantastic for your sex life. While some medical treatments are effective in improving romance, the most important steps to optimizing your sexual function include better fitness, thoughtful nutrient intake, stress management, and building intimacy.

So if you are ready to start the 30-Day Heart Tune-Up, let's focus on the details that will make your next steps to a healthier, stronger, trimmer, and *sexier* you easy, fun, and rewarding!

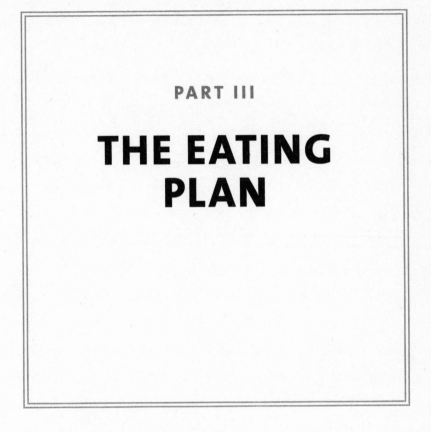

PART III

# THE EATING PLAN

*Chapter Nine*

# Getting Started with the 30-Day Food Plan

During the years I have helped patients transform their lives, I've discovered that they need more than understanding *what* to do. They also need to know *how* to make the changes I recommend. The first and biggest challenge is usually, "Where do I start?" The exercise, stress management, and supplements suggestions in the previous chapters should give you all the tools you need to launch your own 30-Day Heart Tune-Up. Yet adopting and adapting to the new eating plan might present a bigger challenge.

Why? Eating is far more complicated than just putting gas in the car. The social component impacts the people around us, both at home and at work. Our beliefs about what to eat are sometimes as strongly felt as our religious convictions. Also, let's face it, eating well isn't always easy in today's world. If you wait to see what food shows up in front of you, it will probably be junk. It's everywhere—on coworkers' desks, at meetings, after a religious service. You can buy junk food everywhere—the airport, the movie theater, the drug or convenience store, and even the gas station.

You need a plan to succeed with any long-term change. The challenge is to identify healthy foods that you like and can find easily. Then develop a plan to eat more of them more often. One of the keys is being more selective. Instead of eating what might happen to have been set down in front of you, choose to eat something that will help your heart and your overall health.

The first, most critical step is to involve those closest to you. Don't approach this as a plan to change their lives. Just ask for support to help you change yours. Start by explaining your health issues and goals. You want your close friends and family to support you in making the changes required to succeed. If they really care, they will be happy to support you. If you don't seek their involvement, they may sabotage your plans by showing up with pizza, ice cream, cookies, and other special occasion treats you don't want in front of you day after day.

The ten key steps to changing your eating habits are:

1. following our sample eating plan
2. appropriate shopping and meal planning
3. storing food properly
4. having useful kitchen utensils close at hand
5. preparing and cooking food using safe practices
6. eating mindfully
7. knowing how to order when dining out
8. measuring your results
9. having a Plan B
10. sticking with it

## SAMPLE 30-DAY HEART TUNE-UP EATING PLAN

Imagine a buffet that features hearty servings of grilled salmon, scallops, and shrimp along with platters of steamed crab, mussels, oysters, and lobster from pristine waters. There are also platters of sliced chicken and turkey breast seasoned with herbs, pork tenderloin, a roast of free-range bison, sirloin and tenderloin steaks, plus baked quail, pheasant, and other game meats. There are fresh, colorful vegetables and an array of green salads in abundance.

To the left, bowls of blueberries, raspberries, organic peaches, plums, and cherries. To the right, plates laden with luscious red-ripe tomatoes, plump steamed artichokes, and sliced avocados. Here's a tray with almonds, pistachios, pecans, and walnuts and a platter with herb-seasoned wild rice, quinoa with wild mushrooms, and a variety of spicy bean dishes. A golden omelet sprinkled with herbs and sautéed onions decorates yet another plate. Spicy garlic-shrimp kebobs; ceviche tostadas; an artichoke, leek, and mushroom soufflé; curries. What a feast!

For dessert, savor strawberries dipped in dark chocolate, a chocolate-raspberry-orange soufflé, and delicious blueberry-cherry frozen yogurt. To drink with this banquet? Pitchers of iced green tea, elegant red wine, hot cocoa, and pure refreshing water.

Sound fantastic? Too good to be true? Not at all. Welcome to the 30-Day Heart Tune-Up Eating Plan. We will provide you with everything you need including recipes, shopping guides, and food safety recommendations.

The key to changing your eating plan is to choose recipes and food you enjoy and can prepare often. If you don't cook at home, look for equivalents on restaurant menus—say a cioppino at an Italian restaurant—it's mostly fish and seafood in a very tasty tomato broth. Most people only make some variation of 10 to 12 dinner options each month, so don't worry if you don't like everything. Rather, focus on the dishes that appeal to you. If you choose only 8 new dinner recipes and you use them often, you'll change your eating habits by up to 80%!

The following will give you a sample of how the eating plan might look over a week. You'll find that you'll be enjoying fish and seafood 3 times a week and beans 4 or 5 times. You'll get plenty of vegetables and fruit and some nuts each day, although for some dinners, I recommend eating lean protein and vegetables but skipping the starch altogether. You'll be adding a variety of herbs and spices to pack your food with vital nutrients, but also to increase the flavor and fragrance. You'll get to enjoy chocolate and red wine too. If you've got a busy work schedule, you might get into the habit of preparing soups on the weekend. Then you'll have a hearty and quick lunch or snack available whenever you want it. Besides, a soup's flavor often improves with time, so it makes great leftovers. For protein sources in addition to fish, you'll be relying on nonfat dairy products and lean cuts of chicken, beef, and pork. But that shouldn't stop you if you're a vegetarian or vegan. This eating plan is readily adaptable to your eating habits. The 🕐 means "quick and easy."

## SAMPLE MENUS FOR THE 30-DAY HEART TUNE-UP FOOD PLAN

### Day 1

*Breakfast*
  Steel-Cut Oatmeal with Berries (page 287) 🕐
  Tea or coffee

*Lunch*
  Grilled Chicken over Mixed Greens and Vegetables (page 293)
  Masley House Vinaigrette Dressing (page 344), 2 Tbsp 🕐
  Iced tea

*Afternoon Snack*
  An apple, 1 ounce almonds, with pure water or green tea

*Dinner*
  Grilled Salmon with Lemon, Chili, Brown Sugar, and Dill
    (page 312)
  Brown rice, ¾ cup
  Broccoli and Shiitake Mushroom Sauté (page 331), 1 cup 🕐
  Mixed green salad with ½ cup garbanzo beans and 2 Tbsp
    vinaigrette dressing
  Seltzer

*Dessert*
  Protein, Berry, Milk, and Flax Smoothie (page 285) 🕐

*Optional Rescue Snack*
  Hummus with sliced veggies

## Day 2

**Breakfast**
Protein, Berry, Milk, and Flax Smoothie (page 285) 🕐
Tea or coffee

**Lunch**
Turkey breast sliced, 5–6 ounces, wrapped with at least 1 cup of
   sliced tomatoes and lettuce, plus optional mustard or salsa
Two corn tortillas or one whole wheat wrap
Orange
Iced green tea

**Optional Afternoon Snack**
Carrots and/or celery sticks, 1 cup
Pure water

**Dinner**
Chicken Stir-Fry with Orange-Ginger Sauce (page 300)
Decaf green or black tea, or water

**Dessert**
Sliced apple, 1 ounce dry-roasted almonds, 1 ounce dark chocolate

**Optional Rescue Snack**
Black Bean Dip (page 298) with sliced veggies 🕐

## Day 3

**Breakfast**
Protein, Berry, Milk, and Flax Smoothie (page 285) 🕐
Tea or coffee

**Lunch**
Turkey (or vegetarian) Chili (page 323)
Mixed organic salad with Italian dressing (on the side)
Seltzer or iced tea

**Afternoon Snack**
Nonfat cottage cheese, ½ cup, or nonfat yogurt, ½ cup, with fresh
   fruit, 1 cup
Pure water

### Dinner

Cod with Hazelnut Crust (page 321)
Wild Rice with Kale and Wild Mushrooms (page 333)
Mixed green salad, 2–3 cups
Vinaigrette dressing, 2 Tbsp
Seltzer or water

### Dessert

Sliced melon, 1 cup
Hot cocoa

### Optional Rescue Snack

Edamame and Sliced Bell Peppers (page 296), 1 cup 🕐

## Day 4

### Breakfast

Omelet with Artichoke Hearts, Spinach, and Green Onions
(page 286) 🕐
Tea or coffee

### Lunch

Bean Taquitos (page 294) 🕐
Cherries, grapes, or berries, 1 cup
Iced green tea

### Optional Afternoon Snack

Salmon Spread with Hummus (page 296) with carrot and celery
sticks, 1 cup 🕐
Pure water

### Dinner

Mediterranean Sea Scallops (page 304)
Steamed Vegetables with Orange Vinaigrette Dressing
(page 336) 🕐
Organic mixed greens, 2 cups, with Italian dressing, 2 Tbsp
Red wine, 1 serving
Pure water or decaf green or black tea

### Dessert

Yogurt, berries, and dark chocolate

*Optional Rescue Snack*
  Hard-boiled organic, omega-3-enriched egg
  Veggie sticks

## Day 5

*Breakfast*
  Protein, Berry, Milk, and Flax Smoothie (page 285) 🕐
  Tea or coffee

*Lunch*
  Chicken Salad (page 290) with mixed greens 🕐
  Fresh fruit, 1 cup
  Iced green tea

*Optional Afternoon Snack*
  Hummus, ¼ cup, with carrot and celery sticks, 1 cup
  Pure water

*Dinner*
  Italian Seafood Stew (page 315)
  Organic mixed greens with Italian dressing, 2 Tbsp
  Red wine, 1 serving
  Pure water

*Dessert*
  Nonfat yogurt with fresh berries

*Optional Rescue Snack*
  Hard-boiled organic, omega-3-enriched egg
  Veggie sticks

## Day 6

*Breakfast*
  Mexican Scrambled Eggs with Black Beans, Salsa, and Corn
    Tortillas (page 288) 🕐
  Tea or coffee

*Lunch*
  Manhattan Clam Chowder (page 292)
  Orange
  Iced green tea

*Optional Afternoon Snack*
   Dark chocolate, 1 ounce
   Almonds, 1 ounce

*Dinner (Optional Restaurant Night)*
   Mixed green salad with house vinaigrette dressing (served on the
      side; use 1½ to 2 Tbsp)
   Grilled Sirloin and Shrimp (Surf and Turf) (page 308); double the
      vegetables, skip the starch, no butter or margarine product on
      anything
   Red wine, 1 serving
   Water
   Frozen Blueberry-Cherry Yogurt (page 339) 🕐

*Optional Rescue Snack*
   Apple, sliced

## Day 7

*Breakfast*
   2 Oatmeal and Dried Fruit Muffins (page 286)
   Tea or coffee

*Lunch*
   Crab Salad (page 290) 🕐
   Pear, Peach, and Blueberry Crumble (page 341)
   Iced green tea

*Optional Afternoon Snack*
   Split Pea and Barley Soup (page 294)

*Dinner*
   Roasted Chicken with Wine and Rosemary (page 304)
   Roasted Beets and Squash (page 333)
   Tossed green salad with vinaigrette dressing, 1½ to 2 Tbsp
   Wine, 1 serving
   Pure water

*Dessert*
   Chocolate-Raspberry-Orange Soufflé (page 338)

*Optional Rescue Snack*
   Edamame and Sliced Bell Peppers (page 296) 🕐

# SHOPPING AND MEAL PLANNING

Perhaps your biggest challenge in adjusting how you eat is changing how you shop. Your trip down the food aisles with a grocery cart can make the difference between health and vitality, and weight gain and your demise. Assuming you have the support of the people you live with to follow this program, if you don't buy junk, you won't find it in the house, and you won't be able to grab for it when you're hungry.

Most of us shop and buy based on patterns we've established over the years. Before you set off to do your grocery shopping, you probably already know which store you'll visit, what items you'll buy, and where they are in the store. We are creatures of habit. So let's build a better food-buying style.

Check your supplies at home. See what you have in the refrigerator and in the cupboards. Compare that with some of the new recipes you have selected to try. If you plan to ease into this new eating plan, you can finish the food you find on your shelves. However, if you are ready to transform your health immediately for the better, I encourage you to consider the following: *Throw away the bad stuff!* The chips, the candy, the pretzels, the bacon, the fatty cheese spread. Out they go! Yes, I know it's wasteful, but really what's more important: a few dollars lost on heart-damaging processed foods you should not eat, or your health? To me this is a no-brainer.

When you start this program, you will probably need a shopping list, especially for the first 30 days or until the recipes become second nature to you. Clarify which spices, oils, and other staples you have on hand and which ones you'll need to buy. If the ingredients in my recipes are new to you, adding new staples can be a bit pricey, so don't be surprised by your first expenditure. Buying new bottles of spices and containers of protein powder can double your first shopping bill, but look at these as onetime purchases. It will take a while before you need to replenish your stock of balsamic vinegar or bottles of dried Italian herbs and almond oil.

As much as possible, aim to buy organic products. Yes, I know they're more expensive, but again the question becomes, what's in the best interest of your heart and cardiovascular system? If you have access to a health food store, this will make shopping easier, but most national grocery chains do carry organic meat, produce, and canned goods these days.

Speaking of cans, unfortunately, the interior of the cans U.S. food manufacturers use is often coated with a plastic that contains the substance bisphenol A (BPA), a known carcinogen. If you want to avoid ingesting this, I suggest that you soak and cook dried beans yourself rather than relying on canned products. This is less convenient, so I offer recipes with canned as well as home-cooked beans. Italian tomato sauce, whole tomatoes, and other products imported from Europe are typically sold in BPA-free cans, so you may want to look for these brands.

---

### Essentials You'll Need for the Basic Recipes in This Book

**Condiments:** dijon mustard, balsamic and red wine vinegar, salsa, low-sodium tamari sauce (or low-sodium soy sauce), hot sauce, cornstarch, limes and lemons or their juices, low-sodium vegetable or chicken broth, tamarind chutney sauce

**Protein powder:** for breakfast shakes (see "Food Sources and Links," page 364)

**Oils:** virgin olive oil for cooking and extra virgin olive oil for salads; nut oils, such as almond, walnut, or hazelnut oil (in a glass bottle, not plastic); sesame or coconut oil for flavor

**Beverages:** green tea, pure water in glass (not plastic), some form of milk (almond, coconut, soy, or nonfat organic cow's milk)

**Beans:** (canned or dried) black, red, cannellini, garbanzos (chickpeas), lentils, and refried pinto beans. Aim to buy canned products without bisphenol A (BPA), a known carcinogen, if you can.

---

**Spices:** Italian herbs (or fines herbes, or Herbes de Provence), sea salt, whole black peppercorns for a hand grinder, curry spices or red chili flakes, ground cumin, dried oregano, ground paprika, ground cayenne, garlic, cinnamon, fresh gingerroot

**Fresh herbs:** Even if you don't have a backyard, or porch, I highly recommend that you create a patio garden or east-facing window herb garden. Plant parsley, basil, cilantro, rosemary, and dill. Fresh herbs are expensive, and growing them yourself will provide big savings. They also look wonderful in their little pots, and are fairly easy to cultivate from seeds or seedlings.

**Eggs:** Buy omega-3-enriched, organic eggs from free-range, (flaxseed-fed) chickens.

**Chicken and meat:** Rely on free-range, organic chickens and grass-fed, organic beef whenever it is feasible. They are lower in pesticide residues and other toxins.

## OTHER SHOPPING TIPS

Snacks are optional. If you can live happily with three meals a day, then please don't feel obligated to add snacks! Some people can't control their hunger with just three meals, so they need to plan a healthy snack. For the 30-Day Heart Tune-Up, please make an effort to avoid junk foods like chips, crackers, candy, ice cream, cookies, and other prepared desserts. For just 30 days (you can make 30 days!), focus on giving up the junk and nourishing yourself with healthy food. If you need a snack, then keep nuts (almonds, pecans, pistachios, and walnuts), fruit (splurge on berries and other fruits you enjoy), and nonfat yogurt in the house. Don't forget to try some of the snacks in the recipe section too (see pages 296 to 298).

Desserts are optional and are best saved for special occasions or when you're with company. But feel free to have nonfat plain yogurt with fruit, dark chocolate, and nuts every day. Those foods are on the 30-Day Heart Tune-Up eating plan, and they are good for you.

Frozen meals come in handy when your cupboards are bare and you are hungry. But ensure that you have healthy options—see "Helpful Resources," page 363, for details. You should also keep frozen berries for your smoothies and packs of frozen vegetables to add to meals if your supply of fresh vegetables has run out and you don't have time to go marketing.

When you shop for fresh produce, make sure you buy enough. Your goal is to eat at least 5 cups of vegetables and fruits every day, not just for the 30-Day Heart Tune-Up, but forever. Eating more vegetables and fruits daily slows aging, helps with weight control, and is fantastic for your heart. Plan on 2 pieces of fruit (or 1 piece of fruit and 1 cup of berries), plus 3 cups of vegetables a day.

Also be sure to have lean protein stored for your meals. Your refrigerator and freezer should be stocked with chicken and turkey breasts, scallops, shrimp, vacuum-packed salmon. Have something thawing for dinner in the refrigerator along with eggs (organic, from free-range, flaxseed-fed chickens) and nonfat yogurt.

## FOOD STORAGE

This should be the easy part, but there is a critical step for produce. Vegetables and fruits need washing when you first bring them from the store. Far too often, people throw the produce in the bottom of the fridge and plan to wash it later, when they're ready to eat it. Unfortunately, often this doesn't happen. Moreover, your produce crispers may develop a buildup of pesticides and bad bacteria that can make you sick if you continually put unwashed produce in them.

It's best to wash your fruits and vegetables in the kitchen sink before putting them in the fridge. Fill the sink with cold water and add a few drops of hand soap to generate some bubbles. Place the organic produce in the "bath" first. Soak a couple minutes and agitate them in the water. Rinse off the soap and allow to drain. Then swish the remaining produce, rinse, and drain. Put everything in a clean refrigerator. When you wash your produce, you remove up to 90% of the pesticides, and help reduce any rare risk for bacterial contamination as well. However, you shouldn't wash mushrooms or berries because they don't save well when they're wet. Keep these in a container or plastic bag and wash them when you use them. Onions and potatoes are stored in a wire basket, and these are washed before use as well.

Put fresh herbs, celery, and carrots in sealed, airtight containers with a little water. They stay much fresher this way.

## KITCHEN UTENSILS

You do not need a gourmet, high-cost kitchen to create delicious meals. All of the recipes in this book were created in my home kitchen. In addition to testing performed by a few professional chefs with restaurants, several home cooks have retested them in a variety of everyday kitchens with regular ovens, ordinary pots and pans, and simple utensils. But there are a few items that I find essential and time-saving. It goes without saying that all the utensils and surfaces in your kitchen should be washed with hot, soapy water, especially before and after handling meat, fish, chicken, and eggs.

- More than any kitchen tool, you'll need a high-quality, sharp knife. This should last a lifetime, so let yourself splurge at the kitchen equipment store when you buy one. I like a chopping blade (a real chef's knife) that is at least 8 or 9 inches long and 1.5 inches wide at the base. You'll also need a knife sharpener to keep the blade in top condition.
- A large, solid cutting board complements a knife. I always run out of space and have two cutting boards on hand. If you use one that slides out from under the counter, pull it out and place it firmly on a damp hand towel on the counter. Now you have a solid surface to cut on. Make sure

to wash the cutting board with hot soapy water before and after food preparation.

- A good blender is essential for making smoothies and sauces. A food processor is an added tool that makes cooking in quantity much easier. It's terrific for making sauces and for julienning vegetables (cutting them into narrow strips).

- Nonstick skillets and/or sauté pans allow you to cook without using too much oil. You'll need at least one large stainless steel pot for soups and boiling water, as well as a couple of saucepans. I avoid aluminum pots and pans. There is insufficient scientific data to condemn them outright; however, stainless steel or Calphalon hard-anodized pans are clearly superior.

- Extra measuring spoons, measuring cups, and bottles come in handy. A squirt bottle for oil allows me to use much less oil when cooking.

- See-through sealable containers are great for storing food. The best are made of glass with a plastic lid. When you reheat food, don't reheat in plastic, because it literally leaks chemicals into your food. When you're using a microwave, always place your food in glass or ceramic containers.

- Other simple essential tools include a small paring knife, an eggbeater, a peeler, and a grater that can be used to grate cheese but also lemon or lime rind into zest.

## FOOD PREPARATION TECHNIQUES

*Cooking times:* The cooking times suggested in the recipes assume you have all the ingredients in the kitchen and that they are ready to use. They also assume that you are proficient at chopping vegetables. You don't need to be a professional chef. Since most of the recipes were tested by a variety of home cooks, the times are realistic. If cooking is new to you, or you are not handy with a knife, you might need to double the prep times that I have provided in the recipes. You also might use a food processor to speed the job of preparation.

You will note in the recipe section that if a recipe requires less than 20 minutes to prepare and is fairly easy to make, it will be highlighted with an icon of a clock with the hand on 20 minutes.

*Caution when preparing raw animal protein:* Raw animal protein (fish, chicken, beef) has the potential to carry bacteria that can make you sick. Always wash all surfaces well that were in contact with raw animal protein. Don't forget your hands! And be sure not to reuse any marinade as a sauce. If the raw fish or chicken has soaked in it, any bacteria that was on the meat will transfer to it.

*Caution when grilling animal protein:* When you barbecue fish, meat, or poultry, the fat drips out of the flesh, hits the high heat, and is converted into a fine mist of heterocyclic amines. These stick to the animal flesh. This mist is packed with cancer-causing compounds. There is a simple solution to this problem. Marinate all animal protein for 10 to 15 minutes in an acidic solution (lime, lemon, or orange juice; vinegar; Italian dressing; or teriyaki sauce) before grilling. This will sear the flesh surface chemically and will reduce heterocyclic amine formation by 75% to 80%. Not only does this reduce the cancer potential from grilling, but when the fat doesn't drip out, the meat, chicken, and fish stay juicier. This is why restaurants marinate their fish, poultry, and meats and why all of my recipes suggest marinating before barbecuing or grilling.

*Don't smoke the pan:* When heating a pan, you don't want the oil to get so hot that it smokes. Smoked oil is damaged and contains nasty compounds, some of which are carcinogens. But if it does happen, don't fear. Take the pan off the heat, carefully wipe it clean with a paper towel, and start again. To prevent this from occurring, make sure to heat your pan first. Then add the oil and let it spread over the surface of the pan. Place the food in the pan before any smoking occurs. If you add the oil to a room-temperature pan, the oil gradually heats and has a greater chance of being overcooked and smoking.

*Use the right oil:* Extra virgin olive oil smokes easily, so I don't use it when cooking on heat higher than low to medium. Instead, I use virgin olive oil for medium-high to high heat sautéing. I do enjoy using high-quality extra virgin olive oil in salads and drizzled over certain dishes. The extra virgin has more flavor and more nutrients, so it is worth having both in the kitchen. Nut oils, such as almond oil, can also tolerate medium-high heat. Coconut oil has the highest smoke point and is an excellent choice when cooking with high heat. However, how coconut oil impacts your lipid profile is controversial. Yes, it actually improves healthy HDL cholesterol levels and improves the total/HDL ratio, yet there are no scientific publications at the time of this writing clarifying how it impacts the size of LDL or the type of HDL. So for the moment, I only use coconut oil on occasion, relying on olive oil with its proven health benefits, and I use many nut oils as well. On occasion, I'll use sesame oil for the flavor, so I add small amounts after cooking.

It's also important to emphasize that I only buy cooking oil in glass bottles. Avoid those that come in plastic, as the nasty chemicals in plastic will penetrate into the oil.

## MINDFUL EATING

- Do you sometimes overeat, to the point you feel uncomfortably full?
- Do you binge eat?
- Do you overeat when you are stressed, bored, mad, or tired?
- Do you make a healthy eating plan, but then surrender to junk foods that you carefully intended to avoid?
- Do you find yourself sneaking food so others won't notice?

If you answered yes to any of these questions, you may be struggling with the "eat-repent-repeat cycle," a term coined by my colleague and friend Michelle May, MD. Her work is focused on helping people break free of mindless and emotional eating. Until you have a handle on these eating habits, what you eat may be less critical. As Dr. May explains in her book, *Eat What You Love, Love What You Eat*, mindful eating will help you recognize not just what you eat, but why, when, and how you eat, because these factors have a major impact on your decisions about what type of food to consume, and how much. Once you are able to eat mindfully, you can refocus your energy on meeting your nutrient needs. The 30-Day Heart Tune-Up eating plan is a great place to start.

If you don't eat mindfully, then you risk gorging on foods you don't want and feeling worse than you did before you took that first bite. In today's society, we are surrounded by a hostile food environment. Far too often, excessive amounts of food are within reach, the food quality is poor, and our schedules don't allow for proper, nutritious meals.

Here are my suggestions for eating mindfully:

- *Step 1:* Ask yourself prior to placing that first bite in your mouth, "Am I hungry?" Clarify for yourself whether you're about to eat because you need fuel, because it is socially required, or because you are upset or stressed out. This doesn't mean you can't/shouldn't eat, but if you're unclear about "why" you are, you risk uncontrolled eating and subsequent regret. If you are not hungry but are in a situation in which eating socially is required, select a small portion, perhaps the 3-bite taste.
- *Step 2:* Reserve a space for eating, but not in front of the television or the computer, not in your car, and not at your desk. If you are lucky, sit at a proper table with a loved one whom you want to spend time with.

- *Step 3:* To eat mindfully, be sure you look at, smell, taste, and feel each and every bite of food in your mouth. Observe the presentation. Is your plate colorful, and does the amount match your appetite? How does it smell? As you slip the first bite across your lips, how does it feel and taste? Hopefully it's delicious. If not, before taking a second bite, ask yourself, "Do I really want more, or would I like something else?" Switch from one item on your plate to another and appreciate the differences in each bite.
- *Step 4:* If you are eating with another person, talk about the food you are both enjoying.

If you practice mindful eating, you will eat less, enjoy your food more, and make better choices. In contrast, if you eat mindlessly (in front of the television, for example), you may inhale the food without tasting or smelling it. Clearly, this can lead to overeating—perhaps to the point that you are uncomfortable. And without being mindful, you may eat foods you would not have normally chosen. To take care of your heart, the most mindful thing you can do is to pay attention: Stick to the portions of heart-healthy foods that I recommend in the eating plan. Savor each bite. And enjoy!

## DINING OUT

It is a pleasure to eat out. There's nothing to cook, no table to set, no dishes to clean—just sit back and be served. The challenge is being served food the way you want it prepared. Fortunately, it is much easier to customize your meal these days, and some restaurants even advertise that you can have your dish your way.

Fast food is the biggest challenge, because there is little room to modify your order so that it's good for your heart. Perhaps the simplest option is to choose a salad, with a lean protein and a healthy dressing (such as Italian or a vinaigrette dressing) on the side. That way, you can control how much dressing you add.

At a sandwich stop, be sure to request a whole-grain bread (such as whole wheat) and extra lean protein. Skip the cheese. You'll hardly taste it, and sandwich cheese is usually bad quality. *If you are going to treat yourself to a little cheese on occasion, be sure it is good quality, preferably organic, and that you can taste it, such as a little goat cheese crumbled on a beautiful salad.* Say yes to mustard but hold the mayo. Extra veggies (tomato, peppers, lettuce) are encouraged, of course. When offered the "free" bag of chips, buy a piece of fruit or a salad instead. Remember, 350 calories wasted on chips aren't "free." You'll have to spend an extra 30 to 40 minutes exercising in order to burn off that junk. More important than the calories in chips is that they dissolve into sugar when eaten, so they are much more like candy than food. I equate chips with a very occasional treat. And far too often there are those artery-damaging trans fats to reckon with in chips. So if they contain embalming fluid, don't touch them.

In a restaurant, you should have many more options. The most important thing to remember is that you are not limited to the menu—it is just an ingredient list from which you can select what you want to eat. As you scan for what you'd like, avoid anything with the following words attached to the description: *breaded, fried, creamy, crunchy,* or *crispy.* That generally means they've ruined the food as far as you're concerned! When it comes to communicating with the server, follow my favorite tips:

1. When the server tries to put a bowl of chips or bread on your table, pass it up and ask for a salad with the house vinaigrette dressing instead. Be sure to add, "Dressing on the side, please."

2. Read the whole menu to identify what kinds of lean protein they are offering. Decide which you would like. Hopefully you are looking at options such as a chicken breast, pork tenderloin, scallops, shrimp, petite sirloin, or some kind of low-mercury fish. How would you like that protein prepared for you? Baked, grilled, sautéed? They might even have a vegetarian item you'd like to order—but be careful. Even a vegetarian dish could mean

trouble if it's covered in melted cheese or is described as "au gratin." If the lean protein comes with a sauce—especially anything with butter or cream, ask for it "on the side."

3. See what vegetables are available and clarify with your server whether there is a vegetable of the day. Ask for it steamed with a little house vinaigrette on the side (not butter), or sautéed with virgin olive oil. Be sure to *double the vegetable portion!*

4. Skip the starch in exchange for the double vegetable portion. However, if wild rice, quinoa, or baked sweet potatoes are on the menu (without butter or a creamy sauce), then you would be safe ordering these side dishes.

5. It's critical to clarify that you don't want butter or margarine on anything. If an oil is needed for cooking, a little virgin olive oil would be okay.

You should have little problem ordering like this today, whether you've stopped into a casual spot or you're having a festive night out at a high-end restaurant. Many people are health conscious, and the server should be accustomed to special requests like yours.

---

### *What to Say to Your Server*

"Instead of the bread, I'd like a mixed green salad with your house vinaigrette on the side. Then I'll have the surf and turf. Please double the vegetables and skip the baked potato. And please no butter or Crisco on anything, although a little virgin olive oil would be just fine."

The appropriate answer from the server would be, "Excellent choices. What would you like to drink?"

When it comes time for dessert, unless you are celebrating a special occasion or they have a mixed berry dessert option, the best choice is to skip it. Instead, have a piece of dark chocolate when you get home.

---

## MEASURING YOUR RESULTS

One of the most important aspects of your improvement is to measure your progress. With the 30-Day Heart Tune-Up, I propose that you track three key aspects of your health:

- your fitness
- your fiber intake
- your nutrient needs

You should perform the fitness testing as you start the program, when you are ready to jump from Phase Two (your heart recovery rate is 25 beats per minute) to Phase Three, when you begin interval training (burst workouts), and ideally one month after you have begun interval training. With the program, you should see a dramatic improvement in your fitness. Long-term, I'd suggest you retest yourself after three months, six months, and then yearly. Over time it should become easier and easier to do this type of testing. Once again, let your doctor recommend whether you need to do fitness testing with a physician, with an exercise physiologist, in the gym, or on your own.

Measuring your fiber intake is much easier. Use Appendix IV, "Fiber Content of Common Foods" (page 360), or the fiber tool on the www.hearttuneup.com website, to calculate your fiber intake. You should get at least 30 grams of fiber daily; 30 to 50 grams daily is optimal. I recommend you calculate your fiber intake when you start the program, after 30 days, and then yearly.

Next, clarify how you are meeting your key heart nutrient needs. Are you getting an appropriate multivitamin daily? Do you meet your appropriate intake for fish oil, magnesium, vitamin D, vitamin K, and potassium from food, as outlined in Chapter 7? If not, use the information in that chapter to clarify your appropriate supplement requirements.

Measuring your results is a key step to ensuring your success.

# WHAT IF YOU DON'T MEET YOUR GOALS?
# PLAN B IS AN ELIMINATION DIET

At least 80% of my patients achieve their weight, fitness, and laboratory goals by following this program. Since I'm monitoring them, and they check in with me, they are motivated to stay on task. Unfortunately, a few don't. The most common reason people can't meet their goals even when they have given it a serious effort is because they have an unidentified food intolerance. These can cause major health problems.

Perhaps 10% to 15% of my patients have unidentified food intolerances that result in many chronic and unexplained health problems, as well as resistance to weight loss. I uncover these allergies using a 4-week elimination diet.

Far too often, I will meet new patients who have had major, debilitating problems for years. They suffer from brain fog, low energy, terrible gastrointestinal problems, skin rashes, and sometimes even severe neurological problems. They have seen 4 or 5 medical specialists, have had endless testing, but nothing relieved their symptoms. Typically they were labeled "depressed" and treated with anti-anxiety or antidepressant medications that only made them feel worse.

More than half the time, if I ask patients with multiple stubborn chronic health problems to add activity, get enough sleep, and try an elimination diet for one month, their lives are transformed. Most of their symptoms disappear, and their vitality is restored.

So for anyone with unexplained health problems, please consider a one-month trial of an elimination diet. From my functional medicine training, I call this the Comprehensive Elimination Diet, which is a dietary program designed to clear the body of foods and chemicals you may be allergic or sensitive to, and at the same time improve your body's ability to handle and dispose of these substances. It is called an elimination diet because I am asking you to remove certain foods and food categories from your diet. The rationale is that these modifications allow your body's detoxification machinery, which may be overburdened or compromised, to recover and begin to function efficiently again. The dietary changes help the body eliminate or clear various toxins that may have accumulated due to environmental exposure, foods, beverages, drugs, alcohol, or cigarette smoking.

I have found this process to be generally well tolerated and extremely beneficial. There is really no typical or normal response. Most often, individuals on an elimination diet report weight loss, increased energy, mental alertness, decrease in muscle or joint pain, and a general sense of improved well-being. However, some people report some initial reactions to the diet, especially in the first week, as their bodies adjust to a different dietary program. Symptoms you may experience in the first week or so can include changes in sleep patterns, light-headedness, headaches, joint or muscle stiffness, and changes in gastrointestinal function. Such symptoms rarely last for more than a few days.

The simplest form of this diet would be to eliminate all dairy and gluten (gluten sources include wheat, rye, and barley) for four weeks. Since food allergies stimulate your immune system even in minute portions, it doesn't mean cutting down on them. Rather it means *totally avoiding* them for at least one month. The biggest problem with an elimination diet is usually getting people to try it. But fortunately, this has recently changed.

To date, the best and most practical elimination program is one that has been developed by my dear colleague and friend JJ Virgin. Her *Virgin Diet* book has made following an elimination eating plan easy and sexy. And she provides all the tools to succeed.[1]

## YOU HAVE COME SO FAR

As you adopt the 30-Day Heart Tune-Up, you'll find that your life will improve in so many ways. Your new eating habits—including healthy fats, adequate fiber, lean protein, beneficial beverages, and fabulous flavors in your daily menu—will help you feel more energetic and revitalized, even as you lower your blood sugar, improve your cholesterol profile, decrease inflammation, and clear your arteries of dangerous plaque. In addition, following the new recipes I have created can add a sense of adventure to your life. After all, not only is eating the same old artery-damaging foods, week in and week out, bad for your health—it can also be downright boring!

The 30-Day Heart Tune-Up exercise regimen will provide you with much more stamina, strength, and flexibility, not to mention a slimmer and more toned body. As you track your improvements, you'll see how this program is self-reinforcing. The more you can do, the more you'll want to do. And your blood pressure, heart, and arteries will benefit from the change. Just remember to begin within your comfort zone and progress slowly. Those who push forward too enthusiastically can become injured and may abandon the program altogether. I don't want you to go there! So easy does it, as your body adapts to the changes you're asking it to make. Soon enough, you'll be powering forward.

As stress can be damaging to your health in so many ways, you will enjoy the relaxation and peace that comes with the Heart Tune-Up's self-care program. Adequate sleep, daily meditation, exercise, and moments of joy will make your life so much more pleasurable. But I have some ulterior motives here: Stress can lead to habits that injure your cardiovascular system. When you're upset, you may seek out comfort foods, which can set into motion a downward spiral: the worse you feel, the less you exercise, the more poorly you eat, the worse you feel, and so on. So be sure to initiate a stress-reduction program that suits your life—one that also includes a healthy dose of sexual activity, if possible.

Finally, you may have been unfamiliar with the many benefits of a supplement program. No one eats well all the time. The supplements I recommend will enhance and reinforce your new healthy lifestyle by providing some nutrients that you may be lacking. The judicious use of these supplements can improve your heart health in many ways, reducing inflammation and cholesterol levels, protecting your arteries, boosting your energy, and modulating your blood pressure. Just confirm with your doctor that the supplements you're planning to take meet your unique needs for fiber, fish oil, magnesium, vitamin D, vitamin K, and potassium.

## STICKING WITH IT!

The 30-Day Heart Tune-Up is so much more than a 30-day plan. It is a system you can follow your whole life. This isn't a short-term diet, but a life-enhancing strategy that also includes getting fit, managing your stress, and following a personalized supplement regimen. Because you'll be eating delicious foods that nourish your heart, body, mind, and soul, the habit of adding fiber, healthy fats, lean protein, beneficial beverages, and fabulous flavors soon will become a welcome part of your lifestyle. And it will stay that way for decades to come, since you'll feel better and your cardiovascular health will improve.

As we age, we gradually lose aerobic capacity and fitness. The challenge then is to achieve our best fitness level feasible, and maintain that as long as possible, minimizing any decline over time. Now that I'm nearly 60, I'm not trying to beat my fitness scores from when I was 40. But I am trying to hold on to a high level of fitness for as long as I can. The fitness markers you discovered in Chapter 5 are tools you can use regularly the rest of your life.

To make your change as easy as possible, I have added a resource section following the appendices. Please review the list to help you find more options that empower you to follow the 30-Day Heart Tune-Up, not just for 30 days, but for a lifetime.

Be sure to include your physician as a partner in your progress. Many laboratory markers are critical for you to follow in order to clarify how you are aging. Use your physician as a resource to help you make good choices along the way.

The most important step to sticking with this program and ensuring your success is how you involve your family and friends in the process. It's critical to outline your goals with them and identify why these goals are important to you, especially if you live with people who shop and cook for you. The good news is that this program offers optimal health to men and women, young and old, adults and children. So what is good for your health will actually be good for theirs as well.

You can prevent and even reverse heart disease. You can turn back the clock on aging so that you feel younger, trimmer, fitter, mentally sharper, and sexier. You will start feeling the difference in 30 days or less. That's the promise of the 30-Day Heart Tune-Up. I wish you well on your new adventure toward improved health and well-being.

*To your health and bon appétit!*
*Steven Masley, MD*

## Chapter Ten

# 60 Heart-Healing Recipes

**B R E A K F A S T S**

## Protein, Berry, Milk, and Flax Smoothie 🕐

Great with breakfast, for a snack, or as dessert. This is my breakfast 4 to 5 days a week. Yum!

**Prep Time: 2 minutes**

*Serves 1 (makes 2½ cups)*

1½ cups calcium-fortified almond, coconut, soy, or nonfat organic cow's milk

1 cup frozen berries or fruit (blueberries, raspberries, pitted cherries, etc.)

1 Tbsp ground flaxseed (or chia seeds)

1 scoop protein powder (20–30 grams: whey, rice-pea protein, or soy)

Combine ingredients in blender and process at the highest setting. To make your cleanup easier, rinse the blender immediately.

**Nutrient Content per Serving:**

| Calories: | 335 | Fiber: | 7.7 grams | Sodium: | 335 mg |
|---|---|---|---|---|---|
| Protein: | 33.4 grams | Fat: | 11.2 grams | Carbs: | 26.6 grams |
| Saturated Fat: | 1.7 grams | Fat %: | 30% | | |

# Omelet with Artichoke Hearts, Spinach, and Green Onions 🕐

I have fun making this omelet, as it is quick, easy, and fills the kitchen with a lovely herb fragrance—enough to entice family members to join me.

**Prep Time: 10 minutes**
*Serves 2*

1 tsp virgin olive oil, divided

½ cup drained and chopped artichoke hearts packed in olive oil

1 cup fresh spinach

2 green onions, chopped

⅛ tsp sea salt

⅛ tsp ground black pepper

½ tsp dried Italian herbs (oregano, basil, thyme, rosemary) or 1 Tbsp fresh chopped herbs

1 medium red bell pepper, chopped

4 large eggs, omega-3-enriched, free-range, organic

¼ cup chopped parsley

Heat a nonstick sauté pan to medium-high, add ½ tsp oil, and sauté artichoke hearts, spinach, and green onion with salt, pepper, and herbs for 2 minutes.

Add bell pepper and sauté for 1 minute. Meanwhile, whip eggs in a bowl.

When spinach softens and sautéed veggies are nearly cooked, combine them with eggs in bowl. Add parsley. Quickly wipe sauté pan with a paper towel, pour in remaining ½ tsp olive oil, then add egg-and-vegetable mixture back into the hot pan. Lift edges as eggs cook, to allow uncooked egg to get under the edges. When done, fold omelet in half and serve.

Nutrient Content per Serving:

| Calories: | 266 | Protein: | 18 grams | Fat: | 8 grams |
|---|---|---|---|---|---|
| Fiber: | 5.4 grams | Carbs: | 19 grams | Saturated Fat: | 3.7 grams |
| Sodium: | 670 mg | | | Fat %: | 46% |

# Oatmeal and Dried Fruit Muffins

Packed with fiber, nutrients, and flavor, these are equally good for breakfast or a snack. You can also freeze extras in an airtight container for later use.

Prep Time: 20 minutes, plus 30–35 minutes baking time
*Makes 12 muffins*

1 cup oats (rolled or steel cut)

1 cup oat bran

⅓ cup ground flaxseed

1½ tsp baking powder

1½ tsp baking soda

1 tsp ground cinnamon

½ tsp sea salt

1 scoop protein powder (whey or rice-pea protein), 20–30 grams protein

⅔ cup chopped dried fruit (figs, dates, raisins, and/or cherries)

⅓ cup chopped walnuts (or pecans)

⅓ cup molasses

3 large eggs (omega-3, free-range, organic), beaten

4 Tbsp nut oil (walnut, almond)

⅔ cup calcium-fortified almond milk (or soy milk or nonfat organic cow's milk)

1 cup unsweetened applesauce (or 1 cup ripe, mashed bananas)

Muffin pan liners

Preheat oven to 375°F. In a large bowl, combine dry ingredients: oats and oat bran, flaxseed, baking powder, baking soda, cinnamon, salt, protein powder, plus dried fruit and nuts.

In another large bowl, mix molasses, eggs, oil, milk, and applesauce.

Gently fold dry ingredients into wet ingredients. Line muffin depressions with muffin pan liners, which make serving, storing, and cleaning much easier (or simply spray muffin pan with oil) and pour batter into pan. Bake for 30 to 35 minutes, until a wooden toothpick inserted into a muffin comes out clean.

Nutrient Content per Muffin:

| Calories: | 211 | Fiber: | 3.5 grams | Saturated Fat: | 1.7 grams |
|-----------|-----|--------|-----------|----------------|-----------|
| Protein: | 6.8 grams | Sodium: | 318 mg | Total Fat: | 8.5 grams |
| Carbs: | 30 grams | Calories from Fat: | 34% | | |

## Steel-Cut Oatmeal with Berries 🕐

This is an easy and hearty breakfast.

Stove Top Prep Time: 3 minutes, plus 30 minutes simmering time

**Microwave Prep Time: 10 minutes**

*Serves 1*

1 cup water

¼ cup steel-cut oats

2 Tbsp chopped nuts (and/or 1 tsp ground flaxseed)

⅛ tsp ground cinnamon

2 Tbsp diced dried fruit (raisins, dates, and/or cherries; make sure your dried fruit doesn't have added sugar)

½ scoop whey or rice-pea protein, about 15 grams added protein (optional)

½ cup berries, fresh

½ cup calcium-fortified almond milk (or soy milk or organic nonfat cow's milk)

In a heavy saucepan, bring water to a boil. Add oats and reduce to a simmer for 30 minutes. Five minutes before serving, add nuts, cinnamon, dried fruit, and protein powder, if desired. Serve in a bowl with berries and milk.

Microwave: Place water, oats, nuts, cinnamon, and dried fruit (and protein powder, if desired) in a large glass bowl. Microwave for 8 minutes. Remove from the microwave, add fresh berries and milk, and stir.

Nutrient Content per Serving:

| Calories: | 284 | Protein: | 7.4 grams | Fat: | 5.8 grams |
|-----------|-----|----------|-----------|------|-----------|
| Fiber: | 8.4 grams | Carbs: | 54 grams | Saturated Fat: | 0.8 grams |
| Sodium: | 5 mg | | | Fat %: | 17% |

## Mexican Scrambled Eggs with Black Beans, Salsa, and Corn Tortillas 🕐

A flavorful and filling breakfast, packed with nutrients and fiber. For the chili ingredient option below, I prefer poblano chilies for their flavor, but they vary from sweet to very spicy, and not every store carries them. Alternatives are canned green chilies or bell peppers, which are sold everywhere.

**Prep Time: 15 minutes**

*Serves 2*

1 cup black beans, cooked (see Black Bean Dip recipe, page 298)

4 medium corn tortillas

1 tsp virgin olive oil

½ medium sweet onion, diced

¼ tsp sea salt

½ tsp ground paprika

1 medium chili pepper (poblano chili, green chili, or ½ bell pepper)

Dash ground cayenne pepper (or to taste)

4 large eggs, free-range, organic, omega-3-enriched

2 Tbsp fresh cilantro or parsley

¼ cup prepared Mexican salsa

1 Tbsp nonfat plain yogurt

Heat black beans on medium for 5 minutes. In a separate pan, warm tortillas over low heat, flipping occasionally.

Meanwhile, heat a sauté pan to medium-high. Add oil, then sauté onion, salt, and paprika for 1 to 2 minutes, until onion is nearly translucent. Add chili and cayenne pepper, if using, and heat another 1 to 2 minutes, stirring occasionally.

Whip eggs; then pour over vegetables in sauté pan, stirring occasionally, scrambling eggs gently. Garnish eggs with cilantro or parsley.

To serve, place eggs on a plate. Serve salsa and beans on the side. Garnish beans with a dollop of yogurt. Enjoy with warmed tortillas, spooning a mix of beans, eggs, and salsa into each tortilla.

Nutrient Content per Serving:

| Calories: | 422 | Protein: | 26.6 grams | Fat: | 11.7 grams |
|-----------|-----|----------|------------|------|------------|
| Fiber: | 11.8 grams | Carbs: | 54 grams | Saturated Fat: | 2.5 grams |
| Sodium: | 747 mg | Fat %: | 25% | | |

---

## Chicken Salad 🕐

Simple and quick. You can serve this on a bed of greens, in a wrap, or in a sandwich.

**Prep Time: 10 minutes**
*Serves 3*

1½ cups garbanzo beans, cooked, rinsed, and drained

1 Tbsp balsamic vinegar

2 Tbsp extra virgin olive oil

2 Tbsp prepared hummus (or homemade mayo, see Mayonnaise recipe, page 346)

1 tsp tamari sauce, low-sodium

2 Tbsp fresh basil leaves

6 ounces shredded cooked chicken breast (could be grilled, baked, canned, or leftovers), organic, free-range

1 medium celery stalk with leaves, finely diced

Accompaniment: salad; whole-grain tortilla or whole-grain bread

In a food processor, blend the garbanzo beans, vinegar, oil, hummus, tamari sauce, and basil. Then stir in cooked chicken and celery. Serve with a salad, in a whole-grain tortilla wrap, or in a sandwich made with whole-grain bread.

**Nutrient Content per Serving:**

| Calories: | 301 | Fat: | 12 grams | Protein: | 24 grams |
|---|---|---|---|---|---|
| Fiber: | 5.3 grams | Saturated Fat: | 1.8 grams | Carbs: | 24 grams |
| Sodium: | 156 mg | Fat %: | 36% | | |

---

## Crab Salad 🕐

It is so easy to make crab salad with precooked crab. It is colorful, flavorful, and fast! I prepare this when I want a quick, tasty meal my family enjoys. I recommend artichoke hearts from a glass jar because they taste better than canned artichokes. When shopping, look for crab in the frozen or canned refrigerator sections. You can substitute cooked canned salmon or cooked shrimp for crab, as needed.

**Prep Time: 10–15 minutes**
*Serves 4*

### Crab Mixture

- 1 pound cooked, shelled, crab (blue or Dungeness)
- 1 cup chopped celery leaves (leaves with small stems)
- 2 Tbsp canola organic mayonnaise (or homemade mayonnaise, see Mayonnaise recipe page 346)
- 1 Tbsp Dijon mustard
- 2 medium green onions, diced
- 1 medium red bell pepper, diced
- 2 Tbsp lemon juice

### Dressing

- 2 Tbsp walnut oil (or extra virgin olive oil)
- 2 Tbsp balsamic vinegar (or red wine vinegar)
- ⅛ tsp sea salt
- ⅛ tsp ground black pepper
- ½ tsp fines herbes (parsley, chives, tarragon, and chervil) or Italian herbs, dried
- 1 medium garlic clove, diced

### Salad

- 2 cups artichoke hearts (if feasible, buy fresh or from glass container, not canned)
- 8 cups mixed organic greens
- ¼ cup chopped fresh herbs (basil, mint)

Combine crab mixture ingredients in one bowl.

Combine salad dressing ingredients in a separate bowl.

Rinse and drain the artichoke hearts well; then mix with other salad ingredients.

To serve, toss salad ingredients with dressing and divide onto 4 plates. Add crab mixture to the center.

**Nutrient Content per Serving:**

| Calories: | 350 | Protein: | 28 grams | Total Fat: | 14.5 grams |
|---|---|---|---|---|---|
| Saturated Fat: | 1.2 grams | Sodium: | 691 mg | Fiber: | 6.5 grams |
| | | | | Fat %: | 37% |

# Manhattan Clam Chowder

This doubles as lunch or dinner. Buy the best quality clams. They taste better and usually cost more—but they are worth the difference. The baby potatoes have proportionally more nutrients and less sugar load than big potatoes, thanks to their extra skin surface.

Prep Time: 15 minutes (with precooked marinara sauce,
beans, and clams)
Simmering Time: 20 minutes
*Serves 4 (extras make great leftovers)*

2 Tbsp virgin olive oil

1 medium onion, chopped

¼ tsp sea salt

¼ tsp ground black pepper

2 Tbsp oat flour, garbanzo flour, or whole wheat pastry flour

2 medium carrots, diced

2 cups baby potatoes, unpeeled, not more than 1 inch in length, cut into ½-inch cubes

2 cups chopped tomatoes (or 15 ounces of canned tomatoes)

1 cup marinara sauce (no sugar added) or any tomato sauce

2 cups water

2 medium celery stalks, diced (or for a tangier, richer flavor, swap celery for 1 cup chopped artichoke hearts, jarred, rinsed and drained)

15 ounces navy beans, cooked and drained (or butter beans or similar)

12 ounces of clams, canned (drained, rinsed, then soaked in orange juice or milk)*

½ cup chopped parsley

4 Tbsp nonfat sour cream or nonfat plain yogurt (optional)

Hot chili sauce (optional)

*Note regarding clams:* If you can get fresh clams in the shell, even better. Scrub clams thoroughly, steam them for 5 to 7 minutes, and discard shells and any clams that don't open easily.

Heat a pot on medium-high. Add oil and sauté onion with salt and pepper for about 2 minutes. Add flour and heat, stirring, 1 to 2 minutes. Add carrots, potatoes, tomatoes, marinara sauce, and water. Bring to a gentle simmer, add celery, and reduce to low for about 15 minutes. When the potatoes and carrots are nearly tender and still a little al dente (tender but firm with a bite), add beans and clams. Simmer another 5 minutes. If soup is too thick, add water.

Garnish with parsley, and optionally with a spoonful of nonfat sour cream or plain yogurt. If you prefer some heat, add a dash of hot chili sauce to taste.

Nutrient Content per Serving:

| Calories: | 490 | Total Fat: | 10.4 grams | Protein: | 24 grams |
|-----------|------|----------------|------------|----------|----------|
| Fiber: | 11 grams | Saturated Fat: | 1.5 grams | Carbs: | 77 grams |
| Sodium: | 693 mg | Fat Calories %: | 19% | | |

## Grilled Chicken over Mixed Greens and Vegetables

This popular meal option is available nearly everywhere, but you can also make it at home for a quick, delicious, and healthy meal.

### Prep and Marinating Time: 25 minutes
### Serves 1

- 3 Tbsp plus 1 tsp vinaigrette dressing (See Masley House Vinaigrette Dressing, page 344), divided
- 4 ounces skinless, boneless chicken breast (organic, free-range), uncooked
- 2 cups mixed organic salad greens
- 4 cherry tomatoes (or 1 medium tomato, chopped)
- 6 Tbsp garbanzo beans, cooked, rinsed, drained
- ½ cup cooked, quartered, drained artichoke hearts
- 2 Tbsp fresh berries
- 1 Tbsp almond slivers (or chopped nuts)

Set grill at 450°F or turn on the broiler. Mix vinaigrette in a bowl and set aside 4 teaspoons for use as salad dressing.

Marinate chicken breasts in remaining 2 tablespoons dressing for 10 to 15 minutes, turning occasionally.

Shake off and discard excess marinade and grill or broil chicken breasts for 4 to 5 minutes per side. Slice into ½-inch strips.

Meanwhile, combine salad greens, tomatoes, garbanzo beans, and artichoke hearts in a salad bowl and toss with the 4 teaspoons vinaigrette dressing you set aside earlier. Plate salad and lay chicken slices over it. Garnish salad with berries and nuts and enjoy.

Nutrient Content per Serving:

| Calories: | 399 | Total Fat: | 17.5 grams | Total Protein: | 38 grams |
|-----------|-----------|----------------|------------|----------------|----------|
| Fiber: | 10.4 grams | Saturated Fat: | 1.7 grams | Total Carbs: | 30 grams |
| Sodium: | 666 mg | Fat Calories %: | 37% | | |

# Bean Taquitos 🕐

Quick, easy, and flavorful, packed with nutrients and fiber. I love it. *Taquito* means "little taco" and you can have extra fun by varying the ingredients in the different taquitos served.

### Prep Time: 10–15 minutes
### *Serves 2*

1 cup refried pinto beans

⅛ tsp cayenne pepper (or to taste)

¼ cup Mexican salsa (use your favorite brand)

2 medium peppers, roasted (seeds and stems removed), jarred, canned, or see Roasted Peppers recipe, page 337

4 medium corn tortillas (or small whole wheat tortillas)

2 cups shredded cabbage

1 medium avocado, sliced

½ medium lime

4 Tbsp grated low-fat cheese (cheddar, Monterey, Mexican rancho, feta)

Heat beans and cayenne pepper in a saucepan on medium-high. Once the beans bubble, stir in salsa and remove from heat.

Meanwhile, heat peppers for one minute in the microwave, and warm tortillas gently over low heat in a pan.

Spread ¼ of the bean-salsa mixture on each tortilla. Cut peppers in half and place ½ pepper over beans on each tortilla. Add shredded cabbage and sliced avocado. Drizzle lime juice evenly over cabbage. Sprinkle cheese over cabbage. Roll tortilla into a taquito and serve.

Nutrient Content per Serving:

| Calories: | 413 | Total Fat: | 17.2 grams | Total Protein: | 16.8 grams |
|---|---|---|---|---|---|
| Fiber: | 19.6 grams | Saturated Fat: | 2.8 grams | Total Carbs: | 57.5 grams |
| Sodium: | 520 mg | Fat Calories %: | 34% | | |

# Split Pea and Barley Soup

This is a great dish to make for lunch or dinner. Save a couple servings for leftovers—it's even better the next day, though you may have to thin it with water. If you'd like to prepare this soup gluten-free, omit the barley and use 2 cups of split peas—easy.

Prep Time: 10 minutes

Simmering Time: 60 minutes

*Serves 4 (makes 10 cups)*

3 cups low-sodium vegetable broth

4 cups water, plus additional water while cooking as needed

¾ pound (1½ cups) green split peas

½ cup barley, rinsed and drained

1⅔ Tbsp virgin olive oil, divided

1 bay leaf

1 medium onion, diced

¼ tsp sea salt or to taste

4 garlic cloves, crushed or chopped

2 large or 4 small carrots, diced

2 celery ribs, diced

½ tsp fresh thyme sprigs or ¼ tsp dried thyme

Freshly ground black pepper to taste

⅛–¼ tsp red pepper flakes (or to taste)

Combine the broth, water, split peas, barley, 2 tsp olive oil, and the bay leaf in a large stock pot. Bring to a boil, stirring occasionally. Lower to a simmer and cook for 30 minutes, stirring occasionally.

Heat remaining 1 Tbsp of olive oil in a large sauté pan on medium. Add the onions with salt and sauté for 3 to 4 minutes, until translucent. Add the garlic, carrots, celery, thyme, black pepper, and red pepper flakes to the onions. Heat for 2 minutes, stirring occasionally.

Stir the vegetable mixture into the soup. Continue to cook the soup for at least 30 minutes over low heat. The split peas should soften and thicken the soup. Add water as needed and stir often to prevent the soup from sticking to the bottom of the pot.

The soup is ready when the split peas are soft and the vegetables are tender. Discard the bay leaf before serving.

Nutrient Content per Serving:

| Calories: | 269 | Fat: | 5.8 grams | Protein: | 11.1 grams |
|---|---|---|---|---|---|
| Fiber: | 12 grams | Saturated Fat: | 0.8 grams | Carbs: | 43.8 grams |
| Sodium: | 638 mg | Fat %: | 21% | | |

## Salmon Spread with Hummus 🕐

A better option than a tuna spread is this healthier version which is delicious on sandwiches, in pita bread, or served with a tossed salad.

**Prep Time: 5 minutes**

*Serves 2*

6 ounces canned salmon (I prefer wild Alaska pink or red salmon)

2 medium green onions, diced

1 Tbsp Dijon mustard

2 Tbsp prepared organic hummus or mayonnaise (see Mayonnaise recipe, page 346)

1 Tbsp capers

1 tsp lemon juice

1 medium celery stalk, diced

Hot sauce (optional, to taste)

Flake salmon. Mix with the remaining ingredients and serve.

**Nutrient Content per Serving:**

| Calories: | 190 | Total Fat: | 7.8 grams | Protein: | 24.5 grams |
|---|---|---|---|---|---|
| Fiber: | 1.2 grams | Saturated Fat: | 1.6 grams | Carbs: | 2 grams |
| Sodium: | 450 mg | Fat Calories %: | 38% | | |

## Edamame and Sliced Bell Peppers 🕐

You can serve edamame plain—simple and delicious. But I prefer it with the added flavors below. I typically serve edamame in the pods; but don't eat the pod itself, it's far too fibrous. You can buy freshly shelled edamame, but it's easier to find frozen, and it freezes better if it remains inside the pod.

**Prep Time: 5–8 minutes**

*Serves 2*

10 ounces edamame pods, organic (if frozen, microwave 3 minutes, rinse, and drain)

1 small red bell pepper, cut into thin slices

1½ tsp rice vinegar

1½ tsp tamari sauce, low-sodium

Few dashes hot chili pepper sauce (optional, to taste)

Combine the ingredients, toss, and serve.

**Nutrient Content per Serving:**

| Calories: | 215 | Total Fat: | 8.4 grams | Protein: | 18 grams |
|---|---|---|---|---|---|
| Fiber: | 6 grams | Saturated Fat: | 1.7 grams | Carbs: | 18 grams |
| Sodium: | 193 mg | Fat Calories %: | 35% | | |

## Sliced Vegetables

Yes, you could serve vegetables raw, but flash-cooked, these are much tastier, with better texture for dips. If you'd like to avoid the work of slicing vegetables, you can use a food processor, mandolin, or buy presliced veggies.

### Prep Time: 25 minutes
*Makes 5 cups*

1 Tbsp sea salt

1 cup broccoli florets, sliced into thin strips

1 cup sliced cauliflower florets (long strips)

1 cup sliced carrots (3-inch-long strips)

1 cup cut asparagus (3-inch lengths)

1 cup sliced red or orange bell pepper (⅓-inch strips)

1 Tbsp red wine vinegar

1 tsp extra virgin olive oil

1 Tbsp orange juice

¼ tsp dried Italian herbs

⅛ tsp sea salt

Bring 3 quarts of salted water to a boil in a large pot. Keep a large bowl of very cold water and ice nearby.

Add broccoli and cauliflower to boiling water. After 1 minute, veggies should be al dente, tender but still chewy. Remove and immerse in ice water. Bring pot to a boil again and repeat with carrots. (Add ice as needed to the bowl.) Bring pot back to a boil, add asparagus. Thirty seconds later, add bell peppers. After 30 seconds, transfer bell peppers and asparagus to ice water bath. Once all vegetables are blanched and chilled, drain.

In a serving bowl, combine vinegar, oil, orange juice, herbs, and salt, then toss vegetables with the mixture and serve.

# Black Bean Dip 🕐

Quick and easy to prepare, yet packed with fiber and nutrients! Serve as a dip, or add to a tortilla to make a burrito with sliced cabbage and avocado.

### Prep Time: 5–8 minutes
*Makes 2 cups (4 servings)*

15 ounces black beans, cooked
1 medium red bell pepper, roasted
¼ cup prepared Mexican salsa
¼ tsp ground cumin
⅛ tsp red chili flakes (or to taste)
4 Tbsp grated low-fat Monterey Jack or jalapeño cheese (optional)

Rinse and drain beans. In a food processer, combine ingredients and blend until smooth. Heat and serve with julienned vegetables or baked tortillas cut into triangles.

Nutrient Content per Serving (½ cup serving):

| Calories: | 102 | Total Fat: | 0.3 grams | Protein: | 6.5 grams |
|---|---|---|---|---|---|
| Fiber: | 6.8 grams | Saturated Fat: | 0 grams | Carbs: | 18 grams |
| Sodium: | 267 mg | Fat %: | 3% | | |

# Banana-Blueberry Lassi 🕐

A lassi is a yogurt fruit drink, very common in India. It's great for a snack or as a beverage with an Indian meal. Try this with strawberries, mangos, or papaya—whichever fruit is handy and in season.

### Prep Time: 2 minutes
*Serves 2*

1 cup nonfat plain yogurt
1 cup vanilla, almond, soy, or nonfat cow's milk
1 medium banana (ripe)
1 cup blueberries, frozen
1 tsp lemon juice
Garnish: sprig of mint

Combine ingredients in a blender and serve with a sprig of mint.

## Brown Rice Bowl with Veggies and Protein 🕐

This was my basic dinner through medical school and residency. It was easy, quick (assuming I cooked brown rice in advance), flavorful, and nutritious. Heat the rice, steam two cups of veggies per person, add 5 to 8 ounces of lean protein, 2 tablespoons of chopped nuts, plus tamari sauce and/or hot sauce to taste. Enjoy!

Prep Time: 10–15 minutes
Brown Rice Cooking Time: 40 minutes
*Serves 2*

⅔ cup raw brown rice, to make 2 cups cooked brown rice

1⅓ cups water

4 cups veggies (select any that are handy, fresh or frozen)

10–14 ounces lean protein (beans, tofu, grilled chicken breast, sirloin, shrimp, fish)

1 Tbsp nut oil (almond or walnut)

1 Tbsp grated gingerroot

2 medium garlic cloves, minced

2 Tbsp vinaigrette salad dressing (See Masley House Vinaigrette Dressing recipe, page 344, or use prepared)

1 Tbsp tamari sauce, low-sodium (or low-sodium soy sauce)

¼ tsp chili hot sauce (or to taste)

2 Tbsp nuts, chopped (sliced almonds)

You will need: saucepan with steamer basket.

To make rice, combine ⅔ cup raw brown rice with 1⅓ cups water. Bring to a boil. Simmer until cooked, 40 to 45 minutes. I typically make a double or triple batch, and save for another meal.

Assemble your choice of vegetables, protein, and nut oil.

Ten minutes prior to serving rice, slice vegetables into 1-inch pieces. Add water to a saucepan, place steamer basket in it, and bring water to a boil.

Next, heat a sauté pan to medium-high. Add oil to pan, then sauté protein and ginger, stirring occasionally. After 2 minutes, reduce heat to medium and add garlic to sauté pan; heat until protein is fully cooked.

When saucepan is steaming, place vegetables in steamer basket, cover, and steam for 3 to 6 minutes, until veggies are al dente. When vegetables are cooked, remove from heat and drain. Next, mix veggies in a bowl with vinaigrette dressing.

When rice is cooked, combine rice in the sauté pan with protein, season with tamari and chili sauce, and sauté another 1 minute.

To serve, mix rice and protein with veggies in bowls. Garnish with chopped nuts.

Nutrient Content per Serving (using 2 cups broccoli, 2 cups cauliflower, and 10 ounces shrimp):

| Calories: | 588 | Fat: | 22 grams | Protein: | 40 grams |
|---|---|---|---|---|---|
| Fiber: | 8 grams | Saturated Fat: | 3.3 grams | Carbs: | 60 grams |
| Sodium: | 605 mg | Fat %: | 33% | | |

## Chicken Stir-Fry with Orange-Ginger Sauce

Easy to make, delicious flavors, and colorful. To modify this recipe, substitute shrimp or firm tofu for chicken.

### Prep Time: 25–30 minutes
### Rice Cooking Time: 40 minutes
*Serves 4 (leftovers make a great lunch)*

1½ cups raw brown rice

3 cups water

1 Tbsp nut oil (almond or walnut)

1 Tbsp grated fresh ginger root

1 medium onion, diced

1½ pounds boneless, skinless chicken breast (organic, free-range), cut into strips

4 medium garlic cloves, diced

1 medium red bell pepper, sliced

2 cups sliced broccoli

2 cups snow peas

½ tsp ground black pepper

⅛ tsp red chili flakes (or to taste)

⅓ cup low-sodium chicken or vegetable broth

2 medium green onions, roots trimmed and discarded, sliced

1 Tbsp grated orange rind

⅓ cup orange juice, freshly squeezed and seeds removed

1 Tbsp tamari sauce, low-sodium (or low-sodium soy sauce)

1 tsp sesame oil

2 tsp cornstarch

Garnish: 2 Tbsp almond slivers (or chopped cashews), toasted

Bring rice and water to a boil, cover, and reduce heat to simmer. Prepare vegetables and chicken while the rice is cooking.

15 minutes before you are ready to serve, heat wok or large sauté pan over medium-high heat. Add oil, gingerroot, and onion, and stir occasionally until onion becomes translucent, about 2 minutes. Add chicken and stir until opaque, 4 to 5 minutes. *(If cooking shrimp or 1-inch cubed tofu instead of chicken, sauté 2 to 3 minutes, until shrimp turns pink, or tofu is slightly browned.)*

To the wok, add garlic, bell pepper, broccoli, snow peas, pepper, and chili flakes. Stir occasionally for 2 to 3 minutes.

Meanwhile in a bowl, mix the broth, green onions, orange rind, orange juice, tamari sauce, sesame oil, and cornstarch.

When vegetables are brightly colored and tender-crisp, add liquid to wok and stir until chicken and vegetables are coated with the thickened sauce, 1 to 2 minutes.

Toast nuts for 1 minute in a sauté pan on medium-high and sprinkle over stir-fry. Serve immediately, over hot rice.

Nutrient Content per Serving:

| Calories: | 648 | Total Fat: | 16 grams | Protein: | 52 grams |
|-----------|-----|------------|----------|----------|----------|
| Fiber: | 9.0 grams | Saturated Fat: | 2.0 grams | Carbs: | 74 grams |
| Sodium: | 551 mg | Fat %: | 22% | | |

## Chicken, Italian Herbs, and Quinoa 🕐

An easy, delicious meal. Can be served hot or cold.

### Prep Time: 20 Minutes
### Serves 4

2 cups low-sodium vegetable (page 344) or chicken stock

2 cups quinoa, rinsed and drained

24 ounces chicken breast (organic, free-range), uncooked, sliced into thin strips

2 Tbsp virgin olive oil, divided

1 tsp oregano

1 tsp minced fresh rosemary

¼ tsp ground cayenne pepper

1 medium onion, chopped

¼ tsp sea salt

¼ tsp ground black pepper

2 medium carrots, diced

2 medium celery stalks, diced

1 medium red bell pepper, sliced thinly into 1-inch strips

½ cup pistachio nuts, chopped (or sliced almonds)

In a saucepan, bring stock to a gentle boil. Rinse and drain quinoa grain in a sieve. When stock is boiling, add quinoa, cover, and stir. When it begins to boil again, remove from heat and set aside, covered. It should be fully cooked in 15 minutes.

Rinse chicken with water, pat dry with paper, towels, slice into strips, and in a glass bowl rub chicken with 1 tablespoon of the oil (reserve the rest), and the oregano, rosemary, and cayenne pepper, and set it aside.

Heat a sauté pan to medium-high, add the remaining 1 tablespoon of olive oil, the onion, salt, and black pepper. Sauté 1 minute, stirring occasionally. Add chicken with herbs and sauté 2 to 3 minutes, stirring occasionally, until chicken is mostly opaque. Add carrots and celery, and cook another 3 minutes, stirring occasionally. Add bell peppers and heat a final 2 minutes.

Heat nuts in a pan over medium heat for 1 to 2 minutes to warm, but stop before they brown. Stir nuts into quinoa. Serve quinoa with nuts. Then spoon the chicken and vegetable sauté over the quinoa.

Nutrient Content per Serving:

| Calories: | 685 | Fat: | 21 grams | Protein: | 55 grams |
|---|---|---|---|---|---|
| Fiber: | 8.3 grams | Saturated Fat: | 2.9 grams | Carbs: | 70 grams |
| Sodium: | 600 mg | Fat %: | 27% | | |

## Chicken Fajitas

This dish has great flavors and is easy to make. I prefer using poblano peppers, as they have the best flavor, but while some poblanos are sweet, others are spicy hot, and you won't know until you take a bite. So if you don't like "enchiloso" hot, stick to bell peppers. For variety, substitute shrimp or sirloin steak for chicken.

### Prep Time: 30 minutes
*Serves 3*

1 Tbsp virgin olive oil

1 Tbsp red wine vinegar

1 tsp ground paprika

¼ tsp ground cayenne pepper (or to taste)

½ tsp sea salt

½ tsp ground black pepper

1 tsp dried oregano

4 medium garlic cloves, diced

1 Tbsp lime juice

1¼ pounds skinless, boneless chicken breast (organic, free-range), uncooked, cut into thin strips

1 medium onion, cut into thin strips

2 medium peppers (poblanos or bell peppers); remove stem and seeds, and cut into thin strips

2 cups shredded cabbage

15 ounces cooked black beans, rinsed and drained

9 corn tortillas

½ cup prepared Mexican salsa

Garnish: cilantro sprigs (or parsley)

Heat grill to 450°F, or set oven on broil.

Combine oil, vinegar, paprika, cayenne pepper, salt, black pepper, oregano, garlic, and lime juice to make a marinade.

Add chicken, onion, and peppers to marinade, stirring occasionally for 10 minutes.

Meanwhile shred cabbage.

Remove chicken from marinade and discard marinade. Grill or broil chicken, onions, and peppers for 5 minutes on each side, until chicken is cooked. *Depending upon your grill, you may need to use a grilling basket to prevent pieces from falling through the slots.*

Heat beans in a saucepan.

Heat tortillas in a pan.

To serve, place chicken and veggies, beans, cabbage, salsa, and tortillas in separate serving bowls. To assemble, lay one tortilla on each plate. Place chicken, veggies, and beans on tortillas. Sprinkle cabbage and salsa over the top, garnish with cilantro, and enjoy.

**Nutrient Content per Serving:**

| Calories: | 542 | Total Fat: | 11.5 grams | Protein: | 48 grams |
|---|---|---|---|---|---|
| Fiber: | 14.9 grams | Saturated Fat: | 1.7 grams | Carbs: | 67 grams |
| Sodium: | 507 mg | Fat %: | 18% | | |

# Roasted Chicken with Wine and Rosemary

This is simple, juicy, and flavorful. If you prefer crisper skin, be sure to put the chicken on a rack above the wine.

**Prep Time: 10 minutes**
**Baking Time: 60 minutes**
*Serves 4*

2 to 2½ pounds whole chicken (organic, free-range young hen)
2 Tbsp virgin olive oil
½ tsp sea salt
½ tsp ground black pepper
2 tsp dried Italian herbs
4 sprigs fresh rosemary (3-inch sprigs), mince leaves from 1 sprig
8 medium garlic cloves, minced
1 cup dry white wine

Preheat oven to 400°F. Rinse chicken and pat dry with paper towels. Place chicken in an oven roasting pan and rub chicken with olive oil, salt, pepper, Italian herbs, the minced sprig of rosemary, and garlic. Rub about 1 Tbsp of oil-herb mixture inside the cavity.

Pour wine into roasting pan. Place 2 rosemary sprigs in the pan and one inside the chicken. For crisper skin, put chicken on a rack above the wine.

Roast on the middle rack. Measuring with a meat thermometer, you can tell it is done when the thigh and leg temperatures reach 160°F to 170°F, which will be after 60 to 75 minutes. During the last 5 minutes (once it reaches 155°F to 160°F), if the chicken isn't already golden, you can turn on the broiler to brown.

Serve with a vegetable dish, such as Ratatouille (page 329).

**Nutrient Content per Serving:**

| Calories: | 680 | Fat: | 33.5 grams | Protein: | 85 grams |
|---|---|---|---|---|---|
| Fiber: | 0.1 gram | Saturated Fat: | 8.9 grams | Carbs: | 6.5 grams |
| Sodium: | 895 mg | Fat %: | 45% | | |

# Mediterranean Sea Scallops

I love big, juicy, grilled scallops, especially with Mediterranean herbs. They are easy and very quick to prepare. They need high heat to sear the surface so they don't dry out.

**Prep Time: 10 minutes**
**Marinade Time: 20 minutes (up to 24 hours)**
*Serves 2*

1 pound sea scallops, large
1 cup orange juice
4 tsp virgin olive oil
4 Tbsp mixed fresh herbs (basil, rosemary, parsley, thyme)
1 tsp dried Italian herbs or fines herbes (parsley, chives, tarragon, and chervil)
¼ tsp sea salt
¼ tsp ground black pepper
½ tsp paprika

If scallops are frozen, thaw in a bowl of water, changing water every few minutes if you are pressed for time. When thawed, marinate in orange juice for 10 minutes. Drain, discard marinade, and pat dry with a paper towel.

Combine with half the oil and herbs, salt, black pepper, and paprika in a bowl and marinate in refrigerator for at least 20 minutes, up to 24 hours.

To prepare on the barbecue, preheat grill to 450°F. Add scallops once grill is hot. Depending upon your grill, use a grilling basket. After 2 minutes, turn and sear the other side, drizzle remaining oil and herbs, and heat another 2 minutes.

To broil, set oven to broil. Place an ovenproof baking pan under the broiler, on the upper rack, for a few minutes to heat it up. Cautiously pull out rack, place scallops on baking dish, and return to the broiler. After 2 minutes, turn scallops and drizzle any remaining oil and herbs.

Serve with a side vegetable plate.

Nutrient Content per Serving:

| Calories: | 294 | Total Fat: | 11.2 grams | Protein: | 39 grams |
|-----------|-----|------------|------------|----------|----------|
| Fiber: | 0.5 grams | Saturated Fat: | 1.5 grams | Carbs: | 8.3 grams |
| Sodium: | 637 mg | Fat %: | 35% | | |

## Shrimp, Artichoke, and White Bean Salad with Tangerine Vinaigrette

Quick, easy, and tasty. If tangerines are unavailable, use an orange.

**Prep Time: 20 minutes**
*Serves 2*

1 pound shrimp, large, peeled, deveined
1 cup orange juice

3 Tbsp extra virgin olive oil

1 Tbsp white wine

4 medium garlic cloves, minced

¼ cup finely chopped parsley

½ tsp ground paprika

2 medium tangerines: 1 peeled and segmented, the other juiced and
strained to remove seeds

1 Tbsp red wine vinegar

⅛ tsp sea salt

⅛ tsp ground black pepper

¼ tsp dried Italian herbs

4 cups organic, mixed salad greens

1 cup artichoke hearts, quartered, rinsed, and drained (jarred are
better than canned)

1 cup cannellini beans, cooked, rinsed, drained

1 medium cucumber, sliced into bite-sized cubes

10 cherry tomatoes, sliced in half

Set oven to broil. Meanwhile, marinate shrimp in orange juice for 10
minutes. In a roasting pan, combine 1 tablespoon olive oil with the wine,
garlic, parsley, paprika, and tangerine segments (leaving a few segments
aside for garnish). Discard the orange juice. Add drained shrimp to the
olive oil/tangerine mixture and stir to coat. Broil shrimp and tangerine
slices for 4 to 5 minutes until shrimp are pink and cooked.

Mix 2 tablespoons oil with the vinegar, tangerine juice, salt, pepper,
and herbs in a salad bowl. Toss salad greens, artichoke hearts, beans,
cucumber, and tomatoes with dressing. Divide salad onto 2 plates. Top
with warm shrimp and garnish with tangerine sections.

Nutrient Content per Serving:

| Calories: | 741 | Total Fat: | 26.6 grams | Protein: | 58 grams |
|-----------|-----|------------|------------|----------|----------|
| Fiber: | 11.4 grams | Saturated Fat: | 3.8 grams | Carbs: | 68.6 grams |
| Sodium: | 792 mg | Fat %: | 32% | | |

## Roasted Pork Tenderloin with Apples and Sweet Onions

This dish brings memories of pork chops and apple sauce I ate as a child,
yet the pork tenderloin is a much healthier choice, and just as delicious.

**Prep Time: 30 minutes**

**Roasting Time: 30 minutes**

*Serves 3*

1¼ pounds pork tenderloin

2 Tbsp nut oil (almond or walnut), divided

1 medium sweet onion, cut into long, thin slivers

¾ tsp sea salt (divided)

¼ tsp ground black pepper

¼ cup white wine (dry cooking wine)

3 medium apples, cut into ½-inch cubes (about 3 cups)

2 medium yellow squash, cut into ½-inch cubes (about 3 cups)

¼ tsp ground cinnamon

½ tsp ground cumin

¼ tsp red chili flakes (optional)

Preheat oven to 400°F.

Rinse pork under running water and pat dry. Heat a sauté pan to medium-high. Add 2 teaspoons oil, and sear each of the four sides of pork for 60 to 90 seconds, until lightly browned. Remove pan from heat and transfer pork to the center of a 9- x 14-inch ovenproof baking dish.

With a paper towel, clean the sauté pan of any burned oil; then return pan to medium-high heat and add 2 more teaspoons oil. Add onion with salt and black pepper and sauté for 3 minutes, until onion is soft and nearly translucent. Reduce heat to medium and add wine, stirring occasionally for 1 minute, then remove from heat. Cover pork with onions in the center of the baking dish.

If needed, once again clean sauté pan with a paper towel. Return to medium heat and add final 2 teaspoons of oil. Next add apple and yellow squash. Add cinnamon, cumin, and optional red chili flakes. Heat for 2 minutes, stirring occasionally. Spoon apple-squash mixture around the edges of the baking dish, encircling the pork.

Insert a meat thermometer into the thickest portion of the pork tenderloin. Roast until internal heat reaches 145°F, 25 to 35 minutes. Serve with a green salad.

**Nutrient Content per Serving:**

| Calories: | 426 | Fat: | 16 grams | Protein: | 39.5 grams |
|---|---|---|---|---|---|
| Fiber: | 3.3 grams | Saturated Fat: | 2.7 grams | Carbs: | 25 grams |
| Sodium: | 505 mg | Fat %: | 34% | | |

# Roasted Pork Tenderloin with Mediterranean Herbs

The longer this dish marinates, the more flavorful it becomes. It's simple to prepare and goes well with grilled or roasted vegetables.

Prep Time: 15 minutes

Marinating Time: 30 minutes to 24 hours

Baking Time: 35 minutes

*Serves 3*

1¼ pounds pork tenderloin

1 Tbsp plus 2 tsp virgin olive oil

¼ cup finely chopped parsley

1 Tbsp fresh, finely chopped rosemary

1 tsp Italian herbs, dried

3 medium garlic cloves, minced

½ tsp sea salt

¼ tsp ground black pepper

Rinse pork under running water and pat dry with paper towels. Combine 1 tablespoon oil, herbs, garlic, salt, and pepper and rub into pork surface. Seal in a glass container to marinate in the refrigerator, 30 minutes to 24 hours.

Preheat oven to 400°F. Heat 2 teaspoons oil in an ovenproof skillet on medium-high, swirling the oil until just before it smokes. Sear pork on each side for 60 seconds per side, until it is lightly browned. Place the ovenproof skillet on middle rack of the oven and roast until internal heat reaches 145°F on a meat thermometer, 30 to 35 minutes.

Nutrient Content per Serving:

| Calories: | 334 | Fat: | 17.6 grams | Protein: | 38 grams |
|---|---|---|---|---|---|
| Fiber: | 1.5 grams | Saturated Fat: | 4.3 grams | Carbs: | 4.4 grams |
| Sodium: | 665 mg | Fat %: | 48% | | |

# Grilled Sirloin and Shrimp

"Surf and turf" is easy to make, and a good choice if you're looking for the occasional steak dinner. Be sure to buy grass-fed, organic steaks. Serve with a double portion of vegetables and a salad with balsamic vinaigrette, and you have a great meal.

The double marinade process is important, as an acid marinade is critical to sear animal protein before it goes on the grill, but the liquid would drip away during the cooking process, so the second marinade with oil and herbs ensures the flavors stick to the protein.

Prep Time: 10 minutes

Marinade Time: 30 minutes

Cooking Time: 8–10 minutes

*Serves 2*

2 4-ounce sirloin steaks (grass fed, organic), fat trimmed away (each about ¾- to 1-inch thick), or tenderloin steaks if you prefer

8 ounces shrimp, extra-large, shelled, and deveined

2 Tbsp balsamic vinegar

2 Tbsp virgin olive oil

2 Tbsp minced shallots

2 large garlic cloves, minced

½ tsp sea salt

¼ tsp cayenne pepper

¼ tsp ground black pepper

Marinate steaks and shrimp in vinegar for 15 minutes, turning occasionally. Drain and pat dry with paper towels. Combine oil, shallots, garlic, and spices (save 1 tablespoon of this mixture and set aside for brushing later) and rub into steaks and shrimp. Let marinate for 15 minutes, turning occasionally.

Prepare grill or broiler, medium-high heat, or 400°F to 450°F. Grill steaks until cooked to desired doneness, 4 to 5 minutes per side. Grill shrimp until pink, 2 to 3 minutes per side. After turning shrimp and steaks, brush the set-aside 1 tablespoon of marinade over them. Transfer to plates and serve with a double vegetable portion and a salad with balsamic vinaigrette.

**Nutrient Content per Serving:**

| Calories: | 500 | Fat: | 27 grams | Protein: | 57 grams |
|-----------|-----|------|----------|----------|----------|
| Fiber: | 0.1 grams | Saturated Fat: | 6.6 grams | Carbs: | 6.1 grams |
| Sodium: | 777 mg | Fat %: | 48% | | |

## Roasted Tenderloin and Root Vegetables

Be sure to select a grass-fed organic tenderloin beefsteak. This dish is easy to prepare and makes a great meal, but the roasting time varies with every oven, so rely on the meat thermometer to determine doneness.

## Prep Time: 15–20 minutes
## Roasting Time: About 50 minutes
*Serves 3*

1 pound tenderloin (beef tenderloin should be organic, grass-fed)

1 Tbsp virgin olive oil

1 Tbsp herbes de Provence, dried (rosemary, savory, thyme, lavender)

¾ tsp sea salt

½ tsp ground black pepper

4 medium garlic cloves, minced

1 medium red onion, chopped into 1-inch chunks

6 small baby red potatoes (1 inch long), cut in half

3 large carrots, cut into ¾-inch cubes

2 medium turnips, cut into ¾-inch cubes

3 small yams, cut into ¾-inch cubes

1 Tbsp fines herbes, dried (parsley, tarragon, chives, and chervil)

1 Tbsp virgin olive oil

2 Tbsp chopped fresh parsley

Preheat oven to 400°F. Rinse tenderloin and pat dry. In a bowl, rub roast with 1 tablespoon oil and herbes de Provence.

In a separate bowl, mix salt, pepper, and garlic. Rub half the salt-garlic mixture over the roast.

In a separate bowl, mix veggies with the fines herbes and remaining 1 tablespoon olive oil, plus the reserved salt-garlic mixture.

Stick a meat thermometer into the thickest part of the roast. Place the meat in a roasting pan and surround it with the cubed vegetables. Roast in the oven on the middle rack for 20 minutes; then reduce heat to 350°F, and continue roasting until meat temperature reaches 125°F to 130°F. Temperatures vary by oven, but this should take about 15 additional minutes.

Remove the roast and place on a cutting board, covered with foil. Roast vegetables until tender, another 10 to 15 minutes. The meat will continue to cook in the center while resting, covered. When the roast reaches 140°F, remove the foil, slice roast, and check if it is medium-rare (pink). If too rare for your taste, roast another 5 to 10 minutes in the oven. Use caution, as overcooking the roast will toughen it.

Place sliced roast on serving plate, surround with vegetables. Garnish with fresh parsley.

**Nutrient Content per Serving:**

| Calories: | 683 | Total Fat: | 22 grams | Fiber: | 10 grams |
|---|---|---|---|---|---|
| Saturated Fat: | 5.3 grams | Sodium: | 809 mg | Fat %: | 29% |
| Fat Calories %: | 29% | Protein: | 50 grams | Carbs: | 71 grams |

# Roasted Cornish Game Hens

This is a Persian recipe with a lemon marinade, flavored with parsley and mint. It requires an 18- to 24-hour marinade, but otherwise is very easy to prepare.

**Prep Time: 20 minutes**

**Marinade Time: 18–24 hours**

**Roasting Time: 2 hours**

*Serves 4*

2 Cornish game hens (1 to 1¼ pounds each, organic, free-range)

2 medium lemons, juiced

1½ tsp sea salt

¼ tsp ground black pepper

2 tsp virgin olive oil

1 Tbsp finely diced fresh mint

1 Tbsp finely diced fresh parsley

8 medium prunes

Sweet potatoes for accompaniment (optional)

Wash and drain the hens; discard organ meats if present. Place hens in a large bowl. Pour lemon juice over them, turning so that every surface has been covered with juice, and season with 1 teaspoon salt and pepper. Marinate for 18 to 24 hours in the refrigerator, turning every 4 to 8 hours.

To roast, preheat oven to 350°F. Drain lemon juice from hens, but don't rinse them. Rub hens with olive oil, herbs, and the remaining ½ teaspoon salt over their surface, inside and out.

Arrange them, alternating head to toe, in a glass baking dish sprayed with cooking spray to prevent sticking. Tuck one prune under each leg and wing. Place in the middle of the oven. Roast, basting every 20 to 30 minutes, until the juices in the pan run clear—about 2 hours. To serve, cut hens in half down the center vertically. Allow ½ hen per serving. To serve with a vegetable dish and baked sweet potatoes, add sweet potatoes to the oven 45 minutes before hens are done.

Nutrient Content per Serving (without sweet potato):

| Calories: | 351 | Total Fat: | 11 grams | Protein: | 50 grams |
|-----------|-----|------------|----------|----------|----------|
| Fiber: | 1.4 grams | Saturated Fat: | 2.5 grams | Carbs: | 2.5 grams |
| Sodium: | 571 mg | Fat %: | 28% | | |

# Grilled Salmon with Lemon, Chili, Brown Sugar, and Dill

Voila! My favorite grilled salmon recipe. I grew up salmon fishing with my dad, and I now take my sons salmon fishing most summers. Even guests who normally shy away from salmon have enjoyed this recipe. All of their taste buds (sweet, sour, salty, bitter, umami) are stimulated at once!

**Prep Time: 10 minutes**

**Marinade Time: 15 minutes**

**Cooking Time: 8–10 minutes**

*Serves 4*

1½ pounds salmon fillets (preferably wild Alaska Coho or other wild species)

1 cup orange juice

1 medium lemon

½ tsp sea salt

¼ tsp ground black pepper

½ tsp paprika

¼ tsp cayenne pepper (or to taste)

1 tsp brown sugar

1 tsp dried dill weed (or ¼ cup fresh dill weed, cut into 1-inch strands)

Oil spray

Lemon wedges

Fresh dill weed, for garnish

Rinse salmon fillets in cold water. Marinate in orange juice for 15 minutes. Preheat grill to 450°F, or set oven to broil. Drain fillets and pat dry with paper towels.

Sprinkle lemon juice over fillets. Combine salt, pepper, paprika, cayenne, sugar, and dried dill weed, and sprinkle over the salmon. Spray (or finely drizzle) oil over herb-coated fillets.

Transfer salmon fillets to the grill. For a 1-inch-thick fillet, grill 8 to 10 minutes total, 4 to 5 minutes per side (for thinner fillets, grill less time). The timing will be similar if you use the top rack of your oven broiler.

Serve with lemon wedges and garnish with fresh dill weed.

Nutrient Content per Serving:

| Calories: | 245 | Total Fat: | 7.5 grams | Fiber: | 0.5 grams |
| Saturated Fat: | 1.8 grams | Carbs: | 2.5 grams | Sodium: | 382 mg |

## Ceviche-Avocado Tostadas

Easy-to-make, flavorful, and fun to eat. This is a meal that is hard to surpass.

### Prep Time: 15–20 minutes
### Marinating Time: 12–24 hours
*Serves 4*

1 pound white fish, cut into ½- to ¾-inch cubes (my favorite is snapper, but tilapia works well too)

½ medium red onion, diced

1 cup lime juice

½ tsp sea salt

8 medium corn tortillas

½ medium red bell pepper, diced

½ cup chopped fresh cilantro leaves (or parsley)

2 medium green onions, diced

⅛ tsp cayenne pepper (or to taste, or hot sauce, to taste)

1 medium avocado, sliced

½ cup freshly squeezed tangerine juice (about two tangerines or mandarins; strain away seeds; use orange juice or lime juice if tangerines not available)

15 ounces nonfat refried pinto beans

2 cups finely sliced green cabbage

½ cup nonfat sour cream (or nonfat plain yogurt)

Combine fish, onion, lime juice, and salt in a glass container. Make sure lime juice covers fish and onion completely. Marinate at least 6 hours, but preferably 12 to 24 hours (typically overnight) in the refrigerator.

Preheat oven to 425°F. Place tortillas on a baking sheet without any wrapping and bake for 10 minutes.

After marinating, drain fish in a colander. Discard marinade. Return fish to a large bowl and mix gently with red bell pepper, cilantro, green onions, cayenne pepper, avocado, and tangerine juice.

To serve, lay tortilla on a plate, heap 2 tablespoons of beans, a big pinch of cabbage, then ceviche over the top. Garnish with 1 tablespoon of sour cream or yogurt, and enjoy.

Nutrient Content per Serving:

| Calories: | 502 | Total Fat: | 11.1 grams | Sodium: | 672 mg |
|---|---|---|---|---|---|
| Fiber: | 15.8 grams | Saturated Fat: | 1.7 grams | Carbs: | 67 grams |
| Protein: | 37 grams | Fat Calories %: | 20% | | |

# Gumbo

Of the three trio combinations in gumbo, I'll use all three in this dish. The first is the holy trinity of Cajun flavors (onion, celery, and bell pepper). The second is the three gumbo thickeners that include a roux (French) made with flour and fat (although I'm breaking with tradition by using a healthy flour-fat combo), okra (African), and sassafras leaves (Native American). They are typically served with three protein sources (usually shrimp, chicken, and sausage), but here I'll use chicken, scallops, and shrimp, leaving the sausage as optional.

**Prep Time: 25–30 minutes**

**Rice Cooking Time: 40 minutes**

**Simmering Time: 20 minutes**

*Serves 4 (makes great leftovers as the flavors improve with time)*

⅔ cup brown rice

1⅓ cup water

3 Tbsp virgin olive oil

1 medium onion, chopped

¼ tsp sea salt

1 tsp dried oregano

1 tsp ground paprika

¼ cup oat flour

½ pound chicken breast (free-range, organic), rinsed, dried, and cut into ½-inch cubes

2 cups chopped celery (½-inch pieces)

1 large green bell pepper, chopped into ½-inch pieces

1 large red bell pepper, chopped into ½-inch pieces

1 bay leaf

4 cups chopped okra (¾-inch segments, fresh or frozen)

15 ounces diced or stewed tomatoes, canned

4 medium garlic cloves, minced

¼ tsp cayenne pepper (or to taste)

2 cups water (add extra water if desired to modify thickness)

1 cup low-sodium chicken or vegetable broth

½ pound bay scallops

½ pound shrimp, medium, peeled and deveined.

2 cups kidney beans, cooked, rinsed, and drained

¼ pound spicy, cooked turkey sausage, diced (optional)

1 tsp gumbo filé powder (ground sassafras leaves)

½ cup chopped parsley for garnish

In a medium saucepan, bring rice and water to a boil; then simmer 45 minutes until cooked. Set aside.

Heat a large pot on medium-high, add olive oil and onion with salt, oregano, and paprika, stirring occasionally for 1 minute. Add oat flour and chicken while stirring occasionally for 2 minutes. Then reduce to medium heat and add celery, green and red peppers, and bay leaf, and cook another 3 minutes, stirring occasionally.

Add okra, tomatoes, garlic, cayenne pepper, water, and broth. Bring to a gentle boil, then simmer for 10 minutes. Add scallops, shrimp, and kidney beans (and sausage, if desired) and simmer another 10 minutes. Remove from heat and stir in gumbo filé powder.

To serve, remove bay leaf. Mound rice in a bowl, pour in gumbo, then garnish with parsley.

Nutrient Content per Serving:

| Calories: | 598 | Total Fat: | 13.3 grams | Protein: | 45 grams |
|---|---|---|---|---|---|
| Fiber: | 20 grams | Saturated Fat: | 1.9 grams | Carbs: | 78 grams |
| Sodium: | 773 mg | Fat %: | 20% | | |

## Italian Seafood Stew

This is a favorite meal in our home for company. Be sure you buy very fresh fish and shellfish. Vary vegetables and seafood according to availability.

Prep Time: 20 minutes

Simmering Time: 30 minutes

*Serves 4 (makes 8–10 cups)*

1 pound mussels and/or clams in the shell, scrubbed clean

1 Tbsp virgin olive oil

1 medium onion, chopped

¼ tsp sea salt

1 cup sliced mushrooms

1 tsp Italian herbs, dried (rosemary, thyme, oregano, basil)

¼ tsp ground black pepper

3 large carrots, chopped

1 medium-large fennel (or 3 celery stalks)*

1 cup red wine

1 medium red bell pepper, remove seeds, stem, and chop

1 cup chopped tomatoes or tomato sauce

2 cups vegetable or fish broth, low-sodium (prepared, or see
   Vegetable Stock recipe page 344)

1 pound white fish (tilapia, cod, snapper, catfish, whichever is fresh),
   cut into 1-inch pieces

½ pound shrimp, large, peeled and deveined (or crab legs in the shell)

8 large sea scallops

1–2 cups orange juice or milk

½ cup chopped parsley

*Note:* To prepare fennel, cut away any tiny roots from the base, remove stems and leaves. Chop fennel bulb into ½-inch pieces.

Scrub clams and/or mussels with a soap-free brush under fresh water. Set aside. If mussels, remove brown thread material (beard) with fingers or small pliers.

Heat a large stock pot over medium-high heat. Add oil, then onion, salt, mushrooms, Italian herbs, and black pepper, and stir for 2 minutes. Add carrots and fennel and cook another 2 minutes. Add wine to deglaze for 30 seconds, while stirring (the wine helps release the onion's sugars that are stuck to the pan). Add bell pepper, tomato, and broth, and let simmer for 15 to 20 minutes.

Meanwhile, soak fish, shrimp, and scallops in orange juice or milk for 15 minutes. Rinse and drain when ready to add to pot. Discard juice or milk.

Bring another pan with a steamer tray to a boil, add mussels and/or clams, and cook until they open, 5 to 6 minutes. Drain, saving 1 cup of clam-mussel liquid from steaming, and set aside.

Increase temperature under the large stock pot to medium-high and add fish, shrimp, and scallops. Heat 4 to 5 minutes, until shrimp are pink and fish is cooked. Add drained mussels and/or clams, plus 1 cup of clam-mussel liquid, and simmer another minute.

Ladle stew into bowls and garnish with parsley. This stew is fabulous accompanied with heavy, whole-grain bread. It's also great to serve a tossed green salad on the side or as a second course. Be sure to set the table with a second batch of large bowls for discarded shells.

Nutrient Content per Serving:

| Calories: | 852 | Total Fat: | 8.5 grams | Protein: | 51 grams |
|---|---|---|---|---|---|
| Fiber: | 8 grams | Saturated Fat: | 1.7 grams | Carbs: | 30 grams |
| Sodium: | 734 mg | Fat %: | 20% | | |

## Clams with Celery, Baby Potatoes, Carrots, Garlic, and Wine

As a child, I enjoyed digging clams on the beach. Fresh clams cooked with vegetables, herbs, and white wine are wonderful fare and are one of my favorite childhood memories. Enjoy.

### Prep Time: 30 minutes
*Serves 4*

8 pounds fresh clams in the shell

1 Tbsp virgin olive oil

1 medium onion, diced

¼ tsp ground black pepper

1 tsp dried oregano

1 cup white wine (I prefer Chenin blanc or Sauvignon blanc for this dish, most any dry wine will do)

4 medium carrots, chopped

4 medium celery stalks (preferably with leaves), chopped

2 cups baby potatoes (fingerlings, 1–2 inches long)

2 cups vegetable (low-sodium) broth (prepared or see Vegetable Stock recipe, page 344)

½ to 1 cup chopped parsley (if you have ½ cup celery leaves, use only ½ cup parsley, total amount of greens should equal 1 cup)

Scrub clams with a soap-free brush under fresh water and set aside.

Briefly, heat a large pot on medium-high heat, add oil with onion, pepper, and oregano and sauté for about 2 minutes, stirring occasionally until onion is partially translucent. Pour in wine to deglaze (release onion sugars stuck to the pan), add carrots, celery stalks (save celery leaves for serving), potatoes, and broth and bring to a gentle boil. Turn down to low heat and simmer for 20 minutes.

Bring again to a gentle boil, add clams, and reduce to medium heat for 5 to 7 minutes, until most clams have opened. Add parsley and/or celery leaves, stir, and serve. Clams that don't open with a little extra cooking time might be bad, so discard.

**Nutrient Content per Serving:**

| Calories: | 434 | Protein: | 24.5 grams | Fat: | 5.4 grams |
|-----------|-----|----------|------------|------|-----------|
| Fiber: | 8.3 grams | Carbs: | 54 grams | Saturated Fat: | 0.6 grams |
| Sodium: | 606 mg | Fat %: | 11% | | |

## Mussels with Ginger, Lemon Grass, and Coconut Milk

I love this dish, as it is fragrant and delicious, with a Thai twist. The ginger, lemon grass, basil, lime, and veggies add wonderful nutrients to complement the recipe. Since there are many flavors, if a few, such as lemon grass, are unavailable in your area, it will still taste delicious.

### Prep Time: 30 minutes
*Serves 2*

3 pounds mussels (fresh in shell, with beards removed); this is about 40 medium mussels in shell

1⅓ cup water

⅔ cup brown rice

1 Tbsp nut oil (almond or coconut)

1 medium red onion, sliced into 1-inch slivers

2 medium lemon grass stalks*

1½ Tbsp peeled and sliced gingerroot (½-inch slivers)

1 cup sliced, mushrooms

2 medium carrots, cut into 1-inch slivers

⅛ tsp ground cayenne (or 2 red chili peppers, which you can remove before serving—if you don't like heat, skip it)

7 ounces coconut milk (canned)

1 cup vegetable broth, low-sodium

1 medium bell pepper (red, orange, or yellow), sliced into 1-inch strips

1 cup snow peas

2 medium green onions, diced

1 cup green cabbage, cut into very thin 1-inch slices

1 Tbsp lime juice

2 Tbsp chopped fresh basil

*Note:* To prepare lemon grass, use 2 to 3 inches of stalk, trim off the tiny roots, discard the tops, and dice finely to yield about 3 tablespoons.

To clean mussels, scrub with a soap-free brush under fresh water. If brown threads (beards) emerge from shells, pull them off with fingers or small pliers. Plan to cook the mussels immediately after cleaning.

In a pan, bring water to a boil. Add brown rice and reduce heat to a simmer. Cover and cook for 40 minutes. When rice is nearly cooked, turn off heat.

Heat a large pot on medium-high. Add oil, then onion, lemon grass, and gingerroot. Sauté for 1 minute, stirring occasionally; then add mushrooms, carrots, and cayenne pepper (if using), and sauté another 2 to 3 minutes, until onions are translucent. Add coconut milk and vegetable broth. Once the soup reaches a gentle boil, reduce to low heat.

Add bell peppers and snow peas, turn heat back to medium-high and, when gentle boiling resumes, add green onions, cabbage, lime juice, fresh basil, and mussels. Cover and let cook for 4 to 5 minutes, stirring contents every 2 minutes. Once the majority of mussels have opened, turn off the heat and serve. Mussels that don't open with a little extra cooking time might be bad, so discard.

Serve with side bowls of steamed brown rice. Some people enjoy eating mussels from the shell—if so, set the table with empty bowls for shells.

Nutrient Content per Serving:

| Calories: | 851 | Protein: | 50.5 grams | Fat: | 34 grams |
|---|---|---|---|---|---|
| Fiber: | 10.9 grams | Carbs: | 87 grams | Saturated Fat: | 18.4 grams |
| Sodium: | 1,174 mg | Fat %: | 36% | | |

## Lobster Kebobs

Grilling fish or meat with vegetables on a skewer is easy. Just make sure to marinate for at least 10 to 15 minutes in advance. For a special occasion, my wife and I will have lobster, but you can also choose shrimp, large scallops, chicken breast, pork tenderloin, or lean steak. Serve with a mixed green salad with your favorite vinaigrette dressing.

Prep Time: 10–15 minutes
Marinating Time: 15–60 minutes
Grilling Time: 8–11 minutes
*Serves 2*

### Kebobs

12 ounces lobster tails (which would be 16 ounces with the shell; or 12 ounces shrimp, large scallops, or sirloin steak), cut into 18 pieces, about 1 inch each

1 large red bell pepper, cut into 1-inch pieces

1 large yellow or orange bell pepper, cut into 1-inch pieces

8 ounces baby bella mushrooms (or regular small whole mushrooms)

18 cherry tomatoes

1 large red onion, skin removed, and cut into quarters and separated into thin layers

### Marinade

3 Tbsp virgin olive oil

2 Tbsp lemon juice

2 tsp ground paprika

1 tsp Italian herbs

½ tsp sea salt

¼ tsp ground black pepper

⅛ tsp ground cayenne (optional—for those who like heat, but I don't use with lobster as it diminishes the subtle flavors)

4 medium garlic cloves, minced

Prepare seafood and vegetables as noted above. Whisk marinade ingredients together. Set grill at 450°F or turn on the broiler. Combine seafood, vegetables, and marinade in a bowl, turning occasionally for at least 15 minutes while grill/broiler heats.

Grease 6 metal skewers and skewer red and yellow pepper, red onion, and mushrooms, alternating with 3 pieces of seafood and 3 tomatoes per skewer. In truth, you could easily grill or broil without the skewers, but the skewers make it easy to turn everything uniformly, plus they make a great presentation when serving.

Grill or broil for 8 to 11 minutes, until protein is cooked, but not dry, turning 2 or 3 times. Meanwhile toss a mixed green salad with your favorite vinaigrette dressing (see page 344 for an option). Serve the salad on the plates and align the kebobs over the salad.

Nutrient Content per Serving (with lobster, not including salad):

| Calories: | 410 | Protein: | 40 grams | Fat: | 17.2 grams |
|---|---|---|---|---|---|
| Fiber: | 5.7 grams | Carbs: | 26 grams | Saturated Fat: | 2.5 grams |
| Sodium: | 673 mg | Fat %: | 37% | | |

## Cod with Hazelnut Crust

Fish with a nut crust is very tasty. Below, I chose cod and hazelnuts, but also try pecans, pistachios, or almonds. Choose the freshest white fish you can find; flounder, tilapia, snapper, catfish, or sole also works well here.

### Prep Time: 20–25 minutes
### Baking Time: 20–25 minutes
*Serves 4*

1½ pounds cod or other white fish (in 4 fillets)
1 cup orange juice
1 large egg (omega-3, free-range, organic)
1 cup coarsely ground hazelnuts
½ tsp sea salt
1 tsp thyme, dried (or a mixture of Italian or fines herbes)
⅛ tsp ground black pepper
Nut oil (almond or walnut)
4 medium garlic cloves, minced
4 lemon wedges

Preheat oven to 425°F.

Rinse fish fillets, soak in orange juice for 10 minutes, then pat dry. Meanwhile, beat the egg in a bowl.

Heat a sauté pan to medium, sauté the ground hazelnuts with salt, thyme, pepper, and garlic for 2 minutes, enough to toast the hazelnuts slightly, but not brown them.

Transfer ¼ of nut mixture to a plate at a time. Dip the fish first in the egg, then in the hazelnut mixture. When dipping fish coated with egg in the nut flour, some of the flour will become wet and will clump.

When finished coating fish, discard all the excess nut mixture that came in contact with raw fish.

Coat a baking dish with nut oil and place fish on it.

Bake 20 to 25 minutes, until tender and flaky. Garnish with a wedge of lemon.

**Nutrient Content per Serving:**

| Calories: | 286 | Total Fat: | 14 grams | Protein: | 35.5 grams |
|-----------|-----|------------|----------|----------|------------|
| Fiber: | 3.5 grams | Saturated Fat: | 1.1 grams | Carbs: | 6 grams |
| Sodium: | 476 mg | Fat %: | 44% | | |

## Artichoke, Leek, and Mushroom Soufflé

People think of soufflés as being hard to make, but this recipe is fairly easy, and it has a wonderful fluffy texture! You can serve it hot immediately, or save it and serve it cold the next day for brunch. This soufflé won't rise much because of the leek, artichoke, and mushroom filling, yet these nutrient-packed vegetables add structure that prevent the soufflé from falling.

**Prep Time: 35–40 minutes**

**Baking Time: 35 minutes**

*Serves 4*

2 Tbsp virgin olive oil

2 medium leeks, finely diced (use only the white bases and the first inch of light green)

¼ tsp sea salt

⅛ tsp ground black pepper

1 tsp fines herbes, dried (parsley, chives, tarragon)

2 cups diced shiitake mushrooms, woody stems removed

1 cup finely chopped kale

1 cup marinated artichoke hearts (drained), diced

½ cup white wine

¼ cup oat flour (whole grain)

1 cup almond milk (or soy, coconut, or nonfat cow's milk)

½ cup grated part-skim mozzarella cheese

2 Tbsp grated Parmesan cheese

6 large eggs (organic, free-range, omega-3), separated

Virgin olive oil

2 Tbsp chopped fresh parsley (for garnish)

1 Tbsp sliced almonds (for garnish)

Preheat oven to 400°F. Prep the vegetables.

Heat a sauté pan on medium-high. Add oil, then leeks, salt, pepper, and herbs, stirring occasionally.

After 2 minutes, add mushrooms and heat another 3 minutes.

Add kale and artichoke hearts, stir occasionally for 2 minutes; then reduce heat to medium.

Deglaze the pan by adding wine and stirring. Add the flour as the wine evaporates, stirring until the flour coats the vegetables. Continue cooking until mixture is nearly dry.

Add almond milk, stirring occasionally as the mixture forms a sauce. When thickened, but not dry, remove from heat and stir in the grated cheese. Set aside.

Carefully separate the eggs into whites and yolks. Be sure the bowl for the egg whites is absolutely dry, and don't allow any yolk to fall into the whites. Whisk the yolks until blended and then stir into the vegetable mixture.

Whip egg whites at high speed until they are stiff and form peaks. Gently fold ¼ of egg whites into the vegetable/sauce mixture. Then fold ¼ of vegetable/sauce mixture into the remaining egg whites so they blend slowly.

Then combine the two a little at a time so that egg whites remain fluffy and are mixed with vegetables. If you overmix, the air within the whipped egg whites will be lost. The soufflé won't rise, but will still taste delicious.

Spray or wipe a soufflé dish (a 4-inch-high and 9-inch-diameter ceramic casserole dish) with virgin olive oil. Gently pour egg-vegetable mixture into it. Garnish top with fresh parsley and sliced almonds.

Bake for 35 minutes or until a long wooden skewer or thin knife blade inserted comes out clean. Serve immediately. It should be moist but not runny in the center. If runny after cutting, just put back in the oven for 5 minutes. When you serve, it will collapse about 30% in height. Not to worry. It will still taste fabulous.

**Nutrient Content per Serving:**

| Calories: | 299 | Fat: | 16.1 grams | Protein: | 18 grams |
|---|---|---|---|---|---|
| Fiber: | 3.8 grams | Saturated Fat: | 5.1 grams | Carbs: | 15.2 grams |
| Sodium: | 578 mg | Fat %: | 48% | | |

# Turkey Chili

This chili is terrific, with or without the turkey. Serve chili by itself, or serve with a side of brown rice. Makes great leftovers for lunch.

Prep Time: 20–25 minutes

Simmer Time: 5–10 minutes

*Serves 4*

2 Tbsp virgin olive oil

1 medium onion, chopped

½ tsp sea salt

¼ tsp ground black pepper

1 tsp oregano, dried

1 tsp ground paprika

½ tsp cumin powder

1 pound ground turkey breast, organic, free-range (optional)

2 medium carrots, diced

1 medium celery rib, diced

4 medium garlic cloves, diced

2 medium green chilies, roasted (see page 337 for how to roast, or use 4–6 ounces canned or jarred)

¼ tsp crushed red pepper (or to taste)

1 cup water

⅓ cup marinara sauce (or any tomato sauce)

1 medium tomato, chopped

45 ounces pinto beans, cooked, rinsed, and drained (about 5½ cups or three 15-ounce cans)

½ cup chopped fresh cilantro

4 cilantro sprigs (for garnish)

Heat a large saucepan on medium-high, add oil, then onion, salt, black pepper, oregano, paprika, and cumin. Sauté for 1 minute, stirring occasionally. If using ground turkey, add now; sauté for 2 minutes, stirring occasionally, until mostly opaque.

Add carrots and and celery and sauté another 2 minutes while stirring occasionally.

Add garlic, chilies, crushed red pepper, water, marinara sauce, and tomato. When bubbling, add pinto beans, stirring occasionally. When bubbling again, reduce heat and simmer 5 to 10 minutes. Just before serving, add chopped cilantro.

Garnish serving bowls with fresh cilantro sprigs.

Nutrient Content per Serving:

| Calories: | 554 | Fat: | 18.5 grams | Protein: | 41 grams |
|---|---|---|---|---|---|
| Fiber: | 19 grams | Saturated Fat: | 3.9 grams | Carbs: | 57 grams |
| Sodium: | 602 mg | Fat %: | 30% | | |

## Spinach Curry with Tofu and Coconut Milk

Saag panir is a popular dish in Indian restaurants; it is spinach curry with cheese, and is typically loaded with ghee (clarified butter) or cream. Tofu and coconut milk make an easy and healthy substitution.

Prep Time: 30–35 minutes
*Serves 4*

16 ounces cooked spinach (about 3 cups; if frozen, steam and drain; if fresh, you'll need to steam and drain 4 pounds of fresh spinach, washing carefully to remove sand)

1 Tbsp nut oil (almond or coconut), divided

14 ounces tofu, firm (organic), cut into 1-inch cubes

¾ tsp sea salt, divided

½ tsp ground paprika

½ medium onion, diced

1 cup diced mushrooms (button or oyster)

1 Tbsp curry powder

⅛ tsp cayenne pepper (or to taste)

4 large garlic cloves, minced

6 ounces coconut milk

Cook or thaw spinach, drain, and set aside in a bowl.

Heat a sauté pan or skillet to medium. Add 2 teaspoons nut oil (reserve the rest), then tofu. Add ¼ tsp salt and ground paprika. Heat 3 to 4 minutes, stirring occasionally. Turn seasoned tofu into bowl with spinach.

Return pan to medium-high heat, add remaining 1 teaspoon oil, add onion with remaining ½ teaspoon sea salt, and sauté 2 to 3 minutes, until onion softens, stirring occasionally.

Add mushrooms, curry spice, and cayenne pepper; stir, cover, and heat another 2 to 3 minutes, until mushrooms soften.

Reduce heat to medium, add garlic, spinach, tofu, and coconut milk. Stir and heat another 2 to 3 minutes. This dish is typically served with either rice or another curry dish.

Nutrient Content per Serving:

| Calories: | 121 | Fat: | 7 grams | Protein: | 8.2 grams |
|---|---|---|---|---|---|
| Fiber: | 3.2 grams | Saturated Fat: | 1 gram | Carbs: | 9.4 grams |
| Sodium: | 461 mg | Fat %: | 47% | | |

## Tamarind-Tamari Tofu with Broccoli and Shiitake Mushrooms

People think of tofu as bland, yet it absorbs every flavor you can imagine. This sauce makes tofu taste great. If you like, you can use it with chicken, sirloin, pork tenderloin, or seafood. If you can't find tamarind chutney or tamarind sauce, oyster sauce works nicely too.

Prep Time: 15 minutes
Rice Prep Time: 40 minutes
Baking Time: 20 minutes
*Serves 2*

½ cup brown rice
1 cup water
1 pound firm, organic tofu

*Tamarind Sauce*

2 Tbsp tamarind chutney; avoid brands containing MSG
(monosodium glutamate) or more than 5 grams of sugar per
2 Tbsp serving
1½ Tbsp low-sodium tamari sauce (or low-sodium soy sauce)
1 Tbsp lime juice, freshly squeezed
2 Tbsp white wine
1 Tbsp grated gingerroot (or 1 tsp ground gingerroot powder)
4 medium garlic cloves, minced
¼ tsp ground black pepper
⅛ tsp cayenne pepper (or hot chili sauce to taste)
1 tsp sesame oil
½ tsp cornstarch

2 cups (6–7 ounces) sliced shiitake mushrooms, woody stems
removed
4 cups sliced broccoli, florets and stems (1- to 2-inch strips)
½ tsp nut oil (almond or walnut)
2 Tbsp white wine
½ tsp sesame seeds (or chopped nuts)

Put rice and water in a saucepan, bring to a boil, cover, and simmer for
30 to 40 minutes, until cooked.

Preheat oven to 400°F.

Rinse tofu block, then cut into ½- by 2-inch strips. Combine Tamarind
Sauce ingredients and whisk together. Place tofu strips in a baking dish
or on a cookie sheet, covering the bottom of the dish with a single layer
of tofu. Set aside 2 tablespoons of Tamarind Sauce and pour the rest
over the tofu. Bake for 20 minutes.

Meanwhile, slice shiitake mushrooms and broccoli. Five minutes
before removing the tofu from the oven, heat a sauté pan to medium-
high and add oil, then sauté mushrooms in the pan for 2 minutes, until

soft; then add broccoli, white wine, and 1 tablespoon of the remaining Tamarind Sauce. Cover and steam for 2 minutes, until broccoli is barely cooked and still bright green. Remove from heat and uncover.

To serve, mound the rice in the center of the plate, spoon mushrooms and broccoli over rice, creating more height, and add the cooked tofu around the sides. Drizzle remaining sauce over tofu. Sprinkle sesame seeds as a garnish.

**Nutrient Content per Serving:**

| Calories: | 618 | Fat: | 16.6 grams | Protein: | 33 grams |
|-----------|-----|------|------------|----------|----------|
| Fiber: | 10.4 grams | Saturated Fat: | 1.0 gram | Carbs: | 88 grams |
| Sodium: | 652 mg | Fat %: | 23% | | |

## Mushroom-Nut Paté

This dish is incredibly rich, thanks to the nuts and mushrooms. Serve with a lightly steamed vegetable and/or a light salad.

Prep Time: 30 minutes

Baking Time: 50–60 minutes

*Serves 4*

1 Tbsp virgin olive oil

1 medium onion, diced

4 cups diced mushrooms (great with shiitakes, yet button mushrooms are good too)

2 medium carrots, diced

¼ tsp ground black pepper

½ tsp sea salt

1 tsp Italian herbs, dried

½ cup port wine

6 large eggs, omega-3, organic, free-range, beaten

1 cup finely chopped nuts (almonds, pecans, hazelnuts)

Olive oil or parchment paper

Heat a sauté pan to medium-high. Add oil to warm; add onion, and sauté for one minute, stirring occasionally. Add mushrooms, carrots, black pepper, salt, and Italian herbs, and sauté another 5 minutes, stirring occasionally, until the mushrooms have softened. Reduce heat to low, add port wine, and stir. Heat until the bottom of the pan is still moist but most of the port has evaporated. Set aside.

Whisk eggs. Mix eggs, nuts, and veggie-mushroom mixture together; then pour into an oven loaf pan lined with parchment paper (or grease the pan with olive oil). Bake for 50 to 60 minutes at 375° until a toothpick comes out clean. Remove from the oven and let solidify for 5 to 10 minutes prior to serving.

**Nutrient Content per Serving:**

| Calories: | 415 | Fat: | 29 grams | Protein: | 17 grams |
|---|---|---|---|---|---|
| Fiber: | 5.3 grams | Saturated Fat: | 4.3 grams | Carbs: | 18 grams |
| Sodium: | 391 mg | Fat %: | 61% | | |

## Ratatouille

I love this fragrant and delicious side dish from southern France, and it's packed with nutrients. It accompanies chicken or fish, and especially a soufflé. Add 1 pound of cubed tofu or cannellini beans to make a complete meal. Ratatouille can be served hot or cold and usually tastes better when served the next day.

**Prep Time: 10 minutes**

**Cooking Time: 20 minutes**

*Serves 4*

- 1 medium eggplant (remove ends and any damaged skin), cut into 1-inch cubes
- 1 Tbsp virgin olive oil
- 1 medium sweet onion, diced
- ½ tsp sea salt
- ¼ tsp ground black pepper
- ½ tsp oregano, dried
- ½ tsp fines herbes (or Italian herbs), dried
- 3 small zucchini, chopped into ½-inch cubes (about 2½ cups)
- 2 small yellow squash, chopped into ½-inch cubes (about 2 cups)
- 2 Tbsp white wine
- 3 medium tomatoes, chopped (about 2½ cups)
- 4 medium garlic cloves, minced
- 1 Tbsp chopped fresh parsley
- 1 tsp diced fresh rosemary
- 1 Tbsp chopped fresh basil
- ⅛ tsp paprika or cayenne powder (or to taste)
- 15 ounces cubed firm tofu or 15 ounces cooked cannellini beans (optional)
- Fresh herbs for garnish (parsley, basil, and/or thyme)

Steam eggplant on the stove top for 6 minutes or microwave in a glass container for 4 minutes. Cook until tender.

Meanwhile, heat a pan to medium-high and add olive oil. Once hot, add onion, salt, black pepper, oregano, and fines herbes. Sauté for 1 to 2 minutes, or until onions are soft and translucent. Add zucchini, yellow squash, eggplant, and wine, and stir. Cover and heat for 3 minutes, until vegetables soften, stirring occasionally. Add tomatoes, garlic, and fresh herbs; reduce heat to low and cover. Let simmer for 4 to 10 minutes, until squash softens and flavors blend. If you like a touch of heat, add paprika or cayenne pepper.

Garnish with fresh herbs. For a full meal instead of a side dish, add 15 ounces of cubed firm tofu or cooked cannellini beans with the garlic and herbs.

Nutrient Content per Serving:                                    With Cannellini Beans:

| | | |
|---|---|---|
| Calories: | 134 | 210 |
| Protein: | 5 grams | 9 grams |
| Total Fat: | 4.3 grams | 5 grams |
| Saturated Fat: | 0.7 gram | 0.7 gram |
| Sodium: | 353 mg | 384 mg |
| Fiber: | 8 grams | 12 grams |

# Quinoa Salad 🕐

A nutrient-packed side dish everyone will love. It is made with one of the most nutritious grains on the planet and cooks faster than most others. Quinoa is light and very pretty, with a pearly hue. Add a few colorful herbs and vegetables and you have a beautiful dish. Add garbanzo or cannellini beans to the leftovers for an easy lunch.

**Prep Time: 15–20 minutes**
*Serves 6 (makes great leftovers)*

1 cup quinoa
1¼ cup vegetable broth
1 Tbsp olive oil
1 onion, chopped
1 cup sliced wild mushrooms (such as shiitake, crimini, or oyster)
¼ cup chopped fresh herbs (such as basil, parsley, and/or mint)
2 green onions, finely chopped
2 medium tomatoes, diced
¼ cup chopped nuts (walnuts, pecans, and/or almonds)
Salt and pepper to taste
Fresh herb sprigs for garnish

Rinse 1 cup of dried quinoa under running water and drain in a strainer. In a small saucepan, bring vegetable broth to a boil. Add the rinsed quinoa, bring it back to a boil, and then cover and simmer for 10 minutes. Set aside, covered, until liquid has been absorbed (about 10 minutes).

Heat a sauté pan on medium and add oil. Add onion and cook for 1 minute. Add the mushrooms and sauté until they soften, about 2 minutes. Remove from heat and add fresh chopped herbs. In a serving dish, combine with cooked quinoa along with green onions and tomatoes.

In a separate pan, gently roast nuts until slightly browned; remove from heat and sprinkle on quinoa salad. Season to taste with salt and pepper. Garnish with herb sprigs. Serve warm or cold.

**Nutrient Content per Serving:**

| Calories: | 190 | Protein: | 5.4 grams | Total Fat: | 7.3 grams |
|---|---|---|---|---|---|
| Saturated Fat: | 0.5 gram | Sodium: | 206 mg | Fiber: | 3.6 grams |

## Roasted Kale 🕐

Very easy to make and surprisingly crispy and satisfying—the kale will melt in your mouth.

### Prep Time: 5 minutes
### Baking Time: 15 minutes

5–6 large kale leaves (about 8 cups, enough to fill a baking tray)
¼ tsp extra-virgin olive oil or 4 seconds olive oil spray
⅛ tsp sea salt
⅛ tsp ground black pepper
¼ tsp paprika

Preheat oven to 400°F. Remove stems from kale leaves and cut leaves into 3- to 4-inch pieces. Spread on a baking sheet. Spray with oil. Sprinkle with salt, pepper, and paprika. Bake for 15 minutes, until crispy.

**Nutrient Content per Serving:**

| Calories: | 75 | Fat: | 1.8 grams | Protein: | 4.5 grams |
|---|---|---|---|---|---|
| Fiber: | 3 grams | Saturated Fat: | 0.25 gram | Carbs: | 14.5 grams |
| Sodium | 124 mg | Fat %: | 19% | | |

## Broccoli and Shiitake Mushroom Sauté 🕐

This simple side dish is packed with nutrients and flavor.

### Prep Time: 10–15 minutes
*Serves 4*

2 tsp virgin olive oil
½ medium sweet onion, sliced into long slivers

2 cups shiitake mushrooms, sliced into long slices

¼ tsp sea salt

⅛ tsp ground black pepper

1 tsp Italian dried herbs

2 Tbsp white wine (dry cooking wine)

4 cups broccoli, sliced into 2- to 3-inch pieces

Heat a sauté pan to medium-high. Add oil, onion, mushrooms, salt, pepper, and herbs and sauté 2 minutes, stirring occasionally. Add wine and broccoli, and cover as it steams. Heat 2 to 3 minutes, until broccoli is al dente. Serve immediately.

**Nutrient Content per Serving:**

| Calories: | 88 | Fat: | 2.7 grams | Protein: | 2.7 grams |
|-----------|-----------|----------------|-----------|----------|-----------|
| Fiber: | 2.6 grams | Saturated Fat: | 0.4 gram | Carbs: | 14 grams |
| Sodium: | 164 mg | Fat %: | 24% | | |

# Basmati Brown Rice

An easy to make side dish that goes great with curries, fish, or bean dishes.

### Prep Time: 10 minutes
### Simmering Time: 40 minutes
*Serves 4*

1 Tbsp nut oil (almond or walnut)

½ medium onion, chopped

1 cup brown basmati rice, uncooked

1¼ cups water

1 cup low-sodium vegetable or chicken stock (see Vegetable Stock, page 344)

1 cup peas, shelled, frozen

2 Tbsp pistachios

Heat a saucepan to medium-high. Add oil, onion, and sauté for 1 minute. Then add rice and sauté 1 minute, stirring occasionally. Add water and stock, bring to a boil, cover, and then simmer for 40 minutes, until rice is cooked but still firm. Stir in peas, remove from heat, and set aside. Just before serving, heat nuts in a pan for 1 to 2 minutes, until warmed and fragrant, but not browned. To serve, spoon rice onto plates and garnish with nuts.

# Roasted Beets and Squash

Vegetables are sweeter roasted than they are when boiled or sautéed. The herbs and spices make them fragrant. This is an excellent side dish for many entrees. Besides, the colors are gorgeous. I always try to make extra so I have leftovers for the next day.

**Prep Time: 10–15 minutes**

**Baking Time: 45 minutes**

*Serves 6 (yields about 10 cups)*

4 medium beets, cut into ½-inch cubes (about 3 cups)

1 small butternut squash, cut into ¾-inch cubes (about 3 cups); save seeds for a garnish

3 medium yellow scallop squash (or any yellow squash), cut into 1-inch cubes (about 2 cups)

2 medium zucchini, cut into 1-inch cubes (about 2 cups)

3 Tbsp virgin olive oil

½ tsp sea salt

½ tsp ground black pepper

1 tsp Italian herbs, dried

2 cups garbanzo beans, cooked, rinsed, and drained

Preheat oven to 400°F. Put beets into a large baking pan and roast for 10 minutes.

After 10 minutes, remove the baking pan with beets from the oven and add cubed squashes to the hot baking pan. Mix with oil, salt, pepper, herbs, and garbanzos. Sprinkle butternut squash seeds over the top. Bake for about 40 minutes, until all veggies are tender. Serve immediately. Leftovers can be served hot or cold.

Nutrient Content per Serving:

| Calories: | 184 | Protein: | 7.3 grams | Total Fat: | 8.0 grams |
|---|---|---|---|---|---|
| Saturated Fat: | 1 gram | Fat %: | 33% | Sodium: | 375 mg |
| Fiber: | 6.8 grams | | | | |

# Wild Rice with Kale and Wild Mushrooms

This is a flavorful side dish. As a double portion, it makes a light meal. "Wild rice" isn't actually rice, but a grass, which cooks like rice and is loaded with delicious nutrients. And the kale makes it very colorful and healthful!

Simmering Time: 50 minutes

*Serves 4*

- 1 cup wild rice
- 4 cups water
- 1 cup low-sodium chicken or vegetable stock (prepared, or see Vegetable Stock recipe, page 344)
- 1 Tbsp nut oil (almond or walnut)
- 1 medium onion, diced
- ¼ tsp sea salt
- ¼ tsp ground black pepper
- 1 tsp Italian herbs
- 4 cups wild mushrooms (shiitake, crimini, chanterelle, or oyster)
- 4 cups chopped kale, tough stems removed (thin slices)
- 15 ounces garbanzo beans, cooked, rinsed, and drained
- 2 Tbsp chopped pecans

Combine wild rice, water, and stock in a pot; bring to a boil. Simmer for 50 minutes, until rice is barely firm. Drain and set aside.

Ten minutes before rice is ready, heat a large sauté pan to medium-high and add oil, onion, salt, pepper, and herbs. Sauté 1 minute, with occasional stirring. Add mushrooms and sauté an additional 2 minutes until mushrooms soften.

Add kale and garbanzo beans, reduce heat to medium, cover, cook 2 minutes, and remove from heat. When rice is cooked and drained, mix with sautéed vegetables. Serve garnished with pecans.

Nutrient Content per Serving:

| Calories: | 390 | Fat: | 8.3 grams | Protein: | 15.4 grams |
|-----------|-----|----------------|-----------|----------|------------|
| Fiber: | 12 grams | Saturated Fat: | 1 gram | Carbs: | 70.4 grams |
| Sodium: | 326 mg | Fat %: | 18% | | |

## Fiesta Black Bean Salad 🕐

My boys created this salad for me as a surprise. It was delicious! The colors are bright, it is very easy to make, has nice flavors, plus I love the option for a touch of "caliente."

Prep Time: 15 minutes

*Serves 4*

- 1 Tbsp virgin olive oil
- 1 medium onion, diced

¼ tsp sea salt

⅛ tsp ground black pepper

¼ tsp ground cumin

¼ tsp dried oregano

2 medium poblano peppers, de-stemmed, seeds removed, and chopped (poblanos can be sweet to spicy—if you don't want spicy, it's okay to use a bell pepper instead)

4 medium garlic cloves, minced

¼ tsp red chili flakes (or to taste)

1½ cups black beans, cooked, drained, and rinsed (or 15 ounces canned beans)

1½ cups sweet corn (fresh corn steamed, frozen, or canned and rinsed)

2 medium tomatoes, chopped

½ cup fresh cilantro, chopped

1 Tbsp lime juice

Heat a pan to medium-high. Add oil, onion, salt, black pepper, cumin, and oregano, and sauté for about 2 minutes, until onion softens. Add poblano chilis and heat another minute. Reduce heat to medium, add garlic with optional red chili flakes, heat 1 more minute, and set aside.

In a large bowl, combine black beans, corn, tomatoes, cilantro, and lime juice with the onion-spice mixture. Serve immediately, or serve later chilled.

**Nutrient Content per Serving:**

| Calories: | 190 | Fat: | 4.6 grams | Protein: | 8.3 grams |
|---|---|---|---|---|---|
| Fiber: | 8.9 grams | Saturated Fat: | 0.7 gram | Carbs: | 33 grams |
| Sodium: | 290 mg | Fat %: | 20% | | |

---

# Coleslaw 🕐

This cabbage salad is an easy side dish and is made with tasty, healthy ingredients. Most coleslaw recipes add substantial sugar. I decided to try grating an apple with the slaw instead—delicious!

### Prep Time: 15–20 minutes
*Serves 4*

4 cups shredded green cabbage (remove and discard outer couple leaves before shredding)

3 medium carrots, grated

1 medium red apple, grated

2 medium dill pickles, diced

3 medium green onions, diced

1 Tbsp mayonnaise (see Mayonnaise recipe, page 346)

2 Tbsp nonfat yogurt, plain

2 Tbsp red wine vinegar

1 tsp Dijon mustard

Shred cabbage, and grate carrots and apple. Combine in a bowl with pickles and green onion. In a separate bowl, combine mayonnaise, yogurt, vinegar, and mustard; then mix with slaw. Chill and serve.

**Nutrient Content per Serving:**

| Calories: | 127 | Fat: | 5.8 grams | Protein: | 2.4 grams |
|-----------|-----|------|-----------|----------|-----------|
| Fiber: | 5 grams | Saturated Fat: | 0.3 gram | Carbs: | 18.5 grams |
| Sodium: | 541 mg | Fat %: | 39% | | |

## Steamed Green Beans with Vinaigrette 🕐

A simple flavorful side dish.

### Prep Time: 10–15 minutes
*Serves 4*

6 cups green beans, stems removed

1 Tbsp vinaigrette dressing (see Masley House Vinaigrette Dressing, page 344, or use prepared)

2 Tbsp sliced almond

Steam green beans until al dente, 5 to 6 minutes. Toss green beans in a serving bowl with dressing. Garnish with sliced almonds.

**Nutrient Content per Serving:**

| Calories: | 77 | Fat: | 3.3 grams | Protein: | 3 grams |
|-----------|-----|------|-----------|----------|---------|
| Fiber: | 4.5 grams | Saturated Fat: | 0.3 gram | Carbs: | 9.3 grams |
| Sodium: | 72 mg | Fat %: | 38% | | |

## Steamed Vegetables with Orange Vinaigrette Dressing 🕐

I enjoy using this vinaigrette with steamed broccoli, asparagus, and other vegetables.

Prep time: 10 minutes
*Serves 4*

1 pound asparagus (or broccoli, green beans, etc.)

*Orange Vinaigrette*

1 Tbsp extra virgin olive oil

1 Tbsp red wine vinegar

1 Tbsp orange juice

⅛ tsp sea salt

⅛ tsp ground black pepper

Break off woody asparagus stems. Steam asparagus until al dente—tender but still with a firm bite. Mix dressing ingredients, toss with asparagus, and serve.

## Roasted Peppers 🕐

Roasted peppers go very well with Mexican and Latin dishes. They taste much sweeter than raw peppers, and they remain packed with nutrients. You can roast poblano, bell, green, and just about any type of pepper. They make a great side dish all by themselves. Stuff them with cooked brown rice or quinoa and beans and serve as a side dish.

Set oven on broil, or heat up the grill. Cut off pepper crowns and scoop out and discard the seeds. You can roast a dozen peppers at a time and freeze for later use.

Place peppers in a rimmed ovenproof pan on the top rack of the oven. Roast until skin browns, then turn them. When all sides are browned, about 10 minutes, remove from the oven. Allow to cool. Then peel the skin away. You can chop peppers for a stir-fry, bake them in cornbread, or puree them for a dip.

# DESSERTS

---

## Yogurt, Berries, and Dark Chocolate 🕐

---

This is my favorite dessert. It is so healthy that you could enjoy it as often as you want! This isn't a low-calorie dessert, yet it is loaded with nutrients and is very satisfying.

**Prep Time: 2 minutes**
*Serves 1*

½ cup plain nonfat yogurt

1 cup berries (blueberries, blackberries, raspberries, your choice)

1 Tbsp sliced almonds (or other chopped nuts)

1½ Tbsp dark chocolate chips (preferably containing at least 70% cocoa)

1 Tbsp dried cherries (or other dried fruit)

Combine ingredients and enjoy.

**Nutrient Content per Serving:**

| Calories: | 367 | Total Fat: | 12 grams | Protein: | 10 grams |
|---|---|---|---|---|---|
| Fiber: | 6.4 grams | Saturated Fat: | 4.2 grams (but mostly from dark chocolate, which doesn't count as bad) | Carbs: | 55 grams |
| Sodium: | 78 mg | | | | |

---

## Chocolate-Raspberry-Orange Soufflé

---

For an occasional treat, here is a dessert worth celebrating! The combination of chocolate, raspberry, and orange flavors is one of my favorites. You can't taste the yams, but they provide a nice texture and structure along with healthy fiber for the soufflé.

**Prep Time: 25–30 minutes**
**Baking Time: 35 minutes**
*Serves 6*

¾ cup raspberry sauce (prepared, or see Raspberry Sauce, page 345),
½ cup for the soufflé mixture and ¼ cup for the garnish

1 medium yam (or sweet potato)

3 Tbsp Grand Marnier (or other orange liqueur)

⅛ tsp sea salt

½ cup maple syrup

⅓ cup cocoa powder, preferably Dutch processed, sifted

7 large eggs (organic, free-range, omega-3), separated into whites and yolks

4 Tbsp grated orange zest (2 Tbsp for soufflé mixture, 2 for garnish)

Nut oil (almond or walnut)

1 cup fresh berries

Preheat oven to 400°F. Prepare or buy raspberry sauce. Microwave the yam until soft, about 8 minutes. Peel yam, then mash into a puree.

Combine ½ cup of raspberry sauce with baked yam, Grand Marnier, salt, maple syrup, cocoa, egg yolks, and 2 tablespoons orange zest, and whisk until mixed to make the batter.

Beat egg whites until they form soft peaks.

Gently fold the soufflé batter into the egg whites, just enough so that most of the white of the eggs blends with the chocolate-colored batter. Don't overmix or the soufflé won't rise.

Grease a round soufflé dish (9-inch diameter, 4 inches high) with nut oil. Pour the soufflé batter into the dish. (It should fill 90% of the dish, but don't fill it to the brim; use another dish if necessary.) Bake for 30 to 40 minutes, until the top browns slightly and an inserted long wood skewer or thin knife blade comes out clean. If you take it out too soon and the center is too wet when tested, simply put it back in the oven for an additional 5 minutes.

Have guests at the table and serve immediately. The soufflé will drop as it cools and shrink once cut. Garnish each serving with a drizzle of the remaining raspberry sauce and a sprinkle of orange zest and berries.

Nutrient Content per Serving:

| Calories: | 249 | Total Fat: | 6 grams | Protein: | 8.5 grams |
|-----------|-----|------------|---------|----------|-----------|
| Fiber: | 3.3 grams | Saturated Fat: | 2.1 grams | Carbs: | 39 grams |
| Sodium: | 133 mg | Fat Calories %: | 21% | | |

## Frozen Blueberry-Cherry Yogurt 🕐

This is one of my favorite desserts—quick, easy, and delicious. Any ice cream maker will do. Or you can simply put the slurry in the freezer for 5 to 6 hours before serving.

Prep Time: 10 minutes

Set Time: Varies with ice cream maker, 15 minutes with a Donvier ice cream maker

*Serves 4 (makes 4 cups)*

16 ounces nonfat, plain yogurt (or coconut milk beverage from the carton, not canned)

1 cup blueberries, frozen

1 cup cherries, frozen

3–4 Tbsp maple syrup (optional)

4 Tbsp port wine

1/16 tsp sea salt

1 medium lime, grated, zest and juice

1/2 cup fresh berries

Almond slivers (for garnish)

Combine yogurt, frozen blueberries and cherries, maple syrup, wine, and salt in a blender. Add grated lime peel and lime juice. Purée. Place in ice cream maker and follow manufacturer's instructions. Serve garnished with fresh berries and almond slivers.

Nutrient Content per Serving:

| Calories: | 190 | Total Fat: | 0.5 gram | Protein: | 6 grams |
|---|---|---|---|---|---|
| Fiber: | 2.0 grams | Saturated Fat: | 0 gram | Carbs: | 34 grams |
| Sodium: | 78 mg | Fat Calories %: | 2% | | |

## Apricot-Grand Marnier Soufflé

Simply delicious! This soufflé is easy to prepare.

Prep Time: 15 minutes

Baking Time: 40–45 minutes

*Serves 6*

1¼ cup diced dried apricots

1/2 cup Grand Marnier

1/4 cup almond oil (or any nut oil)

1/4 cup oat flour (whole grain)

1 cup almond milk

1/8 tsp sea salt

1/3 cup maple syrup

7 large eggs, free-range, organic, omega-3

2 cups berries, fresh

Combine apricots and Grand Marnier. Let apricots soak up the liquid for 8 to 24 hours in a sealed container.

Preheat the oven to 375°F. Heat a saucepan to medium. To make the flour sauce, mix oil and flour in the saucepan. When mixture bubbles, add almond milk and salt, and stir occasionally for 5 minutes as it thickens. Remove from heat and stir in maple syrup.

Separate egg whites and yolks carefully so only egg whites are in mixing bowl, but save the yolks. Combine apricots, Grand Marnier, and whipped egg yolks with flour sauce.

Whip egg whites until they form stiff peaks. Gently fold together egg whites and apricot–flour sauce mixture. Don't overstir or egg whites will lose their whipped air and the soufflé won't rise. Coat a soufflé baking dish (4 inches high and 9 inches in diameter) with nut oil; then pour batter into the dish. Bake for 40 to 45 minutes, until the top is lightly browned and an inserted skewer comes out clean. Inside, the soufflé should be moist, but not runny. Serve with fresh berries.

**Nutrient Content per Serving:**

| Calories: | 272 | Total Fat: | 11.5 grams | Protein: | 6.7 grams |
|---|---|---|---|---|---|
| Fiber: | 3 grams | Saturated Fat: | 1.9 grams | Carbs: | 30 grams |
| Sodium: | 78 mg | Fat Calories %: | 37% | | |

## Pear, Peach, and Blueberry Crumble

For guests, this is a lovely dish, as it is loaded with nutrients and flavor. Vary the fruit according to varieties that are naturally ripe and fragrant in season. Typically I'll have the fruit mixture and nut crumble prepared separately in advance, so I can quickly assemble the crumble and pop it into the oven.

**Prep Time: 15 minutes**

**Baking Time: 15 minutes**

*Serves 6*

¼ cup water

¼ cup maple syrup

2 medium pears, cored and cut into ½-inch cubes

½ tsp ground cinnamon

2 Tbsp tapioca, quick cooking

1 medium lime, half the skin grated into zest and juiced

1 Tbsp port wine

2 medium peaches, pitted and cut into ½-inch cubes

2 cups blueberries

¼ cup almond slivers (or chopped nuts)

1 cup oatmeal granola (or any low-sugar granola)

¼ cup fresh berries (for garnish)

Preheat oven to 375° F.

In a saucepan, combine water, maple syrup, pears, cinnamon, and tapioca. Bring to a boil; then reduce heat to a simmer. Stir in lime zest and juice, port wine, and peaches; then heat for 5 minutes. Mix in blueberries and remove from heat.

Pour fruit mixture into a pie plate. Just before placing in the oven, mix the nuts and the granola together and sprinkle the mixture over the top. Bake for 15 minutes. Garnish with fresh berries.

Nutrient Content per Serving:

| Calories: | 159 | Fat: | 0.7 gram | Protein: | 2 grams |
|-----------|------|----------------|----------|----------|----------|
| Fiber: | 4 grams | Saturated Fat: | 0.1 gram | Carbs: | 38 grams |
| Sodium: | 45 mg | Fat %: | 3% | | |

## Marinara Sauce

There are endless possible variations to a marinara sauce. When you add the tomatoes, you also have the choice of adding roasted peppers, artichoke hearts, olives, and/or your favorite items. If you want to have a meat sauce, add one pound of ground turkey breast or ground sirloin before adding the mushrooms and cook until browned; avoid using regular ground turkey and ground beef—hard to know what type of meat you're actually getting. For vegetarian protein, add tofu or vegetarian soy-crumbles before adding the tomatoes and garlic.

Prep Time: 20–25 minutes

Simmering Time: 40–60 minutes

*Makes 8 cups*

2 Tbsp virgin olive oil

1 medium onion, finely chopped

½ tsp sea salt

¼ tsp ground black pepper

1 Tbsp Italian herbs, dried

2 cups finely chopped mushrooms (baby portabellos)

2 medium tomatoes, diced

6 medium garlic cloves, minced

2 Tbsp chopped fresh basil

½ cup red wine

12 ounces tomato paste (aim for not more than 100 mg sodium per 2 Tbsp)

28 ounces tomato puree (aim for not more than 15 mg sodium per ¼ cup)

2 large bay leaves

Heat a large saucepan to medium-high. Add oil, then onion, salt, pepper, and Italian herbs, and sauté for 2 minutes, stirring occasionally. Add mushrooms and heat another 3 minutes, stirring occasionally. Reduce heat to medium, add tomatoes, garlic, fresh basil, and stir. Deglaze pan with wine, and stir. Add tomato paste and puree. Reduce heat, add bay leaves, and simmer 40 to 60 minutes, stirring occasionally.

To serve, remove bay leaves and enjoy. In an airtight sealed container, this freezes nicely, or stores in the refrigerator for several days.

Nutrient Content per Serving (1-cup serving):

| Calories: | 110 | Fat: | 3.7 grams | Protein: | 3.5 grams |
|---|---|---|---|---|---|
| Fiber: | 3.5 grams | Saturated Fat: | 0.5 gram | Carbs: | 16.4 grams |
| Sodium: | 336 mg | Fat %: | 27% | | |

## Vegetable Stock

Vegetable stock is essential for cooking. You add it when sautéing vegetables. You mix it with water when cooking rice or quinoa. You could use ready-made varieties, but be sure to select low-sodium, organic brands if you do.

**Prep Time: 15–20 minutes**

**Simmer Time: 1 hour**

1 Tbsp virgin olive oil

4 medium garlic cloves

1 medium onion, chopped

2 medium celery stalks

1 medium russet potato, diced

2 medium carrots

1 medium tomato, chopped

1 cup chopped mushrooms

1 Tbsp Italian herbs, dried

½ tsp sea salt

6 cups water

2 Tbsp low-sodium tamari sauce

Prepare vegetables. Heat a large soup pot on medium-high, and add oil, garlic, vegetables, herbs, and salt. Sauté for 2 to 3 minutes, stirring occasionally. Add water with tamari sauce, turn heat to high, and bring to a boil. Let simmer 1 hour. Strain, discarding vegetables.

In an airtight sealed container, this freezes nicely, or stores in the refrigerator for several days.

## Masley House Vinaigrette Dressing; Raspberry Vinaigrette; and Creamy Vinaigrette 🕐

I use this dressing all the time. I not only love it with salads, but also tossed with steamed vegetables.

**Prep Time: 3–5 minutes**

3 Tbsp balsamic vinegar

2 Tbsp white wine

4 Tbsp extra virgin olive oil (or avocado oil or a nut oil)

1 tsp low-sodium tamari sauce

½ tsp Italian herbs

¼ tsp ground black pepper

2 medium garlic cloves, finely minced

½ tsp Dijon mustard (optional)

Combine ingredients and serve.

**Raspberry Vinaigrette:** Substitute red wine vinegar for the balsamic vinegar, omit the garlic, mustard, and herbs, and add 1 tablespoon Raspberry Sauce (below).

**Creamy Vinaigrette:** Omit the tamari sauce and mustard, and add 1 tablespoon plain nonfat yogurt.

---

## Raspberry Sauce

This sauce is both sweet and tart, and wonderful with chocolate, on frozen yogurt, and with many desserts.

**Prep Time: 10 minutes**

**Simmering Time: 10 minutes**

*Makes ¾ cup*

2½ cups raspberries, frozen or fresh (about 12 ounces)

¼ cup sugar

1 Tbsp Grand Marnier (or any other liqueur)

2 Tbsp orange juice

⅛ tsp sea salt

1 tsp grated orange zest

A few sprigs of mint or whole berries as garnish, mixed

Heat raspberries and sugar on medium in a saucepan until bubbling. Simmer 5 minutes. Push the raspberry pulp through a large sieve with a spatula to remove the seeds. Combine filtered liquid with Grand Marnier or liqueur, orange juice, zest, and salt. Then simmer another 5 minutes to thicken. Set aside to cool. Garnish before serving.

Nutrient Content per Serving (6 servings):

| Calories: | 83 | Total Fat: | 0.3 gram | Protein: | 0.7 gram |
|---|---|---|---|---|---|
| Fiber: | 2 grams | Saturated Fat: | 2.1 grams | Carbs: | 19 grams |
| Sodium: | 55 mg | Fat %: | 3% | | |

# Mayonnaise 🕐

Mayo you make yourself is much more flavorful and vastly healthier, assuming you choose good ingredients.

**Prep Time: 5–10 minutes**
*Makes nearly 1 cup*

1 large egg, organic, free-range, omega-3
1 medium garlic clove, minced
2 tsp lemon juice
1 tsp Dijon mustard
1/16 tsp sea salt
1/16 tsp Italian herbs
¾ cup nut oil (almond or walnut)

Combine the egg, garlic, lemon juice, mustard, salt, and herbs in a food processer or blender; blend until smooth. With the processor running, slowly drizzle oil into the container. The sauce will thicken. Add additional fresh herbs if desired, after the mayonnaise has formed. Refrigerate immediately.

*Caution: Consuming raw egg products has some significant health risks. To reduce the risk, wash the egg with soap and water and sanitize all surfaces that come in contact with the eggshell, including your hands, after food preparation. If you have significant health issues, then buy processed mayo and avoid using raw egg products.*

# Acknowledgments

It gives me pleasure to extend my deepest and most heartfelt appreciation to all the people who have helped me create this book.

First and foremost I want to thank my wife, Nicole. She has been extremely supportive of the work and hours involved in researching and writing this book. She has also helped me test all the recipes and edited several sections. Besides all this, she has been my love and inspiration for 26 years. Thanks are due as well to our sons, Lucas and Marcos, who have been gracious tasters of my meals for years—as well as recipe developers and cooks themselves! They have also participated in data analysis for the research projects in my clinic.

Many thanks are owed to my agent, Celeste Fine, who has been a wellspring of guidance and support throughout the entire production of this book. Likewise, I feel very blessed to have worked with Susan Golant, a talented writer, who has artfully edited this book and helped to transform technical aspects into lively discussion. Susan has been a great source of support throughout the book's creation.

I owe a special thanks to Kate Hartson, senior editor at Center Street with Hachette Book Group, who appreciated what *The 30-Day Heart Tune-Up* had to offer and has endeavored to make my message clear, practical, and powerful. She and her Center Street team have been fantastic to work with, and I'm grateful for their diligent attention and great ideas.

I am very grateful to the medical library staff at Morton Plant Hospital in Clearwater, Florida; I would like to thank Karen Roth, Rachelle Benzarti, and the many hospital volunteers there. They have helped me review thousands of articles over the last ten years, many of which were seminal for the writing of this book.

My Mastermind group, led by JJ Virgin, has been a wonderful source of support, ideas, and collaboration, both for this book and for my www.hearttuneup.com website. They have generously shared their resources to make this book a success. The initial group most involved includes: JJ Virgin, Miriam Zacharias, Anna Cabeca, Alan Christianson, Hyla Cass, Suzanne Bennett, Mikell Parsons, Habib Wicks, Marcelle Pick, Patricia Ptak, Chef Leanne Ely, and Sara Gottfried. I also owe special thanks to Brendon Burchard for his contribution to my educational message, as well as to Roger Love, my voice coach, for restoring my voice and improving how I communicate with people.

Functional medicine helped me to see beyond the simple model of diagnosing and treating disease and directed me toward assessing optimal function. It has become the cornerstone of my clinical practice. In particular, I am indebted to Jeffrey Bland, David Jones, David Perlmutter, Bethany Hayes, and Mark Hyman for their trailblazing efforts in this field.

Over the last 20 years, my clinical research has been sponsored by several organizations, including Group Health Cooperative of Puget Sound, Morton Plant Hospital, the American Heart Association, and my clinic, the Masley Optimal Health Center. Thank you. I have had the opportunity to publish many scientific articles with wonderful colleagues, and in particular I would like to thank Douglas Schocken, Richard Roetzheim, Sharon Phillips, Lucas Masley, Tom Gualtieri, Tim McNamara, Marcos Masley, and Julia Sokoloff for their contributions.

Several medical colleagues critiqued this book and provided valuable feedback. They include Alain Johnson, Joseph Pellicer, Anna Cabeca, Douglas Schocken, Anup Kanodia, Stephen Sinatra, and Gordon Wheat. I have also been blessed by a group of adventurous recipe testers who tried the recipes, confirmed the prep times, and made numerous suggestions to ensure that the finished product would taste fantastic and be easy to prepare. They include: Tamas Ronyai, executive chef at Seattle Mirabella Center; Michelle and Gary Crosby; Kim and Robert Dvorak; Susan Golant; Kelvie Johnson; Peggy and Arpad Masley; Bob McWhorter and Brooke Masley; Evelyn Odegaard; Michelle Piepgrass; and Susan Thomas. Also, special thanks to Stéphan Daigle for his artistry in creating the figures for this book.

My current medical team at the Masley Optimal Health Center has been incredible in their support for this manuscript and to my patients, with a special thanks to Kim Escarraz, Angie Presby, Maryann Miller, and Katherine Reay.

Last, I am grateful to my many patients for their encouragement in creating this book. In addition to agreeing to participate in my studies, which provided incredible data that show which aspects of this program truly shrink arterial plaque, they have also helped me to convert this technical information into everyday words that empower people along a path toward optimal health and vitality. Their struggles and triumphs continue to be my touchstone and my inspiration.

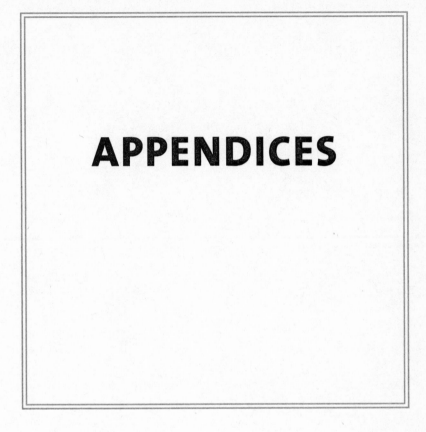

# APPENDICES

# I. Body Mass Index Chart

Male or female—use your height and weight to identify your BMI.

| Weight in lbs | Height in Inches | | | | | | | | | | | | | | | | | | |
|---|---|---|---|---|---|---|---|---|---|---|---|---|---|---|---|---|---|---|---|
| | 58 | 59 | 60 | 61 | 62 | 63 | 64 | 65 | 66 | 67 | 68 | 69 | 70 | 71 | 72 | 73 | 74 | 75 | 76 |
| 100 | 21 | 20 | 20 | 19 | 18 | 18 | 17 | 17 | 16 | 15 | 15 | 15 | 14 | 14 | 14 | 13 | | | |
| 105 | 22 | 21 | 21 | 20 | 19 | 19 | 18 | 17 | 17 | 16 | 16 | 16 | 15 | 15 | 14 | 14 | 13 | | |
| 110 | 23 | 22 | 21 | 21 | 20 | 19 | 19 | 18 | 18 | 17 | 17 | 16 | 16 | 15 | 15 | 15 | 14 | 14 | 13 |
| 115 | 24 | 23 | 22 | 22 | 21 | 20 | 20 | 19 | 19 | 18 | 17 | 17 | 17 | 16 | 16 | 15 | 15 | 14 | 14 |
| 120 | 25 | 24 | 23 | 23 | 22 | 21 | 21 | 20 | 19 | 19 | 18 | 18 | 17 | 17 | 16 | 16 | 16 | 15 | 15 |
| 125 | 26 | 25 | 24 | 24 | 23 | 22 | 21 | 21 | 20 | 20 | 19 | 18 | 18 | 17 | 17 | 16 | 16 | 16 | 15 |
| 130 | 27 | 26 | 25 | 25 | 24 | 23 | 22 | 22 | 21 | 20 | 20 | 19 | 19 | 18 | 18 | 17 | 17 | 16 | 16 |
| 135 | 28 | 27 | 26 | 26 | 25 | 24 | 23 | 22 | 22 | 21 | 21 | 20 | 19 | 19 | 18 | 18 | 17 | 16 | 16 |
| 140 | 29 | 28 | 27 | 26 | 26 | 25 | 24 | 23 | 23 | 22 | 21 | 21 | 20 | 20 | 19 | 18 | 18 | 17 | 17 |
| 145 | 30 | 29 | 28 | 27 | 26 | 26 | 25 | 24 | 23 | 23 | 22 | 21 | 21 | 20 | 20 | 19 | 19 | 17 | 18 |
| 150 | 31 | 30 | 29 | 28 | 27 | 27 | 26 | 25 | 24 | 23 | 23 | 22 | 22 | 21 | 20 | 20 | 20 | 18 | 18 |
| 155 | 32 | 31 | 30 | 29 | 28 | 27 | 27 | 26 | 25 | 24 | 24 | 23 | 22 | 22 | 21 | 20 | 20 | 19 | 19 |
| 160 | 33 | 32 | 31 | 30 | 29 | 28 | 27 | 27 | 26 | 25 | 24 | 24 | 23 | 22 | 22 | 21 | 21 | 20 | 19 |
| 165 | 34 | 33 | 32 | 31 | 30 | 29 | 28 | 27 | 27 | 26 | 25 | 24 | 24 | 23 | 22 | 22 | 21 | 21 | 20 |
| 170 | 36 | 34 | 33 | 32 | 31 | 30 | 29 | 28 | 27 | 27 | 26 | 25 | 24 | 24 | 23 | 22 | 22 | 21 | 21 |
| 175 | 37 | 35 | 34 | 33 | 32 | 31 | 30 | 29 | 28 | 27 | 27 | 26 | 25 | 24 | 24 | 23 | 23 | 22 | 21 |
| 180 | 38 | 36 | 35 | 34 | 33 | 32 | 31 | 30 | 28 | 28 | 27 | 27 | 26 | 25 | 24 | 24 | 23 | 22 | 22 |
| 185 | 39 | 37 | 36 | 35 | 34 | 33 | 32 | 31 | 29 | 29 | 28 | 27 | 27 | 26 | 25 | 24 | 24 | 23 | 23 |
| 190 | 40 | 38 | 37 | 36 | 35 | 34 | 33 | 32 | 30 | 30 | 29 | 28 | 27 | 26 | 26 | 25 | 25 | 24 | 23 |
| 195 | 41 | 39 | 38 | 37 | 36 | 35 | 34 | 33 | 31 | 31 | 30 | 29 | 28 | 27 | 26 | 26 | 25 | 24 | 24 |
| 200 | 42 | 40 | 39 | 38 | 37 | 36 | 35 | 34 | 32 | 32 | 31 | 30 | 29 | 28 | 27 | 26 | 26 | 25 | 24 |
| 205 | 43 | 41 | 40 | 39 | 38 | 37 | 36 | 35 | 33 | 33 | 32 | 31 | 30 | 29 | 28 | 27 | 27 | 26 | 25 |
| 210 | 44 | 42 | 41 | 40 | 39 | 38 | 37 | 36 | 34 | 34 | 32 | 31 | 31 | 30 | 29 | 28 | 28 | 26 | 26 |
| 215 | 45 | 43 | 42 | 41 | 39 | 39 | 38 | 37 | 35 | 34 | 33 | 32 | 32 | 30 | 30 | 29 | 28 | 27 | 26 |
| 220 | 46 | 44 | 43 | 42 | 40 | 39 | 38 | 37 | 36 | 35 | 34 | 33 | 32 | 31 | 30 | 29 | 29 | 27 | 27 |
| 225 | 47 | 45 | 44 | 43 | 41 | 40 | 39 | 38 | 36 | 35 | 34 | 33 | 32 | 32 | 31 | 30 | 30 | 28 | 27 |
| 230 | 48 | 47 | 45 | 44 | 42 | 41 | 39 | 39 | 37 | 36 | 35 | 34 | 33 | 32 | 31 | 30 | 30 | 29 | 28 |
| 235 | 49 | 48 | 46 | 45 | 43 | 42 | 40 | 39 | 38 | 37 | 36 | 35 | 34 | 33 | 32 | 31 | 31 | 29 | 29 |

*continues*

| Weight in lbs | Height in Inches | | | | | | | | | | | | | | | | | | |
|---|---|---|---|---|---|---|---|---|---|---|---|---|---|---|---|---|---|---|---|
| | 58 | 59 | 60 | 61 | 62 | 63 | 64 | 65 | 66 | 67 | 68 | 69 | 70 | 71 | 72 | 73 | 74 | 75 | 76 |
| 240 | 50 | 49 | 47 | 46 | 44 | 43 | 41 | 40 | 39 | 38 | 37 | 36 | 34 | 34 | 33 | 32 | 31 | 30 | 29 |
| 245 | 51 | 50 | 48 | 47 | 45 | 43 | 42 | 41 | 40 | 38 | 37 | 36 | 35 | 34 | 33 | 32 | 32 | 30 | 30 |
| 250 | 52 | 51 | 49 | 48 | 46 | 44 | 43 | 42 | 40 | 39 | 38 | 37 | 36 | 35 | 34 | 33 | 32 | 31 | 30 |
| 255 | 53 | 52 | 50 | 49 | 47 | 45 | 44 | 42 | 41 | 40 | 39 | 38 | 37 | 36 | 35 | 34 | 33 | 32 | 31 |
| 260 | 54 | 53 | 51 | 50 | 48 | 46 | 45 | 43 | 42 | 41 | 40 | 39 | 37 | 36 | 35 | 34 | 34 | 32 | 32 |
| 265 | 55 | 54 | 52 | 51 | 49 | 47 | 46 | 44 | 43 | 42 | 40 | 39 | 38 | 37 | 36 | 35 | 34 | 33 | 33 |
| 270 | 56 | 54 | 53 | 52 | 49 | 48 | 46 | 45 | 44 | 42 | 41 | 40 | 39 | 38 | 37 | 36 | 35 | 34 | 33 |
| 275 | | | 54 | 53 | 50 | 49 | 47 | 46 | 45 | 43 | 42 | 41 | 40 | 38 | 37 | 36 | 35 | 35 | 34 |
| 280 | | | 55 | 54 | 51 | 50 | 48 | 46 | 45 | 44 | 43 | 41 | 40 | 39 | 38 | 37 | 36 | 35 | 34 |

# II. Dr. Masley's Recommended Body Fat Percentage Rates*

| Adult Male | Underweight, Modest Health Risk | Desired Body Fat | Overweight, Mild to Modest Health Risk | Overweight, High Health Risk | Overweight, Very High Health Risk |
|---|---|---|---|---|---|
| Age 18–39 | Less than 10% | 10–20% | 20–25% | 25–30% | More than 30% |
| Age 40–60 | Less than 12% | 12–22% | 22–27% | 27–33% | More than 33% |
| Age over 60 | Less than 13% | 13–24% | 24–29% | 29–35% | More than 35% |
| Adult Female | Underweight, Modest Health Risk | Desired Body Fat | Overweight, Mild to Modest Risk | Overweight, High Health Risk | Overweight, Very High Health Risk |
| Age 18–39 | Less than 18% | 18–24% | 24–30% | 30–37% | More than 37% |
| Age 40–60 | Less than 19% | 19–26% | 26–33% | 33–40% | More than 40% |
| Age over 60 | Less than 20% | 20–27% | 27–35% | 35–42% | More than 42% |
| *% of fat to total body weight | | | | | |

# III. Calcium Requirements

Here is my three-step guideline to calculate your calcium requirements and clarify whether you need a calcium supplement.

### *Step 1: How much calcium do you need?*

Calcium requirements vary by lifestyle. If you do everything right, you could do well with only 800 mg of calcium daily, but if you do most things wrong, 1,500 mg daily won't keep you from fracturing bones later in life. I recommend that you select one of three choices that best matches your lifestyle:

- If you follow an optimal lifestyle for your bones, you only need 800 mg of calcium daily. This means you get 45 minutes of weight-bearing exercise (walking or running) 5 to 6 days a week, you lift weights 2 to 3 times a week, you don't smoke, you do not drink more than 1 to 2 servings of alcohol at a time, you get at least 1,000 IU of vitamin D and 500 mcg of vitamin K daily, you do not eat excessive animal protein or salt (less than 10 ounces meat-poultry-fish daily, less than 2,000 mg salt daily), and you eat at least 5 cups of fruits and vegetables every day. Sadly, this applies to only about 5% of Americans.
- If you don't follow this type of optimal lifestyle, you need 1,000 to 1,200 mg of calcium daily. The less optimal your lifestyle, the more reason to aim for 1,200 mg of calcium daily.

- If you already have osteopenia or osteoporosis, you need 1,200 to 1,500 mg of calcium daily.

***Step 2: Once you know your calcium requirements, calculate how much calcium you get from food. See the "Calcium Content of Some Foods" table, below.***

To simplify it, think of plain yogurt at 400 mg of calcium per 8-ounce cup. Milk and calcium-fortified soy milk, almond milk, and orange juice all have 300 mg of calcium per 8-ounce cup. Leafy green veggies (except spinach) have 100 mg per cup. Beans have 100 mg per cup. On a typical day, how much calcium do you get through your food?

Use the chart below to calculate your typical intake from calcium foods daily. Don't pick your worst or best days; use realistic days to assess your intake.

## Calcium Content of Some Foods

| Item (serving size) | Calcium Content (mg) |
|---|---|
| Yogurt (8 oz) | 415 |
| Cow's milk (8 oz) | 300 |
| Soy or rice milk, calcium-fortified (8 oz) | 300 |
| Almond milk, calcium-fortified (8 oz) | 500 |
| Orange juice, calcium-fortified (8 oz) | 300 |
| Edamame (1 cup) | 261 |
| Sardines in tomato sauce (3.5 oz) | 240 |
| Cheddar cheese (1 oz) | 204 |
| Broccoli, cooked (1 cup) | 175 |
| Kale and other cooked greens (1 cup) | 125 |
| Oatmeal, instant (1 pkt) | 140 |
| Seaweed, hijiki or wakame, dry (1 sheet) | 163 |
| Oatmeal, regular (1 cup) | 20 |
| Tofu (½ cup) | 130 |
| Navy beans, cooked (1 cup) | 128 |
| Garbanzo beans (1 cup) | 80 |
| Almonds (1 oz) | 75 |
| Carrots (1 cup) | 35 |
| Brown rice (1 cup) | 20 |
| Whole wheat bread (1 slice) | 20 |

***Step 3: If your intake doesn't meet your requirements, then plan to add a calcium supplement.***

Now that you know your calcium requirement and your dietary intake, you can calculate how much calcium to add daily to meet your needs. If your dietary intake is lower than your requirement, either add more calcium-rich foods daily or take a supplement.

*What is the best type of calcium supplement?*

* Protein-bound calcium or a calcium chelate (e.g., calcium malate chelate or calcium glycinate chelate) are by far the best absorbed and cause few to no gastrointestinal symptoms.
* Calcium carbonate is the worst type of calcium, as it may contain lead, must be consumed with food, and even then has limited absorption and causes constipation.
* Calcium citrate is normally lead-free, but has limited absorption.

*Should you always take calcium with magnesium?*

Absolutely. Please keep three facts in mind:

**1.** Most people are magnesium deficient.

**2.** Taking a calcium supplement blocks magnesium absorption.

**3.** Magnesium is critical for hundreds of health issues, in particular blood pressure and blood sugar control, preventing constipation and muscle cramps, and preventing fatal cardiac arrhythmias.

So yes, if you take calcium, you should take it with magnesium. Many high-quality calcium supplements come with calcium and magnesium combined in a 2:1 to 3:1 ratio, which is an excellent choice.

My favorite form of calcium and magnesium is OsteoForce, with a nice protein-bound form of calcium and magnesium, plus extra vitamin D and vitamin K too. If you already get your vitamin D and vitamin K from other sources, then try calcium malate chelate and magnesium malate chelate, aiming for a 2:1 ratio.

# IV. Fiber Content of Common Foods (in Grams)

| Fruits | |
|---|---|
| Apple (1 medium) | 3.3 |
| Apple juice (8 oz) | 0.0 |
| Applesauce (⅔ cup) | 2.9 |
| Apricot (3 medium) | 2.4 |
| Apricot, dried (¼ Cup) | 3.0 |
| Banana (1 medium) | 3.0 |
| Blackberries (½ cup) | 3.8 |
| Blueberries (½ cup) | 1.8 |
| Blueberries, frzn (½ cup) | 2.1 |
| Cherries, raw (10) | 1.5 |
| Cherries, dried (⅓ cup) | 2.0 |
| Dates (½ cup) | 7.1 |
| Figs, dried (½ cup) | 10.0 |
| Grapefruit (½) | 1.0 |
| Grapes (1 cup) | 1.8 |
| Mango (1 medium) | 3.0 |
| Melon (1 cup, cubed) | 1.4 |
| Orange (1 medium) | 3.1 |
| Peach (1 medium) | 1.5 |
| Pear (1 medium) | 5.1 |
| Pineapple (1 cup, diced) | 2.2 |
| Plum (2 medium) | 2.0 |
| Prunes (2) | 2.0 |
| Raisins (⅓ cup) | 3.5 |
| Raspberries, raw (½ cup) | 4.0 |
| Raspberries, frzn (½ cup) | 5.5 |
| Strawberries, raw (½ cup) | 1.7 |
| Watermelon, balls (1 cup) | 0.6 |

| Vegetables | |
|---|---|
| Beets (1 cup) | 3.5 |
| Broccoli (1 cup, chopped) | 2.3 |
| Brussels Sprouts (1 cup) | 3.3 |
| Cabbage (1 cup, shredded) | 2.0 |
| Carrots (1 cup) | 3.6 |
| Cauliflower (1 cup) | 2.5 |
| Celery (1 cup, chopped) | 1.6 |
| Eggplant, raw (1 cup) | 2.8 |
| Green beans (1 cup) | 3.7 |
| Lettuce (1 cup, chopped) | 1.0 |
| Mixed vegetable, frzn (1 cup) | 4.0 |
| Okra (1 cup, cooked) | 4.0 |
| Onions (½ cup, chopped) | 1.5 |
| Peas (1 cup) | 7.4 |
| Peas, split (½ cup, cooked) | 8.0 |
| Peppers (½ cup, chopped) | 1.3 |
| Potato (1 med, baked with skin) | 3.8 |
| Potato (1 med, baked no skin) | 2.3 |
| Potato (French fries, 1 med serv) | 4.0 |
| Potato, mashed (1 cup) | 3.0 |
| Potato salad (1 cup) | 2.5 |
| Pumpkin (½ cup) | 3.8 |
| Spinach (1 cup, raw) | 0.7 |
| Spinach (1 cup, cooked) | 4.3 |
| Squash (1 cup, cooked) | 2.5 |
| Sweet potato (1 med, no skin) | 3.0 |
| Sweet potato (1 med, with skin) | 4.0 |
| Tomato (1 medium, raw) | 1.5 |
| Tomato (1 cup, cooked) | 1.7 |

| Vegetables | |
|---|---|
| Artichoke (1 medium whole) | 6.5 |
| Artichoke hearts (½ cup) | 4.5 |
| Asparagus (½ cup/ 6 spears) | 1.7 |
| Avocado (½ medium) | 6.5 |

| Beans (Legumes), Cooked | |
|---|---|
| Baked beans (1 cup) | 10.4 |
| Broad beans (1 cup) | 17.0 |
| Black beans (1 cup) | 15.0 |
| Kidney beans (1 cup) | 16.5 |

*Continues*

| | |
|---|---|
| Lentils (1 cup) | 15.6 |
| Lima beans (1 cup) | 13.2 |
| Navy beans (1 cup) | 19.1 |
| Pinto beans (1 cup) | 15.4 |
| Refried beans (1 cup) | 10.0 |
| Soybeans, green (1 cup, boiled) | 7.6 |
| Soybeans, dry roasted (1 cup) | 13.9 |
| Tofu (½ block) | 2.0 |

| Grain Products, Cooked | |
|---|---|
| Barley, pearled (1 cup) | 6.0 |
| Corn, yellow (1 cup) | 4.6 |
| Gnocchi (1 cup) | 3.0 |
| Popcorn (1 cup) | 1.2 |
| Quinoa (1 cup) | 5.0 |
| Rice, brown (1 cup) | 3.5 |
| Rice, pilaf (1 cup) | 1.2 |
| Rice, white (1 cup) | 0.6 |
| Rice, wild (1 cup) | 3.0 |
| Soba, buckwheat (1 cup) | 7.6 |
| Soba, white noodles (1 cup) | 2.0 |
| Spaghetti, regular (1 cup) | 2.4 |
| Spaghetti, Barilla Plus (1 cup) | 7.0 |
| Tortillas, corn (2 medium) | 3.0 |
| Tortillas, flour (2 white) | 2.8 |

| Breads | |
|---|---|
| Bagel (1) | 0.6 |
| Biscuits, white flour (1) | 0.5 |
| Bread, pumpernickel (1 slice) | 3.0 |
| Bread, 7-grain (1 slice) | 1.8 |
| Bread, white (1 slice) | 0.6 |
| Bread, whole wheat (1 slice) | 2.0 |
| Corn bread, mix (1 piece) | 1.4 |
| English muffin, hearty grain | 3.0 |
| Pita bread, oat flour (1 pocket) | 3.6 |
| Pita bread, regular (1 pocket) | 1.3 |
| Pita bread, whole wheat (1) | 4.7 |
| Roll, (white bread) | 1.5 |
| Roll, (whole wheat) | 3.6 |

| Crackers and Chips | |
|---|---|
| Brown rice cakes (2) | 1.0 |
| Corn chips (2-oz bag) | 1.9 |
| Pita chips, Stacy's (1 oz) | 1.0 |
| Potato chips (2-oz bag) | 2.0 |

| | |
|---|---|
| Rye crisp (3 crackers) | 4.8 |
| Soda crackers (4) | 0.4 |
| Tortilla chips (2-oz bag) | 2.5 |
| Triscuits (6 crackers) | 3.0 |
| Wheat Thins (1-oz serving) | 0.9 |

| Cereal/Breakfast | |
|---|---|
| All-Bran cereal (½ cup) | 10 |
| Cheerios (1 cup) | 3.6 |
| Cocoa Puffs (1 cup) | 0.7 |
| Corn flakes (1 cup) | 0.5 |
| Frosted Wheaties | 0.8 |
| Grits (1 cup, cooked) | 0.5 |
| Honey Nut Cheerios (1 cup) | 1.8 |
| Kashi Go Lean (1 cup) | 10.0 |
| Kashi Go Lean Crunch (1 cup) | 8.0 |
| Kashi Go Lean waffles (2) | 6.0 |
| Kellogg's Raisin Bran (1 cup) | 7.3 |
| Kraft Bran Flakes (1 cup) | 6.7 |
| Oatmeal (1 cup, cooked) | 4.0 |
| Oatmeal, instant (1 cup, cooked) | 2.8 |
| Pancake mix, Bob's Red Mill | 4.0 |
| Pancake mix, Krusteaz | 3.0 |
| Rice Krispies | 0.1 |
| Shredded Wheat | 5.6 |
| Special K | 0.7 |
| Total | 3.5 |
| Wheaties | 3.0 |

| Nuts and Seeds | |
|---|---|
| Almonds (1 oz = 22 kernels) | 3.3 |
| Almond butter (1 Tbsp) | 0.7 |
| Brazil (1 oz = 7 kernels) | 2.1 |
| Cashews (1 oz) | 0.9 |
| Chia seeds (1 Tbsp) | 2.5 |
| Corn-nuts (1 oz ) | 2.0 |
| Filberts, hazelnuts (1 oz) | 2.7 |
| Flaxseeds (1 Tbsp) | 2.5 |
| Macadamia (1 oz = 11 kernels) | 2.3 |
| Mixed nuts (1 oz) | 2.5 |
| Peanuts (1 oz = 28) | 2.2 |
| Peanut butter (1 Tbsp) | 2.6 |
| Pecans (1 oz) | 2.7 |
| Pistachio (1 oz) | 3.0 |
| Sunflower seeds (1 oz) | 2.6 |
| Walnuts (1 oz ) | 1.9 |

*Continues*

| Snacks and Bars | |
|---|---|
| Cascadian Farm Organic Bar | 1.0 |
| Clif Energy Bar | 5.0 |
| Dark chocolate (70%, 40 gm) | 4.0 |
| Fiber One Bar | 9.0 |
| Kashi Granola Bar | 4.0 |
| Kashi 7 Grain Bar | 4.6 |
| Kellogg's All Bran Bar | 5.0 |
| Luna Bar | 4.0 |
| Milk chocolate (<35%, 40 gm) | 0.1 |
| Nature Valley Granola Bar (2) | 2.0 |
| Quaker Crunchy Granola Bar | 1.0 |

| Miscellaneous | |
|---|---|
| Hummus (2 Tbsp) | 2.0 |
| Salsa (2 Tbsp) | 0.5 |
| Soup, Healthy Request veg. | 4.0 |

| Beverages | |
|---|---|
| Almond milk (1 cup)` | 1.0 |
| Cow's milk (1 cup) | 0.0 |

| Hot cocoa (1 cup) | 2.1 |
|---|---|
| Orange juice with pulp (1 cup) | 0.0 |
| Rice milk (1 cup) | 0.0 |
| Soy milk (1 cup) | 1.0 |
| V8 juice (1 cup) | 2.0 |

| Meat, Poultry, Seafood | |
|---|---|
| All meat, poultry, per serving | 0.0 |
| Cheese | 0.0 |
| Eggs | 0.0 |
| Turkey burger | 0.0 |

| Morning Start Veggie Products | |
|---|---|
| Bacon strips (2) | 1.0 |
| Black bean burger (1) | 4.0 |
| Sausage patties (2) | 2.0 |
| Veggie meatballs (5) | 3.0 |

# Helpful Resources

As promised, here is my list of resources to make it easier for you to optimize your life. Please visit www.hearttuneup.com/resources for updated information.

## Websites

www.hearttuneup.com (sign up for Dr. Masley's free vitality tips here)

www.tenyearsyounger.com

## The Masley Optimal Health Center

900 Carillon Parkway
St. Petersburg, FL 33716
(727) 299-9007/www.drmasley.com

## Information Tools

For these DVDs, CDs, and web-videos by Dr. Steven Masley, visit www.hearttuneup.com/resources:

* Heart Tune-Up Introduction
* Shopping for the 30-Day Heart Tune-Up
* Personalizing Your Supplement Plan
* 30-Day Heart Tune-Up Recipe Cooking Demonstrations (from Dr. Masley's Own Kitchen)
* 30-Day Heart Tune-Up Aerobic Fitness Testing and Strength Training Demonstrations
* The Ten Years Younger Program

*Food Sources and Links*

### Organic Foods

Cascadian Farm: www.hearttuneup.com/resources/cfarm
Organic Valley: www.hearttuneup.com/resources/organicvalley
Stonyfield Farm: www.hearttuneup.com/resources/stonyfield
Bob's Red Mill: www.heartttuneup.com/resources
/Bob'sRedMill
Arrowhead Mills: www.hearttuneup.com/resources/
ArrowheadMills

### Seafood

Vital Choice Seafood: www.hearttuneup.com/resources
/vitalchoice

### Protein Powders

www.hearttuneup.com/resources:
For general health and muscle building: whey protein
For treating metabolic syndrome and abnormal cholesterol
profiles: UltraMeal Plus 360
When following an elimination diet: the Virgin Diet Shake
www.heartshakes.com

### Oils

Spectrum Naturals: www.hearttuneup.com/resources/spectrum

### Free-Range, Organic, Frozen Meals

Artisan Bistro: www.hearttuneup.com/resources/artisanbistro

## Exercise Tools

Heart rate monitors: www.hearttuneup.com/resources
/heartratemonitor
Exercise ball: www.hearttuneup.com/resources/exerciseball

# Recommended Reading and Information Sources

- *Ten Years Younger*, by Steven Masley, MD: www.tenyearsyounger.com
- The Institute for Functional Medicine (IFM): www.functionalmedicine.org
- American Academy of Family Physicians medical topic search link: www.aafp.org/online/en/home/internal /advanced-search.html
- *Change Your Brain, Change Your Life*, by Daniel G. Amen, MD
- *8 Weeks to Vibrant Health*, by Hyla Cass, MD, and Kathleen Barnes
- *The Complete Idiot's Guide to Thyroid Disease*, by Alan Christianson, ND, and Hy Bender
- *The Great Cholesterol Myth: Why Lowering Your Cholesterol Won't Prevent Heart Disease—and the Statin-Free Plan That Will*, by Jonny Bowden, Phd, and Stephen Sinatra, MD
- *The Hormone Cure*, by Sara Gottfried, MD
- *The Blood Sugar Solution*, by Mark Hyman, MD
- *Life Is Your Best Medicine: A Woman's Guide to Health, Healing, and Wholeness at Every Age*, by Tieraona Low Dog, MD
- *Eat What You Love, Love What You Eat*, by Michelle May, MD
- *You: The Owner's Manual*, by Mehmet C. Oz, MD, and Michael F. Roizen, MD

- *The Better Brain Book*, by David Perlmutter, MD, and Carol Colman
- *Power Up Your Brain*, by David Perlmutter, MD, and Alberto Villoldo, Phd
- *Is It Me or My Hormones?* by Marcelle Pick, MSN, OB/ GYN NP
- *The Sinatra Solution: Metabolic Cardiology*, by Stephen T. Sinatra, MD, and James Roberts, MD
- *The Virgin Diet*, by JJ Virgin, CNS, CHFS (my favorite elimination diet)

# Supplement Companies I Use

- Thorne: www.thorne.com
- Metagenics: www.metagenics.com
- Designs for Health: www.designsforhealth.com
- ProThera: www.protherainc.com
- Xymogen: www.xymogen.com
- Skin Medica (skin care products): www.skinmedica.com

View www.hearttuneup.com/supplements for details on how to personalize your supplement plan.

# References

## Chapter 1

1. Yusuf S, Hawken S, Ounpuu S, Dans T, Avezum A, et al. Effect of potentially modifiable risk factors associated with myocardial infarction in 52 countries (the INTERHEART study). *Lancet* 2004;364:937–52.
2. Smith SC. Need for a paradigm shift: the importance of risk factor reduction therapy in treating patients with cardiovascular disease. *Am J Cardiol* 1998;82:10–13.
3. Forrester JS. Role of plaque rupture in acute coronary syndromes. *Am J Cardiol* 2000;86:15–23; Falk E. Why do plaques rupture? *Circulation* 1992;86:30–42.
4. Dobs A, et al. Effects of high-dose simvastatin on adrenal and gonadal steroidogenesis in men with hypercholesterolemia. *Metabolism* 2000;29: 1234–38; Corona G. The effect of statin therapy on testosterone levels in subjects consulting for erectile dysfunction. *J Sex Med* 2010;7:1547–56; Akduman B, et al. Effect of statins on serum prostate-specific antigen levels. *Urology* 2010;76:1048-51.
5. Masley SC, Weaver W, Peri G, Phillips S. Efficacy of exercise and diet to modify markers of fitness and wellness. *Altern Ther Health Med* 2008;14:24–29; Masley SC, Roetzheim R, Gualtieri T. Aerobic exercise enhances cognitive flexibility. *J Clin Psychol* 2009;16:186–93.
6. Olshansky SJ, Passaro DJ, Hershow RC, Layden J, Carnes BA, et al. A potential decline in life expectancy in the US in the 21st century. *N Engl J Med* 2005;352:1138–45.
7. Sterigiopoulos K, Brown DL. Initial coronary stent implantation with medical therapy versus medical therapy alone for stable coronary artery disease. *Arch Intern Med* 2012;72:312–19; Boden WE, O'Rourke RA, Crawford MH, Blaustein AS, Deedwania PC, et al. Outcomes in patients with acute non-Q wave myocardial infarction randomly assigned to an invasive as compared with a conservative management strategy. (VANQWISH). *N Engl J Med* 1998;338:1785–92; Pitt B, Waters D, Brown WV, Van Boven AJ,

Schwartz L, et al. Aggressive lipid-lowering therapy compared with angioplasty in stable coronary artery disease. *N Engl J Med* 1999;341–46.

8. Newman MF, Kirchner JL, Phillips-Bute B, Gaver V, Grocott H, et al. Longitudinal assessment of neurocognitive function after coronary-artery bypass surgery. *N Engl J Med* 2001;344:395–402.

9. Yusuf S, Hawken S, Ounpuu S, Dans T, Avezum A, et al. Effect of potentially modifiable risk factors associated with myocardial infarction in 52 countries (the INTERHEART study). *Lancet* 2004;364:937–52.

## Chapter 2

1. Masley SC, Roetzheim R, Masley LV, Schocken DD. Emerging lifestyle factors that predict carotid IMT scores. Accepted as an abstract, American College of Nutrition Annual Conference, November 2013.

2. Gregg EW, Chen H, Wagenkneckt LE, Clark JM, Delahanty LM, et al. Association of an intensive lifestyle intervention with remission of type 2 diabetes. *JAMA* 2012;308:2489–96.

3. Masley SC, Roetzheim R, Masley LV, Schocken DD. Emerging lifestyle factors that predict carotid IMT scores. Accepted as an abstract, American College of Nutrition Annual Conference, November 2013.

4. Van Sant Crowle C, Phillips S, Masley SC. Efficacy of a high-fiber, low-fat diet and exercise for the metabolic syndrome. Abstract for the American Academy of Family Physician Scientific and WONCA Meeting, October 2003.

5. Barzilai N, Atzmon G, Schechter C, Schaefer EJ, Cupples AL, et al. Unique lipoprotein phenotype and genotype associated with exceptional longevity. *JAMA* 2003;290:2030–40.

6. Ortega FB, Lee DC, Katzmarzyk PT, Ruiz JR, Sui X, et al. The intriguing metabolically healthy but obese phenotype: cardiovascular prognosis and role of fitness. *Eur Heart J* 2012;34:389–97.

7. Lee IM, Djousse L, Sesso HD, Wang L, Buring JE. Physical activity and weight gain prevention. *JAMA* 2010;303:1173–79.

8. Ridker PM, Hennekens CH, Buring JE, Rifai N. C-reactive protein and other markers of inflammation in the prediction of cardiovascular disease in women. *N Engl J Med* 2000;342:836–43; Sesso HD, Buring JE, Rifai N, Blake GJ, Gaziano JM, Ridker PM. C-reactive protein and the risk of developing hypertension. *JAMA* 2003;290:2945–51; Ridker PM, Cannon CP, Morrow D, Rifai N, Rose MS, McCabe CH, Pfeffer MA, Braunwald E. C-reactive protein levels and outcomes after statin therapy. *N Engl J Med* 2005;352:20–28.

9. Berry JD, Dyer A, Cai X, Garside DB, Ning H, et al. Lifetime risks of cardiovascular disease. *N Engl J Med* 2012;366:321–29.

10. Wilkins JT, Ning H, Berr J, Zhao L, Dyer AR, Lloyd-Jones DM. Lifetime risk and years lived free of total cardiovascular disease. *JAMA* 2012;308:1795–801.

## Chapter 3

1. Forrester JS. Role of plaque rupture in acute coronary syndromes. *Am J Cardiol* 2000;86:15–23; Falk E. Why do plaques rupture? *Circulation* 1992;86:30–42.

2. Ikeda N, Kogame N, Iijima R, Nakamura M, Sugi K. Carotid artery intima-media thickness and plaque score can predict the SNYTAX score. *Eur Heart J* 2012;33:113–19; Morito N, Inoue Y, Urata M, Yahiro E, Kodama S, Fukuda N, Saito N, et al. Increased carotid artery plaque score is an independent predictor of the presence and severity of coronary artery disease. *J Cardiol* 2008;51:25–32; Kablak-Ziembicka A, Tracz W, Przewlocki T, Pieniazek P, Sokolowski A, Konieczynska M. Association of increased carotid intima-media thickness with extent of coronary artery disease. *Heart* 2004;90:1286–90.

3. Lorenz MW, Markus HS, Bots ML, Rosvall M, Sitzer M. Prediction of clinical cardiovascular events with carotid intima-media thickness. A systemic review and meta-analysis. *Circulation* 2007;115:459–67; O'Leary DH, Polak JF, Kronmal RA, Manolio TA, Burke GL, Wolfson SK. Cardiovascular Health Study Collaborative Research Group. Carotid artery and media thickness as a risk factor for myocardial infarction and stroke in older adults. *N Engl J Med* 1999;340:14–22; Van der Meer IM, Bots ML, Holfman A, Iglesias del Sol A, van der Kuip DAM, Witteman JCM. Predictive value of noninvasive measures of atherosclerosis for incident myocardial infarction—the Rotterdam Study. *Circulation* 2004;109:1089–94.

4. Aminbakhsh A, Mancini GB. Carotid intima-media thickness measurements: what defines an abnormality? A systematic review. *Clin Invest Med* 1999;22:149–57; Tonstad S, Joakimsen O, Stensland-Bugge E, Ose L, Bonaa KH, Leren TP. Carotid intima-media thickness and plaque in patients with familial hypercholesterolaemia mutations and control subjects. *Eur J Clin Invest* 1998;28:971–79; Polak JF, Pencina MJ, Pencina KM, O'Donnell CJ, et al. Carotid-wall intima-media thickness and cardiovascular events. *N Engl J Med* 2011;365:213–21; O'Leary DH, Polak JF, Kronmal RA, Manolio TA, et al. Carotid-artery intima and media thickness as a risk factor for myocardial infarction and stroke in older adults. *N Engl J Med* 1999;340:14–22.

5. Greenland P, Abrams J, Aurigemma GP, Bond MG, Clark LT, Criqui MH, Crouse JR, et al. Beyond secondary prevention: identifying the high-risk patient for primary prevention. *Circulation* (AHA Conference Proceedings) 2000;101:e16–22.

6. Masley SC, Roetzheim R, Masley LV, Schocken DD. Emerging lifestyle factors that predict carotid IMT scores. Accepted as an abstract, American College of Nutrition Annual Conference, November 2013.

7. Schwartz J, Allison M, Wright CM. Health behavior modification after electron beam computed tomography and physician consultation. *J Behav Med* 2011;34:148–55; Orakzai RH, Nasir K, Orakzai SH, Kalia N, Gopal A, et al. Effect of patient visualization of coronary calcium by electron beam computed tomography on changes in beneficial lifestyle behaviors. *Am J Cardiol* 2008;101:999–1002.

8. Bonow RO. Should coronary calcium screening be used in cardiovascular prevention strategies? *N Engl J Med* 2009;361:990–97; Miller JM, Rochitte CE, Dewey M, Arbab-Zadeh A, Niinuma H, et al. Diagnostic performance of coronary angiography by 64-row CT. *N Engl J Med* 2008;359:2324–36; Polonsky TS, McClelland RL, Jorgensen NW, Bild DE, Burke GL, Guerci AD, Greenland P. Coronary artery calcium score and risk classification of coronary heart disease prediction. *JAMA* 2010;303:1610–16.

9. Masley SC, Roetzheim R, Masley LV, Schocken DD. Emerging lifestyle factors that predict carotid IMT scores. Accepted as an abstract, American College of Nutrition Annual Conference, November 2013.

10. Cole CR, et al. Heart rate recovery after submaximal exercise testing as a predictor of mortality in a cardiovascularly healthy cohort. *Ann Intern Med* 2000;132:552–55.

11. Aktas MK. Global risk scores and exercise testing for predicting all-cause mortality in a preventive medicine program. *JAMA* 2004;292(12):1462–68.

## Chapter 4

1. Theobold M, Masley SC. *A guide to group visits for chronic condition affected by overweight & obesity.* American Academy of Family Physicians, Americans in Motion (AIM) Monograph, 2008; Masley SC, Copeland JR, Phillips S. The D.I.E.T. study (Dietary Intervention & Evaluation Trial), group office visits change dietary habits of patients with coronary artery disease, *J Fam Pract*, 2001;50; Masley SC, Sokoloff J, Hawes C. Planning group visits for high-risk patients. *Fam Pract Manag*; 2000:33–37; Masley SC. Dietary therapy for preventing and treating coronary artery disease. *Am Fam Physician* 1998;57:1299–306.

2. Estruch R, Ros E, Salas-Salvado J, Covas MI, Corella D, et al. Primary prevention of cardiovascular disease with a Mediterranean diet. *N Engl J Med* 2013;368:1279–90.

3. Masley SC, Weaver W, Peri G, Phillips S. Efficacy of exercise and diet to modify markers of fitness and wellness. *Altern Ther Health Med*, 2008;14:24–29.

4. Van de Laar RJJ, Stehouwer CDA, Van Bussel BCT, Velde SJT, Prins MH, Twisk JWR, Ferreira I. Lower lifetime dietary fiber intake is associated with carotid artery stiffness. *Am J Clin Nutr* 2012;96:14–23.

5. Streppel MT, Arends LR, Veer PV, Grobbee DE, Geleijnse JM. Dietary fiber and blood pressure. *Arch Intern Med* 2005;165:150–56.

6. Jenkins DJA, Kendall CWC, Augustin LSA, Mitchell S, Sahye-Pudaruth S, et al. Effect of legumes as part of a low glycemic index diet on glycemic control and cardiovascular risk factors in type 2 diabetes mellitus. *Arch Intern Med* 2012;172:1653–60.

7. Bloedon LT, Balikai S, Chittams J, Cunnane SC, Berlin JA, et al. Flaxseed and cardiovascular risk factors. *J Am Coll Nutr* 2008;27:65–74.

8. Hu FB, Stampfer JM, Manson JE, Rimm EB, Colditz GA, et al. Frequent nut consumption and risk of coronary heart disease in women. *BMJ* 1998;17:1341–45; Kris-Etherton PM, Ahao G, Binkoski AE, Coval SM, Etherton TD. The effects of nuts on coronary heart disease risk. *Nutr Rev* 2001;59:103–11.

9. Estruch R, Ros E, Salas-Salvado J, Covas MI, Corella D, et al. Primary prevention of cardiovascular disease with a Mediterranean diet. *N Engl J Med* 2013;368:1279–90.

10. Spiller GA, Miller A, Olivera K, Reynolds J, Miller B, et al. Effects of plant-based diets high in raw or roasted almonds or almond butter on serum lipoproteins in humans. *J Am Coll Nutr* 2003;22:195–200; Sabate J, Fraser GE, Burke K, Knutsen SF, Bennett H, Lindsted KD. Effects of walnuts on serum lipoid levels and blood pressure in men. *N Engl J Med* 1993;328:603–7.

11. Foster GD, Shantz KL, Vander Veur SS, Oliver TL, Lent MR, et al. A randomized trial of the effects of an almond-enriched, hypocaloric diet in the treatment of obesity. *Am J Clin Nutr* 2012;96(2):249–54.

12. Rimm EB, Ellison RC. Alcohol in the Mediterranean diet. *Am J Clin Nutr* 1995;61:1378–82; Solomon CG, Hu FB, Stampfer MJ, Colditz GA, Speizer FE, et al. Moderate alcohol consumption and risk of coronary heart disease among women with type 2 diabetes. *Circulation* 2000;102:494–99; Berger K, Ajani UA, Kase CS, Gaziano JM, Buring JE, et al. Light to moderate alcohol consumption and the risk of stroke among US male physicians. *N Engl J Med* 1999;341:1557–64; Thun MJ, Peto R, Lopez AD, Monaco JH, Henley SJ, et al. Alcohol consumption and mortality among middle aged and elderly US adults. *N Engl J Med* 1997;337:1705–14.

13. Wan Y, Vinson JA, Etherton TD, Proch J, Lazarus SA, Kris-Etherton PM. Effects of cocoa powder and dark chocolate on LDL oxidative susceptibility and prostaglandin concentrations in humans. *Am J Clin Nutr* 2001;74:596–602.

14. Fraga CG. Cocoa, diabetes, and hypertension: should we eat more chocolate? *Am J Clin Nutr* 2005;81:541–42; Rein D, Paglieroni TG, Wun T, Pearson DA, Schmitz HH, Gosselin R, Keen CL. Cocoa inhibits platelet activation and function. *Am J Clin Nutr* 2000;72:30–35.

15. Steiner M, Khan AH, Holbert D, Lin RI. A double-blind crossover study in moderately hypercholesterolemic men that compared the effect of aged garlic extract and placebo on blood lipids. *Am J Clin Nutr* 1996;64:866–70; Silagy CA, Neil HA. A meta-analysis of the effect of garlic on blood pressure. *J Hypertens* 1994;12:463–68.

16. Taubert D, Roesen R, Lehmann C, Jung N, Schomig E. Effects of low habitual cocoa intake on blood pressure and bioactive nitric oxide. *JAMA* 2007;298:49–60; Grassi D, Lippi C, Necozione S, Desideri G, Ferri C. Short term administration of dark chocolate is followed by a significant increase in insulin sensitivity and a decrease in blood pressure in healthy persons. *Am J Clin Nutr* 2005;81:611–14; Faridi Z, Njike VY, Dutta S, Ali A, Katz DL. Acute dark chocolate and cocoa ingestion and endothelial function. *Am J Clin Nutr* 2008;88:58–63.

## Chapter 5

1. Masley SC, Roetzheim R, Gualtieri T. Aerobic exercise enhances cognitive flexibility. *J Clin Psychol* 2009;16:186–93; Lee IM, Djousse L, Sesso HD, Wang L, Buring JE. Physical activity and weight gain prevention. *JAMA* 2010;303:1173–79; Hambrecht R, Wolf A, Gielen S, Linke A, Hofer J, et al. Effect of exercise on coronary endothelial function in patients with coronary artery disease. *N Engl J Med* 2000;342:454–60; Myers J, Prakash M, Froelicher V, Do D, Partington S, Atwood JE. Exercise capacity and mortality among men referred for exercise testing. *N Engl J Med* 2002;346:793–801; Gregg EW, Chen H, Wagenknecht LE, Clark JM, Delahanty LM, et al. Association of an intensive lifestyle intervention with remission of type 2 diabetes. *JAMA* 2012;308:2489–96.

2. Masley, SC. "Measuring Physical Fitness." Chapter 16 in Evans C, White R, et al. *Exercise Testing for Primary Care and Sports Medicine*. New York: Springer, 2009.

3. Masley, SC. "Measuring Physical Fitness." Chapter 16 in Evans C, White R, et al. *Exercise Testing for Primary Care and Sports Medicine*. New York: Springer, 2009.

## Chapter 6

1. Post, SG. *Altruism and Health: Perspectives from Empirical Research*. New York: Oxford University Press, 2007.


## Chapter 7

1. Gaziano JM, Sesso HD, Christen WG, Bubes V, Smith JP, et al. Multivitamins in the prevention of cancer in men. *JAMA* 2012;308:1871–80.
2. Muhammad KI, Morledge T, Sachar R, Zeldin A, Wolski K, Bhatt DL. Treatment with omega-3 fatty acids reduces serum C-reactive protein concentration. *Clin Lipidol* 2011;6:723–29.
3. Torfadottir JE, et al. PLoS One 2013 April 17;8(4).
4. Masley SC, Roetzheim R, Masley, LV, Schocken D. Emerging lifestyle factors that predict carotid IMT scores. Accepted as an abstract, American College of Nutrition Annual Conference, November 2013.
5. Chiuve SE, Korngold EC, Januzzi JL, Gantzer ML, Albert CM. Plasma and dietary magnesium and risk of sudden cardiac death in women. *Am J Clin Nutr* 2011;93:253–60.
6. Larsson SC, Orsini N, Wolk A. Dietary magnesium intake and risk of stroke. *Am J Clin Nutr* 2012;95:362-66.
7. Paul, C. "Vitamin K." Chapter 136 in Pizzorno JE, Murray MT. *Textbook of Natural Medicine*. 4th edition. St. Louis, Missouri: Churchill Livingstone, 2012.
8. Wade L, Nadeem N, Young IS, Woodside JV, McGinty A. Alphatocopherol induces proantherogenic changes to HDL2 and HDL3: an in vitro and ex vivo investigation. *Atherosclerosis* 2013; 226:392–97; Brown BG, Zhao XQ, Chait A, Fisher LD, Cheung MC, et al. Simvastatin and niacin, antioxidant vitamins, or the combination for the prevention of coronary disease. *N Engl J Med* 2001;345:1583–92; Cheung MC, Zhao XQ, Albers JJ, Brown BG. Antioxidant supplements block the response of HDL to simvastatin-niacin therapy in patients with coronary artery disease and low HDL. *Arterioscler Thromb Vasc Biol* 2001;21:1320–26; Hodis HN, Mack WJ, LaBree L, Mahrer PR, Sevanian A, et al. Alphatocopherol supplementation in healthy individuals reduces low-density lipoprotein oxidation but not atherosclerosis: VEAPS. *Circulation* 2002; 106:1453–59.
9. Ridker PM, Danielson E, Fonseca FAH, Genest J, Goto AM. Rosuvastatin to prevent vascular events in men and women with elevated C-reactive protein. *N Engl J Med* 2008;359:2195–207.
10. Dobs A, et al. Effects of high-dose simvastatin on adrenal and gonadal steroidogenesis in men with hypercholesterolemia. *Metabolism* 2000;

29:1234–38; Corona G. The effect of stain therapy on testosterone levels in subjects consulting for erectile dysfunction. *J Sex Med* 2010;7:1547–56; Akduman B, et al. Effect of statins on serum prostate-specific antigen levels. *Urology* 2010:76:1048-51.

11. Becker DJ, Gordon RY, Halbert SC, French B, Morris PB, Rader DJ. Red yeast rice for dyslipidemia in statin-intolerant patients: a randomized trial. *Ann Intern Med* 2009;150(12):830–39.

## Chapter 8

1. Miner MM. Erectile dysfunction and the "window of curability": a harbinger of cardiovascular events. *Mayo Proc* 2009;84:102–4.
2. Dording CM, Fisher L, Papakostas G, Farabaugh A, Sonawalla S, Fava M, Mischoulon D. A double-blinded, randomized pilot dose-finding study of maca root for the management of SSRI-induced sexual dysfunction. *CNS Neurosci Ther* 2008;14:182–91.
3. Vaillant, GE. *Aging Well*. New York: Little Brown and Company, 2002.
4. See the following website for more details: http://nutritiondata.self.com /foods-000089000000000000000.html.

## Chapter 9

1. Virgin, JJ. *The Virgin Diet*. New York: Harlequin, 2012.

# Index

# About the Author

Steven Masley, MD is a Fellow with the American Heart Association, the American Academy of Family Physicians, and with the American College of Nutrition. He has devoted his medical career to the study of heart disease and aging, and has published significant research on these subjects in leading medical journals. His passion is empowering people to achieve optimal health through comprehensive medical assessments and lifestyle changes.

Currently he is the president of the Masley Optimal Health Center in St. Petersburg, Florida. Dr. Masley is also a clinical assistant professor at the University of South Florida and teaches programs at Eckerd College and the University of Tampa. In 2010, he received the physician Health Care Hero Award from the *Tampa Bay Business Journal*, and he has received several awards for his lifestyle-related research. Dr. Masley sees patients from across North America at his clinic.

Dr. Masley has published several health books, including *Ten Years Younger*, and numerous scientific articles. His work has been featured on the Discovery Channel, Public Broadcasting Service (PBS), the *Today* show, and in more than 250 media interviews. He completed a chef internship at the Four Seasons Restaurant in Seattle, Washington, and he has performed cooking demonstrations at Canyon Ranch, the Pritikin Longevity Center, and for multiple television appearances.

For additional information, visit his websites: www.hearttuneup.com, www.tenyearsyounger.com, and www.drmasley.com.